RECENT ADVANCES IN MEDICINE

CLINICAL LABORATORY THERAPEUTIC

RECENT ADVANCES IN MEDICINE

Clinical Laboratory Therapeutic

BY

G. E. BEAUMONT

M.A., D.M. (Oxon.), F.R.C.P., D.P.H. (Lond.)

Physician to the Middlesex Hospital: Physician to the Hospital or Consumption and Diseases of the Chest, Brompton: Lecturer in Medicine, Middlesex Hospital Medical School.

AND

E. C. DODDS, M.V.O.

D.Sc., Ph.D., M.D., F.R.C.P., F.R.I.C., F.R.S. (Edin.), F.R.S.

Courtauld Professor of Biochemistry in the University of London: Director of Courtauld Institute of Biochemistry, Middlesex Hospital.

THIRTEENTH EDITION

With 59 Illustrations

THE BLAKISTON COMPANY

PHILADELPHIA—NEW YORK

1952

First Edition . . .	1924
Second Edition . . .	1925
Third Edition . . .	1926
Fourth Edition . . .	1928
Fifth Edition . . .	1929
Sixth Edition . . .	1931
Seventh Edition . . .	1934
Eighth Edition . . .	1936
Ninth Edition . . .	1939
Tenth Edition . . .	1941
Eleventh Edition . .	1943
,, ,, *Reprinted*	1944
,, ,, ,,	1945
Twelfth Edition . . .	1947
,, ,, *Reprinted*	1948
Thirteenth Edition . .	1952

Translated into Spanish.
,, ,, *Italian.*
,, ,, *Roumanian.*

Printed in Great Britain and published in London by J. & A. Churchill Ltd. 104 Gloucester Place, W.1.

PREFACE TO THE THIRTEENTH EDITION

This edition contains about two hundred pages of new material and twenty-nine new figures. As the size of the book has not been increased, it has been necessary to omit completely certain chapters together with sections of others. The chapters we have discarded are those dealing with Chemotherapy, Glycosuria and Diabetes Mellitus, The Treatment of Addison's Disease, and The Sex Hormones.

New Chapters have been written on The Collagen Diseases, The Antihistamines, and The Use of Isotopes in Medicine. The last Chapter, on Biochemical Methods, has been rewritten. The Antibiotic Chapter has been revised and expanded to include an account of Aureomycin, Chloramphenicol, Streptomycin and Terramycin.

Other additions include sections on Vitamin B_{12}, a general consideration of hepatitis, and liver puncture biopsy. The description of the tests for liver function has been rewritten. The medical treatment of gastric ulcer has been brought up to date, and an article added on vagotomy. In the Chapter dealing with The Cardiovascular System sections have been added on Unipolar Lead Electrocardiography, Cardiac Catheterisation, and the use of methonium salts and the rice diet in hypertension.

Further, accounts are given of Q Fever in Great Britain, and the methods which may be adopted for the prevention of tuberculosis, including the B.C.G. vaccine. Artificial pneumoperitoneum and the streptomycin and P.A.S. treatments of tuberculosis are also considered. The section on Bronchography has been rewritten to include the various techniques which may be adopted for adults and children. The description of the use of thiouracil drugs has been revised and a section added on radioactive iodine in the diagnosis and treatment of thyrotoxicosis. The Hæmopoietic System Chapter has been brought up to date and an account given of the intravenous administration of iron. The section dealing with the blood groups has been completely rewritten.

Medicine has advanced so rapidly during the past few years that it is difficult to keep apace, but it is hoped that nothing of major importance has been omitted from this edition.

We have received much help in its preparation from our colleagues and we take this opportunity of gratefully acknowledging our indebtedness. Sir Weldon Dalrymple Champneys kindly supplied us with information on milk supplies. Dr. S. Oram not only read the article on Unipolar Electrocardiography, but also supplied all the electrocardiograms which illustrate this section. For his valuable suggestions, criticisms and amendments we are deeply grateful. Dr. F. H. Scadding rewrote the article on Bronchography, and gave helpful information for the account of Cardiac Catheterisation. Dr. J. M. Gardiner also read the latter article and made various useful suggestions. To Dr. A. M. Jelliffe we are obliged for the two figures illustrating Liver Needle Biopsy, and for assistance in describing the technique of the method.

Dr. D. N. Baron and Mr. C. F. M. Rose have played a major part in the revision of the biochemical sections of the book, and have assisted with the sections on antihistamines and the liver, and the methods, respectively. To Drs. Johnstone, Palmer and Tait we are much obliged for assistance with the sections on blood groups, antibiotics and isotopes, respectively.

We also wish to acknowledge with thanks permission to reproduce the following figures and diagrams: Fig. 4, Dr. Myron Prinzmetal and *The Journal of the American Medical Association.* Fig. 5, Dr. Edith H. Quimby and *Radiology.* Fig. 6, Dr. G. F. Green, Dr. J. F. Tait, Mr. R. Worsnop and Professor B. W. Windeyer and *The British Journal of Radiology.* Fig. 48, Mr. R. C. Brock, and *Thorax.* Fig. 56, Professor J. P. Peters and Dr. Donald D. Van Slyke, and The Williams and Wilkins Company. Fig. 59, Dr. Franklin C. McLean and *The American Journal of the Medical Sciences.*

Our publishers have once again given us every help in the production of this edition, and we wish especially to thank Mr. J. Rivers for his ready assistance at all times. To Mr. J. Shields we owe the index of this volume and indeed of all the previous editions.

G. E. B.
E. C. D.

LONDON.

PREFACE TO THE FIRST EDITION

During the last decade changes have taken place in medicine, especially in the routine methods adopted in the clinical and laboratory investigation of disease, and also in certain forms of treatment.

This book has been compiled with the following objects: to assist practitioners who have not had the opportunity of recent post-graduate study, to familiarise themselves with some of these advances; to provide a reference book for those who are working for the higher examinations in medicine; to give candidates studying for the primary examination for the Fellowship of the Royal College of Surgeons an account of the application of physiological and biochemical principles to medicine. It is also hoped that it will prove of assistance to the laboratory worker in that the recent chemical methods are dealt with in detail. It should also form a link between the wards of a hospital and the laboratories, giving fuller details of methods which are alluded to in medical textbooks, but often omitted from the handbooks on clinical methods. The recent work of American and Continental authorities has also been incorporated.

One of the chief difficulties has been to decide the actual scope of the contents, which of necessity encroach upon the domains of theoretical medicine, therapeutics, biochemistry and bacteriology. The guiding principle has been to confine the subject-matter to a description of such methods of diagnosis and treatment as are used for medical patients in a general hospital, and which can be justly termed "recent advances in medicine."

Great care has been taken to give a workable description of each procedure, all techniques described have been performed personally by one or other of us, and the accounts are taken from our notebooks. Although these may differ slightly from the original descriptions, the methods described have been used by us as a routine for some time, and have given very satisfactory results. We have attempted to state the value of the results obtained by the various tests.

The authors wish to express their indebtedness to the numerous writers whose works have been consulted, and an endeavour has been made to acknowledge them by the list of references.

We have pleasure in thanking Sir Thomas Lewis for permission to reproduce the electrocardiograms taken from his book entitled "Clinical Electrocardiography." Dr. D. E. Bedford has supplied the polygraph tracings, and has also read through the proofs of the chapter dealing with the heart. We are grateful for his valuable suggestions and help. Further, we wish to express our thanks for the loan of certain blocks: to Messrs. Hawksley & Sons for the one illustrating the Jacquet polygraph; to Messrs. Down Bros. for those illustrating the pneumothorax needles; and to Professor Harris for the diagram of the electrocardiograph from Anrep and Harris' "Practical Physiology".

In conclusion we wish to acknowledge the unfailing help which we have received from the publishers of this volume.

G. E. BEAUMONT
E. C. DODDS

LONDON, 1924.

CONTENTS

RECENT ADVANCES IN MEDICINE

CHAPTER I

COLLAGEN DISEASES

RECENT developments concerning rheumatic diseases are extremely difficult to describe in any logical or chronological sequence. This is due to the fact that three main groups of workers, proceeding quite independently, have developed more or less independent conceptions of the group of rheumatic diseases and have tried amongst themselves to reconcile their views and to consolidate a comprehensive theory. An attempt to treat the matter chronologically yields such a confusing picture that this will not be attempted. The three main groups are as follows :—

The first group is that headed by Hench (1) of the Mayo Clinic, who was responsible for the introduction of the cortisone and A.C.T.H. treatment of rheumatoid diseases in the year 1949. The second group, headed by Klemperer (1942) (2) attempted to classify a number of diseases under the heading of the collagen group, thereby hoping to unify under a single " pathology " a whole series of diseases which had hitherto been regarded as unconnected with each other. Finally, as the leader of the third group, there is Selye, who has attempted to fit the views of Hench and Klemperer into his own conception of the general adaptation syndrome. It will be necessary to consider the work of each of these three groups separately.

1. The Hench Group at the Mayo Clinic. Hench and his collaborators have been studying the problem of the rheumatic diseases for a prolonged period. Hench (1938) (3) showed that the symptoms of rheumatoid arthritis frequently underwent a remission during an attack of jaundice or during pregnancy. From careful observations on a large number of cases, it was proved conclusively that these remissions were genuine though temporary. Hench speculated as to the possible cause and felt that the circulation of some steroidal substance in pregnancy and in jaundice might be responsible for the alleviation of the joint symptoms. After consultation with E. C. Kendall, Professor of Biochemistry in the Mayo

Clinic, they decided together to investigate the activity of certain steroidal substances isolated from the suprarenal cortex and identified by Kendall. One of these was the now familiar compound " E " which will be dealt with from the chemical point of view at a later stage of this chapter. Hench (1949b) (4) made the astonishing observation that the administration of compound " E " daily in 100 mg. doses resulted in a dramatic improvement in the general symptoms of rheumatoid arthritis. They were also able to show that the same results could be obtained by the injection of A.C.T.H. (which again will be dealt with in detail at a later stage). The improvement resulted in some cases in a complete disappearance of general symptoms and was attended by a feeling of well-being or euphoria in most of the patients. Unfortunately they found that interruption of the treatment was attended by a rapid return of the symptoms and in a few days the patient was in just as bad a condition as before the treatment. In some later observations the results appeared in a limited number of patients to be of a little more permanent character.

There is no doubt that these classical observations stimulated all the recent interest in the rheumatic diseases.

2. Klemperer, Pollack and Baehr (1942) (5) **at New York** introduced a generalisation into pathology by combining a number of disease processes as an entity which they called the diffuse collagen disease. The underlying pathological process was found to be a fibrinoid degeneration of collagen in this series of diseases, which include disseminated lupus erythematosus, rheumatoid arthritis, periarteritis nodosa, thrombo-angiitis obliterans and scleroderma—all having the same fundamental pathology. An alternative name has been suggested of " para-rheumatic disease " for the above mentioned group.

The group of collagen diseases is constantly being added to and there is, naturally, considerable controversy. At the time of writing the following are regarded as being members of this group:— serum sickness, periarteritis nodosa, disseminated lupus erythematosus, rheumatic fever, rheumatoid arthritis in its various forms, scleroderma, dermatomyositis and, according to some workers, calcinosis. Others would like to include Buerger's disease and malignant nephrosclerosis.

General Pathology of the Collagen Diseases. In the first place the chemistry of collagen itself is incompletely understood. It forms the basis of bone and cartilage and the interfibrillary connective tissue. It can be broken down to gelatin and various mucopolysaccharides, such as chrondroitin-sulphuric acid. Another constituent is hyaluronic acid which is again a highly complicated substance whose behaviour is controlled by an elaborate system of enzymes of which hyaluronidase, or the spreading factor, is one. From the histological point of view a study of the diseases mentioned above will show that there are in all similar changes in the fibroblasts, which are largely composed of collagen. They become stained, very refractile ; and the general term for such changes is fibrinoid degeneration. The ætiology of this condition is very largely speculative. Leaving out for the moment Selye's conception that these diseases are related to stress, we can say that various theories have been favoured from time to time. Thus bacterial infection has attracted a number of workers from the time of Poynton and Paine in 1900 and 1901 (6, 7, 8), to the present day work on β-hæmolytic group A streptococcus infection.

Another suggestion has been that these diseases might be associated with allergy and with immunity. Thus Rich and Gregory (1943) (9) claimed to have produced periarteritis nodosa lesions in rabbits by injection of heterologous serum.

The role of hormones in the production of this group of diseases will be discussed in relation to Selye's views.

In a brief review of the varied collagen diseases we may start with *serum sickness,* which made its first appearance after the production and use of diphtheria antitoxin in 1890. The symptoms commence within a week or so of the administration of the serum and consist of enlargement of the lymphatic glands with underlying tenderness, and skin lesions such as urticaria, itching, and macular erythemas may also develop. Joint pains may or may not occur. The symptoms usually clear up in the course of a few weeks.

Periarteritis Nodosa. This condition was first described by Kussmaul and Meier in 1866 ; its clinical diagnosis is extremely difficult and its pathology is essentially a degeneration of the media and intima of the small and medium-sized blood vessels. Thrombosis, hæmorrhage etc. can occur, again rendering the condition very difficult to diagnose except at post mortem.

Disseminated Lupus Erythematosus. This is a disease occuring in young women and frequently initiated by exposure to sunlight. The skin lesions characteristically have the well known "butterfly" distribution on the face and may consist of confluent red eruptions; and a swinging pyrexia associated with pains of a rheumatic character in the joints frequently occurs.

Scleroderma. This condition occurs in the fingers but may involve the whole body. There is a characteristic thickening of the skin together with an infiltration of the subcutaneous tissue by collagenous material.

Dermatomyositis. This is a vary rare disease in which it is claimed by many that the underlying pathology is the characteristic collagen degeneration. The clinical features consist of pain in the muscles, with or without pyrexia. Occasionally there may be skin reactions.

Calcinosis. In this condition calcification of the subcutaneous tissues and connective tissues occurs. Its pathology is similar to that of scleroderma, but proof that this condition is a collagen disease is not definite.

Gout. Attempts have been made to include gout in the collagen diseases group, but this appears to be hardly justifiable as any collagen changes that occur are more likely to be due to the primary metabolic defect associated with purine metabolism.

3. Selye at Montreal has developed a very complex theory to explain the ætiology of the collagen diseases. No attempt will be made to give a detailed account of this work as at the present time the views of most workers on this subject are in a state of flux. For those requiring a full statement, the reader is referred to the massive work entitled "Stress" by this author (10).

Selye developed the idea that animals react to stress or injury by a certain sequence of physiological reactions, which is termed the "general adaptation syndrome" (or G.A.S.). This consists of a number of phases, of which perhaps the most important is the discharge of hormones from the pituitary to act on the suprarenal. According to this theory, when an animal is subjected to stress or injury the anterior pituitary pours out adreno-corticotropic hormones, and the stimulated cortex secretes hormones which Selye divides into two more or less clear-cut categories, namely those regulating the electrolyte metabolism which he calls "mineralo-corticoids" and those which influence carbohydrate metabolism and which he calls "gluco-corticoids". According to Selye it is the interplay of the action of these hormones which provides the rheumatoid phenomenon. The experimental evidence on which this rests has been clarified by a number of workers. The fundamental observation was by Selye and Pentz (1943) (11) who showed that unilaterally nephrectomised rats treated with a high sodium chloride intake developed lesions similar to periarteritis nodosa when they are injected with very heavy doses of deoxycorticosterone.

Selye extended this work and showed that giving heavy doses of deoxycorticosterone to animals that had been damaged in various ways, such as by adrenalectomy, thyroidectomy, exposure to cold etc., would cause arthritic changes similar to those in man. On the basis of this Selye put forward the view that the fundamental underlying pathology of the collagen diseases was an upset of the suprarenal cortex produced by the pituitary secretion as a result of stress. This pituitary secretion caused cortical stimulation leading to the outpouring of the mineralo-corticoids which were responsible for the syndrome.

Selye's main work on G.A.S. was prior to the discoveries of Hench and his colleagues and this accounts for the extraordinary confusion of the literature, and also for the difficulties of anyone attempting to give an orderly summary. As Marrian puts it in his review of the subject (12) :—

"Following the announcement in 1949 by the Mayo Clinic group of the effects of cortisone and of A.C.T.H. in rheumatoid arthritis and rheumatic fever, Selye (1949) (13) re-interpreted his earlier findings concerning the effect of adrenalectomy on the production of experimental arthritis by D.O.C.A. He suggested that 'it was reasonable to assume that adrenalectomy sensitizes to the toxic effects of D.O.C.A. because it removes the source of endogenous gluco-corticoids and thereby predisposes to the development of a particularly unfavourable gluco-corticoid–mineralo-corticoid balance'. In support of this hypothesis he cited a number of earlier observations made by himself and his co-workers suggesting that certain of the effects on living animals of 'mineralo-corticoids' such as deoxycorticosterone are 'diametrically opposed to those of gluco-corticoids'. It may be noted, however, that this earlier work did not include any observations that 'mineralo-corticoid' induced rheumatic lesions in animals could be cured by the administration of gluco-corticoids. In the same communication Selye showed that an experimental 'arthritis' could be produced in rats by the injection of formaldehyde into the vicinity of the joints. This experimental arthritis, he found, could be aggravated by pre-treatment of the animals with D.O.C.A. and inhibited by cortisone or A.C.T.H."

The whole position of Selye's theory is very difficult to assess today. It is, for instance, very doubtful whether his clear-cut distinction between "mineralo-corticoids" and "gluco-corticoids" is justifiable. Very carefyl observations on the pharmacology of compounds such as deoxycorticosterone and so forth tend to show that this clear-cut distinction does not hold.

Up to the present it has been possible to isolate and identify those substances capable of prolonging the life of adrenalectomised animals. These are as follows :— (1) 11-deoxycorticosterone ; (2) 11-deoxy-17-hydroxycorticosterone ; (3) Corticosterone ; (4) 17-hydroxy-corticosterone ; (5) 11-dehydro-corticosterone ; (6) 11-dehydro-17-hydroxycorticosterone (cortisone). In addition to these six substances, adrenal extracts contain the so-called "amorphous fraction", the constitution of which is quite unknown, and which will also maintain life. According to Selye's (1950) views the pharmacology of these compounds can be considered under two headings : (*a*) compounds 1 and 2 and the amorphous fraction are concerned with the regulation of electrolyte metabolism and water balance, whilst (*b*) compounds 3–6 are concerned almost entirely with the carbohydrate effect. Recent investigation has shown that the pharmacological actions of these substances overlap very considerably.

Whilst an interpretation of Selye's view must await much more experimental work, it is interesting to note that Marrian (1951) (12) and his colleagues have very definitely demonstrated that in established rheumatoid arthritis progesterone metabolism is modified. It is known that progesterone is excreted mainly in the form of pregnanediol, and when progesterone is administered to a patient with rheumatoid arthritis an abnormally high amount of pregnanediol is excreted. The actual interpretation of these results, as Marrian points out, must be cautious, but it would certainly seem to be interesting evidence that the disease rheumatoid arthritis is associated with some abnormality of steroid metabolism.

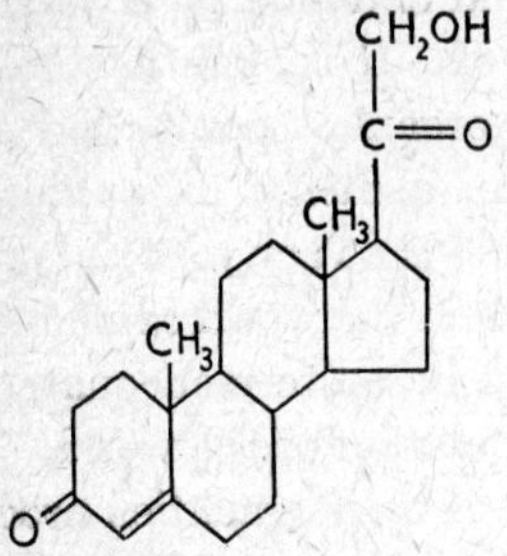

11-deoxycorticosterone

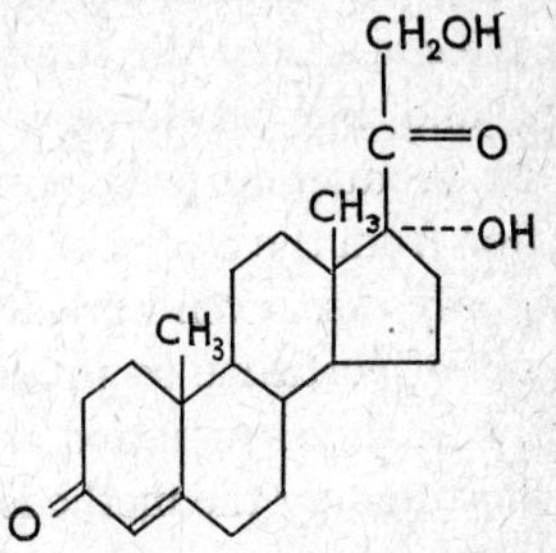

11-deoxy-17-hydroxycorticosterone

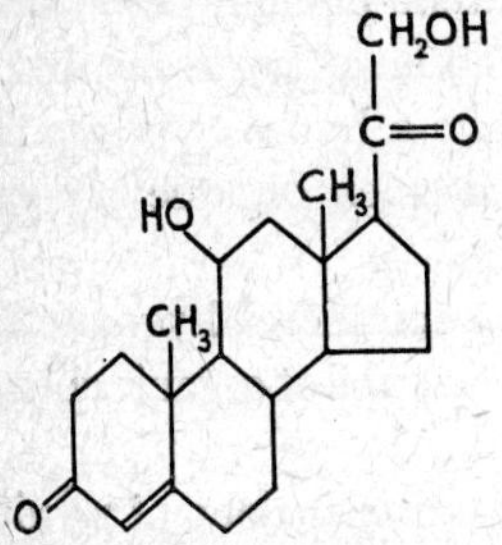

Corticosterone

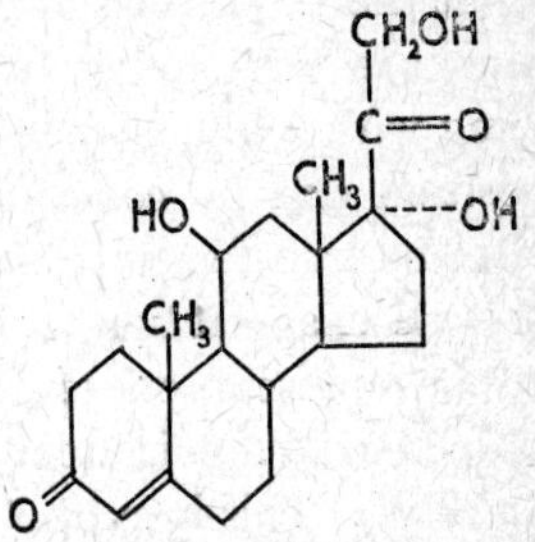

17-hydroxycorticosterone

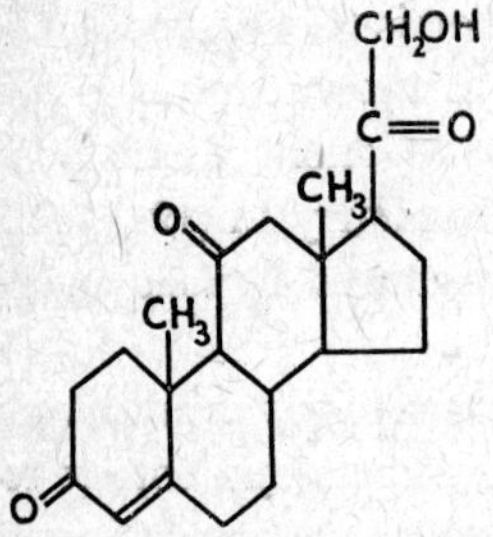

11-dehydrocorticosterone

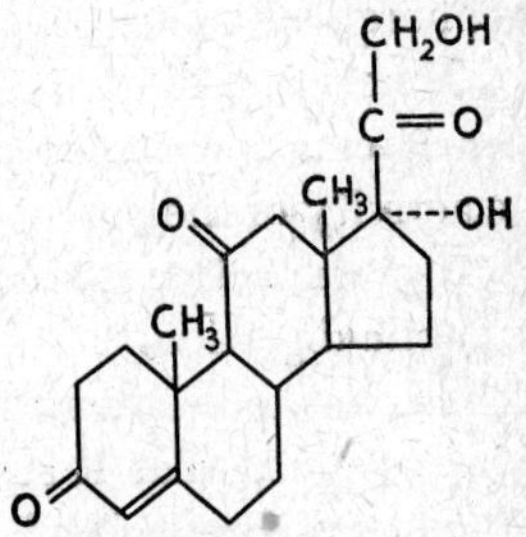

11-dehydro-17-hydroxycortico-sterone (cortisone)

Practical considerations. Whatever may be the final outcome of the theories which have been discussed above the fact remains that two substances, cortisone and A.C.T.H., are capable of causing a remission in the symptoms of patients with collagen diseases, particularly rheumatoid arthritis. It is proposed to review briefly the chemistry of the two substances.

Cortisone. This substance is a steroid obtained by Kendall and his colleagues from the suprarenal cortex. It is slightly soluble in water, and, like all steroids, soluble in organic solvents and in oil, and its production presents problems of immense difficulties. Its isolation from the cortex of the suprarenal is a very wasteful process and in any case, even were all the glands in the world available, the amount of cortisone so produced would be quite inadequate for a fraction of the rheumatoid arthritis population of the world.

Unfortunately the methods of synthesis by degradation processes from cholesterol cannot be applied as, at the time of writing, there is no practical method of introducing either an oxygen or a hydroxy group at the 11 position of the cyclopenteno-phenanthrene ring. A solution has been found to the production of cortisone by commencing with a bile acid. Bile acids have a hydroxy group at the 12 position and by considerable and complex organic procedures this can be transferred to the 11 position.

It is no exaggeration to say that the commercial production of cortisone represents one of the greatest triumphs of organic chemistry in its industrial application.

A.C.T.H. This is extracted from the anterior lobe of pituitaries obtained from the slaughter house. It is a protein and its constitution is unknown despite the fact that it has been obtained electrophoretically pure. The work of Morris (Cortis-Jones, Crooke, Henly, Morris and Morris, 1950) (14) has shown that it is possible to ultra-filter a low molecular weight component which possesses all the activity of the parent material. Similarly Li (1949) (15) has shown that the active extract may be produced by acid hydrolysis or by peptic digestion.

A.C.T.H. has to be administered intramuscularly or intravenously and it is assumed that it stimulates the suprarenal cortex to produce "mineralo-corticoids", and the "gluco-corticoids" including cortisone.

Physiological Action of Cortisone and A.C.T.H. in Man

A detailed account of the action of cortisone and A.C.T.H. in man is found in a comprehensive article by Sprague (1950) and his colleagues (16). The material used in this investigation was cortisone acetate administered usually in doses of 100 mg. (being equivalent to 89 mg. of free cortisone) in the form of a suspension in saline, or A.C.T.H. obtained in ampoules (containing 25 mg.) of which the pressor content and the oxytocin content were known. The anti-rheumatic effect is not described in this paper except that the authors state that the results of Hench and his colleagues have been confirmed. The following are the principal effects of the substances :—

Body weight. Due to the euphoria and increased appetite produced, the body weight was invariably increased in the use of both substances ; and a marked feature in some cases was a characteristic moon-shaped face.

Effects on the skin. Acne and hairiness were produced in a number of subjects, but it is interesting to note that there was no masculinisation of females as is obtained by the use of testosterone in the treatment of inoperable carcinoma. Keratosis and the development of cutaneous striæ has been noted, and in some instance deep pigmentation occurred.

Muscular weakness. This developed in a considerable number of patients undergoing prolonged treatment.

Changes in electrolyte and metabolism balance. A negative balance in nitrogen and potassium was produced by A.C.T.H. whilst cortisone caused relatively slight changes. It would appear that A.C.T.H. produces more of the mineralo-corticoid effect than does cortisone. Details of individual experiments with these substances will be found in the paper referred to.

Effect on menstruation. This was very variable in the series of 10 women treated. Three became amenorrhœic, a fourth missed a period and others remained unaffected. In general, treatment with both cortisone and A.C.T.H. appeared to reduce sexual activity in both male and female patients.

Euphoria. This again was very variable, but occurred very regularly with high dosage, consisting of a general feeling of well-being with a very definite improvement in mental activity, particularly in patients who were seriously ill either with arthritis or some similar condition. For example, the authors quote the case of a man in the terminal stages of myelogenous leukæmia who, when treated with cortisone, took a constructive interest in his future despite the fact that he was to die in a very few days' time.

Blood pressure. The general consensus of opinion is that the materials have little effect on blood pressure. In a small number of cases there was a significant rise. The authors feel, however, that the substances may induce hypertension is some circumstances.

Excretion of urinary steroids. Treatment with A.C.T.H. causes an increase in the excretion of urinary steroids, whereas in the case of cortisone administration the excretion of 17-ketosteroids usually falls unless high doses are given. Persistent low levels were observed after very prolonged treatment.

Leucocytes. Cortisone produced very little consistent change in the circulating leucocytes on prolonged treatment, whereas A.C.T.H. produces a characteristic disappearance of eosinophils.

Effect on cortical function. There appears to be evidence that treatment with cortisone produces depression of animal adrenal function. It is suggested that this depression is the cause of the lowered excretion of 17-ketosteroids on and after treatment with cortisone.

Treatment of Rheumatoid Arthritis with Cortisone and A.C.T.H.

The dosage is still mainly unstandardised and arbitrary. In the first instance Hench and his colleagues maintained that 100 mg. per day in divided doses of 25 mg. were necessary to produce an effect, though recent workers have found that smaller doses are capable of producing remissions.

The actual regimen is not yet established, but it is usual to continue the treatment for seven to fourteen days and then to reduce the dose in the hope that the good effects will not pass off. With regard to A.C.T.H., it is usual to find the effect developing after the administration of the substance for some four to five days and similarly the effect is prolonged for that length of time after the drug has been withdrawn. With regard to dosage, this again is a matter for experimentation, but usually between 40–80 mg. are recommended (Prunty, 1951) (17). With regard to the type of case treated, any member of the collagen group, including rheumatic fever, is suitable for treatment. Contra-indications are observed in the following conditions:— Myocardial insufficiency, diabetes mellitus, Cushing's syndrome, tuberculosis and advanced renal disease. One of the most important contra-indications is tuberculosis, for the administration of A.C.T.H. and cortisone to patients with tuberculous lesions is frequently followed by dissemination of lesions throughout the body.

Treatment of Skin Diseases with A.C.T.H.

A very good review of this subject together with an account of a number of cases treated will be found in the paper by Brodthagen, Reymann & Schwartz (1951) (18). Pemphigus vegetans was favourably affected and the patient remained clear of symptoms for three months after the treatment had been stopped. A case of pemphigus vulgaris was also affected, but relapsed almost as soon as the treatment was interrupted. In the case of scleroderma, improvement was shown in a few cases, but some proved to be resistant. It is interesting to note that these authors found one patient with periarteritis nodosa resistant, despite prolonged treatment. The dosage in most of the cases consisted of 75 mg. per day for the first week and then a reduction to 25 mg. later. Frenkel, Hellinga and Groen (1951) (19) have described a successful treatment by A.C.T.H. of the rare condition known as Sjögren's disease. This condition occurs in middle-aged women and consists of chronic inflammatory changes in the lachrymal and salivary glands with a diminution in the production of tears and saliva. Joint lesions occasionally occur and these are usually of a rheumatoid character. The condition relapsed and during treatment the patient appeared to be quite well.

Clinical Use of Cortisone

Cortisone acetate is put up in 20 ml. vials ready for intramuscular injection, each ml. containing 25 mg. It must be shaken before use and must not be stored in a refrigerator. It is injected deeply into the gluteal muscles. Before and during treatment of any case certain investigations must be carried out. The chest must be X-rayed to exclude the presence of tuberculosis. An electrocardiogram should be taken with the three standard and nine unipolar leads in case an electrocardiogram is required later to indicate a potassium deficiency. Further an abnormal electrocardiogram may return to normal under treatment. The patient should be weighed daily. The serum sodium and potassium content should be estimated weekly in Addison's disease to check a rise in the sodium or fall in the potassium level, as this is indicative of an overdosage. The erythrocyte sedimentation rate should be determined weekly. Daily blood pressure readings and tests of the urine for glucose should be made. The patient's grip should be tested twice a week, by seeing the height to which he can raise the column of mercury in a sphygmomanometer, when compressing the rolled-up cuff into which a little air has been pumped. The joint sensitivity can be tested in cases of rheumatoid arthritis by firm pressure over the affected hands or wrists. Grade 0 indicates no pain, Grade 1 some pain, Grade 2 wincing, and Grade 3 the patient pulls his hand away. The usual dose for rheumatoid arthritis is 100 mg. every eight hours for 3 doses, than 100 mg. every twelve hours for 2 doses, then 100 mg. every twenty-four hours for seven to fourteen days, followed by 100 mg. every forty-eight hours for fourteen to twenty-eight days. It may now be possible to give 50 mg. in water by mouth for six days, with a weekly intramuscular injection of 100 mg. in order to maintain the improvement. In Addison's disease smaller doses are usually required, such as 12·5 to 25 mg. daily intramuscularly.

Results. We have treated a series of cases including rheumatoid arthritis, disseminated lupus erythematosus, sarcoidosis, Sjögren's disease, and Addison's disease. The case of Sjögren's disease appeared to do best and maintained the improvement after the cortisone was discontinued. The lupus erythematosus and rheumatoid arthritis cases, although treated for two to three months, quickly relapsed when the treatment was discontinued. In sarcoidosis the uveal tract lesions, and the salivary gland swellings rapidly improved with the intravenous administration of A.C.T.H. in small doses (20), but the X-ray shadows in the lungs were not affected.

REFERENCES

(1) Hench, Kendall and Slocumb. *Proc. Staff Meet. Mayo Clinic*, 1949(a), **24**, 181.
(2) Klemperer. *Journ. Amer. Med. Assocn.*, 1942, **119**, 331.
(3) Hench. *Proc. Staff. Meet. Mayo Clinic*, 1938, **13**, 161.
(4) Hench. *Proc. Staff. Meet. Mayo Clinic*, 1949(b), **24**, 277.
(5) Klemperer, Pollock and Baehr. *Journ. Amer. Med. Assocn.*, 1942, **119**, 331.
(6) Poynton and Paine. *Lancet*, 1900, *ii*, 861.
(7) Poynton and Paine. *Lancet*, 1900, *ii*, 932.
(8) Poynton and Paine. *Brit. Med. Journ.*, 1901, *ii*, 779.

(9) Rich and Gregory. *Bull. Johns Hopkins Hosp.*, 1943, **73**, 239.
(10) Selye. *Stress*, 1950. Acta Inc. Publications, Montreal.
(11) Selye and Pentz. *Canad. Med. Assocn. Journ.*, 1943, **49**, 264.
(12) Marrian. *Practitioner*, 1951, **166**, 43.
(13) Selye. *Brit. Med. Journ.*, 1949, *ii*, 1129.
(14) Cortis-Jones, Crooke, Henly, Morris and Morris. *Biochem. Journ.*, 1950, **46**, 173.
(15) Li. Abstracts of Communications, 1st International Congress of Biochemistry, 1949, 386.
(16) Sprague, Power, Mason, Albert, Mathieson, Hench, Kendall, Slocumb and Polley. *Arch. Int. Med.*, 1950, **85**, 199.
(17) Prunty. *Practitioner*, 1951, **166**, 33.
(18) Brodthagen, Reymann and Schwartz. *Act. Endocrinol.*, 1951, *vi*, 110.
(19) Frenkel, Hellinga and Groen. *Act. Endocrinol.*, 1951, *vi*, 161.
(20) Jelliffe, Stewart and Beaumont. *Lancet*, 1951, *i*, 1260.

CHAPTER II

ANTIBIOTIC SUBSTANCES

Penicillin

The last few decades have witnessed the introduction of an increasing number of compounds which, whilst showing toxicity of a high order against pathogenic organisms, exercise little or no harmful effect upon their human hosts. Penicillin was discovered by Fleming in 1929 (1). It is an extracellular product of the metabolism of the mould *Penicillium notatum* and represents one of the first of a series of antibacterial compounds obtained from moulds and bacteria. Many of these compounds display potency of a very high order when tested *in vitro*; relatively few are sufficiently free of toxic effects on the host to permit their therapeutic application.

Antibiotic Activity. Penicillin is most active against gram-positive and gram-negative cocci and gram-positive bacilli. It is active against spirochætes and possibly some of the larger viruses. Sensitivity of various strains of organisms varies widely, so that it is important to know the organism responsible for the infection and its sensitivity to penicillin.

Administration. Penicillin is now available in large quantities and at a fraction of its original cost. The yellow amorphous sodium penicillin has been largely superseded by the pure crystalline penicillin G, or by pure penicillin G combined with procaine. Increasing purification has led to fewer side reactions and there is a general tendency to employ very much larger doses.

It is necessary in treating infections with penicillin to maintain an effective bacteriostatic level in the plasma, which varies from 0·02–0·20 units per ml. This may be achieved by injecting intramuscularly aqueous solutions of penicillin three-hourly. The rapid elimination of penicillin in the urine prevents this figure being maintained except by very frequent injections.

Several attempts have been made to delay the absorption of penicillin from the site of injection. This was done by suspending penicillin in sterile white beeswax and arachis oil, but the solution was difficult to suck up into a syringe on account of its viscosity and the beeswax frequently excited undesirable foreign body reactions locally. A great advance has been achieved by the introduction of procaine penicillin (2, 3) which is an equimolecular compound of penicillin and procaine in a suspending agent. It is sometimes combined with a water-repellent substance, aluminium monostearate, which is said to even out absorption. A single dose of procaine penicillin of 300,000 units gives an assayable blood level for twenty-four hours. Commercially procaine penicillin is often combined with sodium or potassium penicillin G to ensure a satisfactory initial blood level.

Excretion of penicillin by the kidney can be delayed by some substances which are excreted by the tubules. Caronamide (4, 5) diminishes renal tubular excretion of penicillin, and 3 g. by mouth three-hourly produces a plasma caronamide level of 15 mg. per 100 ml. Since the development of preparations such as procaine penicillin there is little general use for caronamide except possibly in treating infections due to resistant bacteria, where it is necessary to maintain exceptionally high penicillin blood levels.

Penicillin is rapidly destroyed by acid and by organisms, such as those found in the gut which produce penicillinase. These factors prevent penicillin being administered orally or rectally as a routine. Penicillin has been combined with a number of vehicles to neutralise gastric acid, and enclosed in capsules to aid absorption from the gut. Oral administration is possible, and satisfactory blood levels and therapeutic effects have been reported (6, 7) but the dose should be about ten times that for intramuscular injection. It may be used in children and infants, or where the organism is highly sensitive to penicillin.

Toxic Effects. Penicillin has maintained its promise of being almost non-toxic in therapeutic doses. Skin reactions, especially urticaria, are the commonest effects although drug fever and swelling of the joints may occur. The reactions usually come on after treatment has been maintained for some time, but some patients may develop allergic reactions very rapidly. When penicillin is given by mouth, glossitis and stomatitis may occur, and there is often secondary invasion with saprophytic fungi. These reactions may be reduced by giving the Vitamin B complex to patients who are taking penicillin by mouth. When penicillin is used topically for skin diseases a sensitisation dermatitis may occur, and it is important to discontinue penicillin should this happen.

There is usually no indication to discontinue treatment on account of the milder allergic effects, and they may be controlled by the administration of one of the anti-histamine groups of drugs. For the rare severe general reactions desensitisation may be attempted by giving very small doses of penicillin subcutaneously, such as 400 units three times a week, and increasing the dose gradually until a full therapeutic dose can be injected without any side effects (8).

Preparations of Penicillin. Many of the earlier preparations of penicillin have been replaced by the more recently developed ones. Penicillin cream and solutions of penicillin should be kept in a refrigerator. Aqueous solutions of procaine penicillin retain their potency for seven days at room temperature and twenty-one days in a refrigerator. The other preparations of penicillin keep for up to two years in the dry state in cool dry conditions. The date of expiry is usually printed on the vial.

Powder. Sodium or potassium penicillin G is put up in rubber-capped vials containing 100,000, 200,000, 500,000, and 1,000,000 international units. Calcium penicillin which is used for surface applications is put up in containers of 1, 10 or 50 Mega units. (1 Mega unit = 1,000,000 units).

Procaine Penicillin. This is put up as :— Penicillin G procaine salt (300,000 units per ml.). Penicillin G procaine salt in aqueous suspension (300,000 units per ml.). Penicillin G procaine salt + penicillin G (300,000 units of procaine penicillin G per ml. + 100,000 units of penicillin G.)

Tablets for Oral Use. 10,000, 20,000, 50,000 and 1,000,000 units of penicillin G per tablet.

Lozenge. 500 units calcium penicillin per lozenge.

Chewing Gum. 5,000 units calcium penicillin.

Creams. 500 mg. calcium penicillin/g.Lanette wax base with 1·1% phenoxetol.

Ointments. Calcium penicillin 50,000 units and ointments of alcohols 100 g. They contain 500 units penicillin/g.

Powder for Local Application. 5,000 units/g. of calcium penicillin combined with a sulphonamide or starch or talc base.

Eye Drops. 500–2,500 units per ml.

Eye " Tabloids ". 250 units per " tabloid ".

Eye Ointment. 25,000 units penicillin G per g.

Clinical Applications

Intramuscular Injection. A dose of 50,000–250,000 units of penicillin is given every three hours.

The dose is prepared by adding 1–2 ml. of sterile pyrogen-free water to the powder. The vial should then be gently rotated, vigorous shaking is unnecessary and may cause frothing. The syringe and needle should be boiled in plain water and kept in distilled water. They must never be placed in antiseptic or spirit as these substances destroy penicillin. The skin round the site for intramuscular injection may be prepared with soap-water, ether or Cetrimide. For ordinary intramuscular injection an Arnold No. 6 serum needle may be used.

Procaine penicillin is administered by intramuscular injection only. The dose is 300,000–600,000 units of procaine penicillin every twelve hours. A 5 ml. syringe fitted with a No. 20 S.W.G. needle is suitable, and 2–4 ml. of sterile distilled water are injected through the rubber cap at the base of the vial. This is unnecessary with the aqueous suspension of procaine penicillin. The vial is shaken vigorously to suspend the particles. It is advantageous to build up a positive pressure by injecting a syringe-full of air into the vial. The required dose (1–2 ml.) is withdrawn and injected into the patient.

Powder for Local Treatment. Dry penicillin powder made up with sterile sulphathiazole is used for wounds and abrasions. The powder is blown on to the surface with an insufflator to form a thick hoar frost. The application should be repeated every twenty-four hours, but must not be continued for longer than five days, owing to the risk of the development of skin reactions due to sensitivity to the sulphonamide. This method is of most use in relatively dry surfaces, as blood or exudate tends to wash away the powder.

Ointments and Creams. These are used for local application in certain skin or eye infections.

Lozenges or Pastilles. These are useful in treating infections of the mouth and throat. One pastille should be sucked every hour for 8 hours.

Eye Drops. In certain eye infections drops containing 500–2,500 units per ml. every one or two hours are beneficial.

Inhalation. Penicillin may be given by inhalation, in the treatment of bronchitis and bronchiectasis, by means of an inhaler, such as the Collison. 20,000 to 100,000 units in 2 ml. of distilled water are put into the bulb for each inhalation, and the "mist" inhaled every two hours daily through the oro-nasal mask furnished with an expiratory valve. The vaporisation is effected by oxygen and takes about fifteen minutes. The rubber tubing of the apparatus should not be a synthetic preparation, which inactivates the penicillin.

Solutions. These can be made up with distilled water or saline, at 1,000 units per ml. for instilling twelve-hourly through fine rubber tubes into wounds which have been closed, for injecting into abscess cavities after aspiration, and as a spray for skin and mucous membrane infections. Solutions of a strength of 1,000 to 2,000 units per ml. are suitable for injecting into the cerebro-spinal, pleural, pericardial and joint cavities, and 10,000 units per ml. for intratracheal injection.

Septicæmia. Successful treatment of septicæmia, whether of staphylococcal or streptococcal origin, necessitates not only the complete sterilisation of the blood, but also the elimination of primary and secondary foci of infection. It is recommended that 100,000–250,000 units of penicillin G should be injected intramuscularly every three hours.

Sub-Acute Bacterial Endocarditis. Patients should be given at least 2,000,000 units of penicillin G a day for six weeks by intermittent intramuscular injection every three hours. If there is a relapse or an increase in resistance of the organism 5,000,000 units a day for eight weeks or more should be given (9).

Meningitis. Successful treatment of meningitis by the administration of penicillin and sulphonamides has been reported by many workers including Rosenberg and Arling (10) and Daniels et al. (11). Staphylococcal infections of the meninges are usually secondary to mastoid and sinus foci. Immediate surgical drainage of such centres, followed by local treatment with penicillin solution, is of considerable value in reducing the chance of reinfection. Smith, Duthie and Cairns (12) advise the treatment of uncomplicated pneumococcal meningitis as follows : After finding pneumococci in the cerebro-spinal fluid 8,000 to 16,000 units of penicillin are injected intrathecally, with smaller doses for infants. The penicillin is in pyrogen-free saline solution, 2,000 units per ml. Fifteen thousand units of penicillin are injected intramuscularly every three hours to control any primary infection or septicæmia. Sulphadiazine is also given by mouth or nasal tube, first 4 g., and then 2 g. every four hours, an adequate fluid intake being ensured to prevent renal block. After twelve hours a second intrathecal injection of penicillin is given. If the fluid is now thicker a third puncture should be made twelve hours later to detect any incipient ventricular block, which might require intraventricular injections of penicillin. Daily injections of penicillin into the theca must be continued for five days, the intramuscular injections are discontinued after five days, and the sulphadiazine reduced to 1 g. four-hourly after five days and maintained at this dose for a week.

If the cerebro-spinal pathway becomes blocked by pus, in sites such as the aqueduct, penicillin should be injected into the lateral ventricles through parietal burr-holes. After draining the pus the penicillin can be injected through an indwelling catheter. In all cases in which intrathecal injections are required non-irritating preparations of penicillin should be used, and great care taken in the aseptic technique. In meningococcal and streptococcal meningitis similar amounts of penicillin are injected intrathecally every twenty-four hours until the cerebro-spinal fluid is free from organisms, and intramuscular injections of 100,000 units are given every three hours for seven days.

Pneumonia. In the treatment of pneumonia there is little to choose between penicillin and the sulphonamides, except in cases of sulphonamide resistance especially those due to staphylococci, or where the lower toxicity of penicillin is advantageous. The usual dose for an adult is 50,000–100,000 units every three hours for seven days; for a child 5,000 units per year of age. Primary atypical (virus) pneumonia does not respond to penicillin.

Empyema. In the treatment of empyemata due to pneumococci, streptococci or staphylococci, but not in cases of Bact. coli infections, also in infected hæmothorax following injury, intra-pleural instillation is the method of choice. Penicillin solution containing 1,000 units per ml. should be injected into the pleural space following aspiration of pleural fluid. The amount of penicillin injected depends on the size of the empyema cavity. Cavities holding 10 to 20 oz. of fluid should receive 60,000 units of penicillin, total empyemata 120,000 units, and 30,000 units for small pockets. Three to four aspirations and instillations generally suffice. Thoracotomy is usually required to evacuate blood clot, fibrin and pus. Local penicillin treatment after rib-resection is often unsatisfactory and penicillin is then best given by eight-hourly intramuscular injections of 100,000 units.

Bronchiectasis. The cavities are emptied as far as possible by postural drainage, followed by the intratracheal injection of penicillin. The skin and subcutaneous tissues are anæsthetised in the neck, between the cricoid cartilage and the first ring of the trachea, with 2 ml. of 2% procaine. Two ml. of 2% Amethocaine are then injected rapidly through a No. 14 needle into the trachea and the patient told to avoid coughing. The syringe is detached from the needle, the patient placed in the optimum position for fluid to run down the trachea to the affected part of the lung, and then 8 ml. of penicillin solution containing 10,000 units per ml. are rapidly injected through the needle which has been left *in situ* in the trachea. This treatment, repeated daily for seven days, has resulted in considerable clinical improvement. Alternatively the penicillin can be given every two hours by inhalation.

Chronic Bronchitis. In some cases the amount of sputum can be very considerably reduced and the breathing made easier, by the inhalation of penicillin, as described above.

Infections of the Skeletal System. Osteomyelitis and coccal infections following compound fractures respond well to both penicillin and sulphonamide therapy. It is on record that cases of chronic osteomyelitis of some years' duration have been cleared in a relatively short period by penicillin treatment. Sterile blood cultures may be obtained following intravenous, supported by intramuscular injection, but the intramedullary route is obviously recommended for resistant strains. Grace and Bryson (13) treated 7 cases of chronic osteomyelitis, with 1 failure. The penicillin was given intramuscularly in doses of 30,000 units every three hours for ten to twenty-one days, and simultaneously 4,000 to 20,000 units of penicillin per ml. were applied locally into the sinus tract. In open wounds, aspiration of exudate and local administration of penicillin and sulphonamide powder accelerate the recovery. Kirby and Hepp (14) have emphasised the risk of secondary meningococcal infection from osteomyelitis of the facial bones, and recommend penicillin rather than sulphonamides in order to reduce the risk of reinfection. Penicillin treatment of osteomyelitis should be followed by surgical removal of infected or necrotic bone. Infections by streptococcal and staphylococcal organisms located in bone, joints and synovial membranes respond well to prolonged penicillin treatment. In contrast, chronic rheumatoid arthritis, even when associated with recognised coccal strains known to be penicillin-sensitive, fails to respond to what must be regarded as massive doses of the drug. Boland, Headley and Hench (15), who have given careful attention to classical cases of arthritis, report complete failure.

Florey and Florey (16) recommend the daily application of penicillin in the wound following mastoidectomy.

Gonorrhœa in the Male. The efficacy of penicillin treatment in gonorrhœa has been established beyond doubt. Even when examined over a period of several weeks, patients show no recurrence of symptoms. Welch et al. (17) report the superiority of penicillin X in the treatment of gonorrhœa by single intramuscular injections of 25,000 units, but many other workers suggest that 100,000 units of penicillin or even more are essential to ensure a permanent cure in all cases. Most strains of the organism are sensitive to sulphathiazole treatment, but are prone to develop sulphonamide resistance. Fortunately the sulphonamide-resistant strains which are encountered show no penicillin resistance. Five injections of 20,000 units every two hours are usually sufficient to effect a cure. The difficulty of maintaining a sufficiently high blood concentration by one injection in out-patients who cannot attend for the five injections, has been overcome by Romansky and Rittman (18) who recommend a beeswax-peanut oil mixture as the medium for injection. By this means they cured 11 out of 12 patients suffering from gonococcal urethritis with a single injection of penicillin of 40,000 to 66,000 units. Romansky et al. (19) obtained 100% of cures in 75 cases of gonorrhœa in males, by a single oil injection of 175,000 units of penicillin. Whatever treatment is given the patient should be re-examined for infection after two and four months. A single dose of 600,000 units of procaine penicillin is usually effective.

Gonorrhœa in the Female. This responds equally well to

penicillin therapy, symptoms disappearing in the majority of cases following the administration of 100,000 units.

Syphilitic Infections. In primary and secondary syphilis penicillin therapy has proved equally satisfactory. The results obtained by many workers compare well with those using massive arsenical therapy, without exposing the patient to the toxic effects and idiosyncrasies of the latter drugs. Whether penicillin is given intramuscularly or intravenously, a continuously high concentration in the blood must be maintained. Mahoney et al. (20) in an early communication, showed the disappearance of the spirochætes and clearing of serological reactions following the administration of 25,000 units every four hours for eight days. Moore et al. (21) and Norcross (22) confirm this finding and have reported apparent recovery from primary and secondary syphilis following treatment with much lower quantities of penicillin. Leifer (23) from his experience in treating 96 cases, concluded that early syphilis can be cured by intramuscular injections of 20,000 units every three hours for seven and a half days, giving a total of 1·2 million units. Lourie et al. (24) have reported favourably on a method for the ambulatory treatment of early syphilis. Three intramuscular injections of 600,000 units were given at hourly intervals on five consecutive days. The penicillin was dissolved in 5 ml. water. The treatment of cardio-vascular syphilis with penicillin has proved unsatisfactory in the hands of Dolkart and Schwemlein (25), the injections having to be abandoned owing to cardiac pain. The simultaneous administration of arsenicals and penicillin has been claimed to have a synergistic effect and to be superior to straightforward penicillin therapy. The Committee on Medical Research and the United States Public Health Service (26) reported in 1946 on the treatment of early syphilis with penicillin. They found that the percentage failure at the end of eleven months after treatment varied from 15% when 2,400,000 units of penicillin had been given, to 62% with 600,000 units. Patients treated during the first week of disease did twice as well as those treated after two months or later. Simultaneous treatment with arsenic or bismuth increased the number of patients cured when total amounts of penicillin were given varying between 300,000 to 1·2 million units. Crystalline penicillin G is superior to amorphous penicillin in both experimental animals and man. McElligott (27) recommends for primary and early secondary syphilis a course of 8 daily injections of procaine penicillin followed by 10 weekly injections of bismuth suspension, each injection being equivalent to 0·2 g. of bismuth metal.

Gas Gangrene. The administration of penicillin to subjects with wounds infected by organisms producing gas gangrene has been reported from several sources. No clear indication of the effectiveness of penicillin alone is possible, since the administration has always been accompanied by injections of antitoxin, local administration of sulphonamides, and, where necessary, by surgical operation. Although Cutler (28) has reported 4 cases of gas gangrene infections following compound fractures which failed to respond to intravenous injection of penicillin, the consensus of opinion in this matter is that local administration of penicillin is at least as effective as any preceding method, and that intravenous administration of the drug prior to operation is an effective means of localising the area of attack.

Tetanus. *In vitro,* Cl. tetani is sensitive to penicillin. Altemeier (29) did not find that penicillin had any beneficial influence on the course of established clinical tetanus. This is to be expected, as penicillin has no known effect on the tetanus toxin.

Agranulocytosis. Boland et al. (30) have shown that penicillin is of value in treating agranulocytosis due to various causes, as death generally results from secondary infections rather than from the suppression of bone marrow function. If the infection can be checked the bone marrow is given a chance to recover. The agranulocytosis may be due to such causes as sulphonamides, mapharsen, gold salts, thiouracil, etc.

Actinomycosis. Hamilton and Kirkpatrick (31) successfully treated 2 cases of cervical actinomycosis with three-hourly intramuscular injections of penicillin, the dose varying from 25,000 to 33,000 units, and a total of between 5 and 6 million units being given. We treated a case of actinomycosis of the pleura, in which the organism was penicillin-sensitive *in vitro*, with intramuscular and intrapleural injections of penicillin, but the disease proved fatal in a few weeks.

Wounds and Burns. The low toxicity of penicillin together with its high bacteriostatic action makes it pre-eminently suitable for local administration at the wound sites, especially when combined with a sulphonamide.

Skin Diseases. Penicillin may be used as a cream, or a spray containing 500 units of penicillin per ml. It is of value in skin infections caused by staphylococci and streptococci. Impetigo and sycosis barbæ respond well to local treatment, but if cases relapse a course of intramuscular injections is useful in reaching the deeper parts of the hair follicles. Eczema with secondary infection is improved by penicillin locally. When the infection has cleared up it is important to treat the underlying eczema. Blepharitis responds well to penicillin cream. The spray or cream should be applied three or four times daily. The cream must be smeared on with a sterile spatula, or the handle of a spoon which has been boiled. Carbuncles, cellulitis, erysipelas and cavernous sinus thrombosis are best treated by intramuscular injection of 20,000 units every three hours for five days. Good results have followed the use of penicillin cream in pemphigus neonatorum, but intramuscular injections are needed in severe cases.

Eye Infections. Superficial eye infections caused by penicillin-sensitive organisms can be treated by instillation every one to two hours of drops containing 500–2,500 units of penicillin per ml., by the application of penicillin ointment, or by ophthalmic "Tabloids" containing 250 units. Blepharitis, conjunctivitis, ophthalmia neonatorum, infective keratitis and corneal ulcers respond well. Penicillin is especially of value in the treatment of sulphonamide-resistant staphylococcal infections.

Throat Infections. For streptococcal tonsillitis penicillin lozenges may be sucked every hour for 8 doses or the throat sprayed two-hourly with a solution containing 1,000 units per ml. In Vincent's infections it is usually necessary to give a course of intramuscular injections.

Aureomycin

Aureomycin was discovered in 1948 by Duggar (32). It is produced from a fungus, *Streptomyces aureofaciens* which forms a golden yellow pigment during its growth. The chemical formula of aureomycin has not yet been determined nor has it been synthesised; its molecular weight is known to be about 500.

Pharmacology. Aureomycin is a yellow crystalline substance which is soluble in acid or alkaline solution but is sparingly soluble in water. A 2% aqueous solution of aureomycin hydrochloride has a pH of 4·5. In the dry state the drug is stable, but in solution it rapidly loses its activity, especially in the presence of serum or blood. When given by mouth or per rectum aureomycin is rapidly absorbed into the blood and passes into the cerebro-spinal, peritoneal and pleural fluids. It is found in bile, urine and milk and probably crosses the placental barrier (33). Doses of 5–10 mg. per kg. body weight of aureomycin given orally at six-hourly intervals maintain measurable blood levels. It appears rapidly in the urine in high concentration, and has been detected fifty-five hours after a single dose of 0·5 g.

Dosage and Administration. Aureomycin is supplied in capsules containing 25, 50 or 100 mg. and in vials for intravenous use containing 100 or 500 mg. For adults give either 25 mg. per kg. body weight every twenty-four hours in divided doses; or 500 mg. every six hours. This dosage should be maintained until there is a satisfactory clinical response, and it should be continued for three to five days afterwards. If there is no improvement within forty-eight hours of starting treatment with aureomycin the dose should be increased to 500 mg. every three hours, and reduced to 500 mg. every six hours when the patient becomes afebrile. The dosage for children is 30 mg. per kg. body weight every twenty-four hours, in divided doses every six hours.

Aureomycin may be injected intravenously as an emergency measure in a severely ill patient, but this route should be discontinued when the patient can take the drug orally, as there is a risk of thrombophlebitis at the site of injection. For intravenous use 500 mg. of aureomycin may be injected twice daily. This dose is dissolved in 50 ml. of physiological saline and should be prepared immediately before use. The drug must be injected slowly. In eye infections aureomycin may be applied locally as a 0·5 % solution of aureomycin borate, 1–2 drops being instilled into each conjunctival sac every two hours.

Toxic Effects. Aureomycin is relatively non-toxic and side reactions have decreased with the production of purer preparations. It may cause nausea, vomiting, diarrhoea and flatulence. There is seldom any indication for discontinuing the drug, and the side effects may be reduced by giving half the six-hourly dose every three hours. As with chloramphenicol, patients receiving aureomycin may develop mucous membrane and dermal lesions of the type seen in deficiency of the Vitamin B complex. Women may develop vaginitis and vulvitis, which responds well to synthetic oestrogens by mouth. Soreness of the mouth and tongue, and perianal exudation and fissuring (which is probably due to secondary invasion with *Candida albicans*) can be prevented or minimised by giving adequate doses of the B complex (34).

Antibiotic Activity. Aureomycin has been shown to act bacteriostatically and at higher concentrations as a bacteriocide *in vitro* and *in vivo* against a wide variety of pathogens. In general it is effective against gram-negative and gram-positive cocci, gram-negative and gram-positive bacilli, the rickettsiæ and some viruses.

Organisms do not normally become resistant to aureomycin except the Proteus vulgaris, which has been shown to do so readily.

Clinical Applications

Staphylococcal Infections. During the past few years staphylococci have been encountered which are resistant, or relatively so, to penicillin. Such strains of staphylococci are found especially in patients with infections developing from ward cross-infection, and in patients who have had penicillin therapy. These penicillin-resistant staphylococci can cause epidemics in hospital communities. Penicillin-resistant staphylococci are susceptible to aureomycin (35). Some strains of staphylococci have shown an increase in resistance to aureomycin (36, 37, 38) and aureomycin-resistant staphylococci may be a problem of the future. Staphylococcal infections in general, whether treated by penicillin or aureomycin, should be treated by full courses of the antibiotic in maximum dosage. Staphylococcal septicæmia, meningitis, endocarditis, pneumonia, osteomyelitis, pyodermia, mastitis and other miscellaneous infections caused by staphylococci, or where staphylococci were playing a part in the disease, have been shown to respond rapidly and effectively to aureomycin therapy.

Streptococcal Infections. Aureomycin is effective in infections caused by β-hæmolytic streptococci. Streptococcal pneumonia, erysipelas, cellulitis, scarlet fever, tonsillitis, endocarditis, meningitis, and septicæmia respond satisfactorily to aureomycin. Aureomycin is very valuable in treating infections caused by Str. fæcalis and Str. viridans.

Pneumococcal Infections. Pneumococcal infections involving lungs and meninges in children and adults respond satisfactorily to aureomycin in standard dosage.

Bacterial Pneumonias. Aureomycin is of great value in the treatment of bacterial pneumonia. Infections where the predominant organism is a pneumococcus, staphylococcus, streptococcus, H. influenzæ, or K. pneumoniæ (Bact. friedländeri) respond well. It is especially valuable in treating pneumonia due to penicillin-resistant staphylococci and in mixed viral and bacterial pneumonias. Herrell (39) states that since aureomycin produces good results in bacterial and non-bacterial pneumonia it is the treatment of choice for all types of pneumonia. Aureomycin is given in doses of 500 mg. six-hourly by mouth. There is rapid symptomatic improvement in twelve to forty-eight hours and this is followed in three to five days by radiological resolution.

Primary Atypical (Non-Bacterial) Pneumonia. Several authors have reported the favourable effect of aureomycin in primary atypical pneumonia (40, 41, 42, 43). The temperature falls in forty-eight hours and there is symptomatic improvement with radiological resolution in 3–7 days. The effect of aureomycin has been dramatic in cases which were alarmingly ill with high fever, cyanosis, dyspnœa and delirium. Penicillin and sulphadiazine had not improved these patients.

Psittacosis. Experimental and clinical reports of treatment of psittacosis have been favourable.

Rickettsial Infections. Epidemic and murine typhus, scrub typhus, Rocky Mountain Valley fever (44, 45, 46) and Q fever, have all been shown to respond very effectively to aureomycin (47).

Urinary Tract Infections. In the absence of impaired renal function aureomycin is excreted in the urine in high concentration two to eight hours following oral administration. It is effective in infections of the urinary tract due to Bact. coli, Bact. aerogenes, K. pneumoniæ (Bact. friedländeri), Str. fæcalis and Pseudomonas pyocyanea. It has some action against Proteus vulgaris but this organism may become highly resistant during treatment. A combination of streptomycin and aureomycin is valuable in treating mixed infections. 500 mg. of aureomycin are given every six hours until the infection is controlled, and this dose should be continued for several days to prevent recurrence. Acute infections respond well. Chronic infections tend to recur unless mechanical obstruction to the outflow of urine and calculi is dealt with surgically. Aureomycin has been shown to be effective when other antibiotics and urinary antiseptics have failed, and it is especially valuable when strains of bacteria have developed resistance to other antibiotic agents (48, 49, 50, 51).

Brucellosis. Many clinical reports have indicated the value of aureomycin in the treatment of brucella infections. Acute infections with Br. abortus, Br. melitensis or Br. suis respond promptly to 250 mg. every three hours for twelve to fourteen days. If there is a relapse a further course may be given, but 89% of 110 cases of chronic brucellosis treated by Harris resulted in complete recovery (52). Debono (53) has drawn attention to an initial rise in temperature lasting one to two days which is followed by a fall in pyrexia and clinical improvement. Herrell and Barber (54), and Rosenbaum and Reveno (55), believe that aureomycin combined with dihydrostreptomycin is the treatment of choice in brucella infections. During the treatment of brucellosis with aureomycin where rather larger doses are needed than for other infections, Vitamin B complex should be given by mouth, as this reduces the incidence of mucous membrane and dermal side effects which may develop.

Salmonellæ and Shigellæ Infections. Aureomycin has not been shown to have an important place in the treatment of these infections. Most reports have been equivocal although isolated good reports have appeared.

Whooping Cough. Bradford and Day (56) found that aureomycin had a bacteriostatic effect on Hæmophilus pertussis and that daily doses of 10–100 mg. per kg. body weight protected mice, given intranasal installations of 250 M.L.D. of the organism. Clinical reports (57, 58) have shown that aureomycin brings about symptomatic improvement with reduction in frequency and intensity of paroxysms, vomiting and cyanosis.

Skin Infections. Aureomycin has been reported of value in treating herpes simplex, Kaposi's varicelliform eruption, eczema vaccinatum, dermatitis herpetiformis, molluscum contagiosum, pemphigus, and herpes zoster. Aureomycin is given by mouth in usual dosage and this may be combined with aureomycin locally.

Liver Disease. In a controlled series aureomycin did not appear to have any effect in acute viral hepatitis (59), but some authors consider it of value in treating chronic hepatic disease following viral hepatitis, and in hepatitic coma from various causes (60, 61). Aureomycin prevented the development of cirrhosis in rats which had been fed on a diet (*i.e.* high fat, low protein) which produces cirrhosis experimentally (62).

Acute Amœbiasis. Aureomycin has been shown to be of value in acute intestinal amœbiasis (63) but more work is needed to assess the place of aureomycin in the treatment of amœbiasis.

Gonorrhœa. Chen et al. (64) reported cure of acute gonorrhœa in males and females in 98% of cases: 3–6 g. was given daily for three days.

Syphilis. Clinical work on aureomycin in syphilis is still in the experimental stage. It appears to produce a satisfactory initial decline in serological titre and sterilises surface lesions in about forty hours (65). Willcox (66) has obtained gratifying clinical results and recommends further trials of aureomycin in syphilis.

Lymphogranuloma Venereum. Good results have been obtained in a number of cases of this infection treated with aureomycin. There is retrogression of buboes and marked clinical improvement after four days' therapy. Runyan et al. were unable to demonstrate the virus in the healing buboes after three days' treatment (67).

Chancroid. Willcox reports aureomycin to be of value in the treatment of chancroid (68).

Other Infections. Aureomycin has been reported to be of value in the treatment of the following diseases :— Rat-bite fever, leptospirosis, fusospirochetosis, trichomonas vaginalis, ulcerative colitis, mumps, infective mononucleosis, lymphocytic choriomeningitis, actinomycosis, epidemic keratoconjunctivitis, dendritic keratitis, conjunctivitis and peritonitis.

Chloramphenicol

Chloromycetin (as first called) was produced from cultures of *Streptomyces venezuela* in 1947 by Burkholder and his colleagues at Yale University (69). It was subsequently synthesised by Crooks and his co-workers at the Parke Davis Laboratories, and the substance is now known as Chloramphenicol, and is the first antibiotic to have been prepared synthetically.

Chemical Composition. Chloramphenicol is D (–) *threo* - 1 - *p* - nitrophenyl - 2 - dichloracetamido - propane - 1 : 3 - diol.

NO_2

$HO-C-H$

$H-C-NH-CO-CHCl_2$

CH_2OH

Pharmacology. Chloramphenicol is a white crystalline powder which is sparingly soluble in water. It is stable in aqueous solution at room temperature for twenty-four hours. It is rapidly absorbed from the gastro-intestinal tract. An oral dose of 3 g. of chloramphenicol produces a maximum blood level in two hours ; after eight hours this level is approximately halved and the drug is not detectable after 24 hours (70). Chloramphenicol is absorbed per rectum, and may be administered by this route in infants or patients who cannot swallow. The capsule is pricked at both ends before being introduced into the rectum.

Chloramphenicol is found in bile, cerebro-spinal fluid and body fluids and it crosses the placental barrier (71). It is principally excreted in the urine.

Dosage. Chloramphenicol is supplied in capsules each containing 0·25 g. For adults the average dose is 50 mg. per kg. of body weight daily (in divided doses). The interval between doses should not exceed eight hours, to ensure the maintenance of effective therapeutic levels in the blood. When the patient has become afebrile and there is a satisfactory clinical response the dose may be halved *i.e.* 25 mg. per kg. body weight per day. This dose should be continued for two to seven days after the infection has been controlled clinically. In infants and children 100 mg. per kg. body weight should be given at four- to six-hourly intervals, followed by 50 mg. per kg. body weight for two to seven days.

Toxic Effects. Chloramphenicol is generally well tolerated. The drug has a bitter taste and may cause anorexia, nausea, vomiting, diarrhœa, sore tongue and muscle fatigue. Transient ophthalmoplegia has been reported in children. No serious or permanent toxic effects have occurred, and the gastro-intestinal upset clears in a day or two when the drug is discontinued. In children the bitter taste may be masked by mixing the drug with honey, jam or blackcurrant purée. Chloramphenicol inhibits the growth of the normal intestinal flora which may be responsible for the bio-synthesis of the B_2 group of vitamins, therefore it is advisable to give the patient a preparation containing all the B_2 complex. The normal bacterial flora of the intestinal and respiratory tract inhibit the growth of yeasts, so children suffering from thrush should not be given chloramphenicol. Chloramphenicol may be given with sulphonamides, penicillin, streptomycin and aureomycin without incompatibility, and it is effective against organisms within its range which have become resistant to other antibiotics.

Antibiotic Activity. Chloramphenicol is effective against gram-positive and gram-negative pathogens, the rickettsiæ and certain of the larger viruses.

Clinical Applications

Typhoid Fever. Chloramphenicol has been shown to have a rapid curative action in this infection. Woodward et al. (72) in a controlled series of patients suffering from typhoid fever showed the effectiveness of chloramphenicol. Defervescence of fever occurs in two to three days, the urine and stool cultures become negative for S. typhi and the titre of the Widal reaction falls within ten to fourteen days. Perforation of the bowel or bleeding from a typhoid intestinal ulcer may occur although the infection is well controlled clinically. Convalescence therefore should be careful and prolonged. If stool or urine cultures become positive for S. typhi during this period, or if there is a clinical relapse, a further course of chloramphenicol should be given. The use of chloramphenicol has been disappointing in chronic carrier states, with or without gall-bladder involvement. Negative stool cultures are produced temporarily, but relapse invariably occurs.

For an average adult patient an initial loading dose of 3–4 g. is given over a period of one hour. This is followed by 3–4 g. daily in divided doses at eight-hourly intervals until the patient becomes afebrile, then 1·5 g. daily eight-hourly for fourteen days. Bacteriological or clinical relapse can be treated by a further course (3 g. daily at eight-hourly intervals for 3–5 days).

Paratyphoid Fever. Paratyphoid fever responds to chloramphenicol (73) in a manner similar to typhoid fever save that larger doses *i.e.* 100 mg. per kg. body weight daily in adults are recommended. Results with chronic carriers have been disappointing.

Salmonellæ Infections. This group of organisms is extremely sensitive to chloramphenicol and it has been found effective in gastroenteritis due to S. oranienburg, S. newport, S. typhi-murium S. choleræ-suis and S. san-diego in children and adults. 50–75 mg. per kg. body weight per day eight-hourly for three to five days produces clinical and bacteriological cure.

Shigellæ Infections. This group of organisms is responsible for bacillary dysentery, and although results of treatment with chloramphenicol have been encouraging, the more recently developed members of the sulphonamide group of drugs remain the first choice.

Rickettsioses. Chloramphenicol represents an important advance in the treatment of the Rickettsioses, which include epidemic and endemic or murine typhus fever, scrub typhus, rickettsial pox, Rocky Mountain spotted fever and Q fever.

Smadel et al. (74) treated cases of epidemic typhus, murine typhus and scrub typhus successfully with doses of chloramphenicol of 50–60 mg. per kg. body weight, followed by 0·2–0·3 g. two- to four-hourly for twelve days. Q fever has been reported in England recently (75), and this is the only one of the Rickettsioses likely to be found in the British Isles. A case of Q fever in a pathologist was successfully treated by Whittick (76), who gave an initial dose of 3·5 g. of chloramphenicol followed by 0·25 g. every three hours for thirty-six hours.

Primary Atypical Pneumonia. This infection, characterised by fever, malaise, myalgia, headache, pleuritic pain, cough and often blood-stained sputum with patchy consolidation in the lungs, has been successfully treated by chloramphenicol. There is rapid symptomatic improvement in one to two days, which is followed by radiological resolution. 50–75 mg. per kg. body weight should be given daily in divided doses at eight-hourly intervals for three to five days (77, 78, 79).

Whooping Cough. Clinical observations have shown that chloramphenicol reduces the cough plate count, controls the pyrexia and toxæmia, and converts an intractable and lengthy disease into a mild ailment. Gray (80) observed that chloramphenicol limited the course of the infection irrespective of the stage at which treatment is started. The initial dose is 50–100 mg. per kg. body weight followed by maintenance doses of 0·125–0·3 g. six-hourly for seven days (81, 82, 83).

Brucellosis. Acute brucellosis due to Br. abortus, Br. melitensis and Br. suis responds well to chloramphenicol in doses of 50–100 mg. per kg. body weight, followed by 50 mg. per kg. body weight six-hourly until the fever subsides, then 0·25 g. three-hourly for five days. If there is a relapse this course should be repeated. Chronic brucellosis responds satisfactorily initially, but careful follow-up studies are necessary before complete cure can be proved (84, 85, 86).

Bacterial Pneumonia. Lobar pneumonia and bronchopneumonia due to Str. pneumoniæ, K. pneumoniæ (Bact. friedländeri), Staph. pyogenes, hæmolytic streptococci and H. influenzæ respond to chloramphenicol, especially in infants and children. The patient becomes afebrile in forty-eight hours and radiographic findings usually resolve in a week. Bronchial obstruction, sterile effusion, and empyemata should be treated by the appropriate methods. For adults dosage is 3 g. daily for five to eight days. For children 100 mg. per kg. body weight should be given at four- to six-hourly intervals, followed by 20–30 mg. per kg. body weight for seven days or more when the fever has subsided (87, 88).

Urinary Infections. A high concentration of chloramphenicol is found in the urine after the usual doses by mouth, and it has been found of value in treating chronic and acute infections of the urinary tract due to the coli-aerogenes group of bacteria. K. pneumoniæ (Bact. friedländeri) and many other strains of enterococci and streptococci, Proteus vulgaris and Pseudomonas infections may not respond. In mixed infections due to gram-positive cocci and gram-negative bacilli, chloramphenicol may be combined with penicillin, streptomycin or sulphonamides. Recurrence of infection is likely to occur unless mechanical obstruction and anatomical defects are dealt with surgically. The doses recommended are an initial daily dose of 2–3 g. divided into 2 or 4 doses, followed by 0·25 g. 4 times a day for five to seven days after the urine has become sterile (89).

Gonococcal Infections. Acute gonorrhœa in males and females is satisfactorily treated by 3 g. of chloramphenicol initially, followed by 1 g. eight-hourly for two to three days.

Syphilis. Chloramphenicol has a weak action against Treponema pallidum *in vitro*, but it has been found effective in treating acute primary and secondary syphilitic lesions. It is not yet possible to state that the antibiotic is effective in treating syphilis, as many years are necessary before final cure can be pronounced (90, 91).

Lymphogranuloma Venereum. Chloramphenicol in doses of 3 g. every eight hours has produced clinical cure.

Granuloma Inguinale. Chloramphenicol, in doses ranging from 20–40 g. given over a period of twelve days heals large lesions. If Donovan bodies persist for five to seven days after chloramphenicol is started, therapy should be continued until healing is complete (92).

Chancroid. Willcox reported 2 cases of chancroid which were successfully treated with chloramphenicol. Fluctuant buboes still required aspiration (93).

Surgical Infections. Chloramphenicol is valuable in treating infection with gram-negative organisms, and where mixed infections are found it may be used in conjunction with other antibiotics.

Other Infections. Chloramphenicol has been found to be of value in treating the following diseases: Psittacosis, trachoma, ulcerative colitis, herpes zoster, infective hepatitis, acute laryngo-tracheo-bronchitis in children, infantile gastro-enteritis in which a serologically specific type of colon bacillus (Bact. coli, B.C.T.) was found, chicken-pox, mumps, infective mononucleosis and relapsing fever.

Streptomycin

Following the discovery of penicillin, Waksman, a soil micro-biologist, tested many thousands of soil fungi for antibiotic properties. He paid especial attention to species which inhibited the growth of gram-negative organisms. He discovered a substance called streptothricin which had considerable antibiotic activity against gram-negative organisms, but it proved too toxic for clinical use. This was followed by an announcement that streptomycin, which is derived from a soil actinomycete, *Streptomyces griseus,* possessed a bacteriostatic action against many organisms *in vitro* (94). Streptomycin has since been proved to be a very valuable antibiotic clinically against a wide range of bacteria, including Myco. tuberculosis.

Chemical Composition and Pharmacology. Streptomycin is a water soluble base, whose salts with mineral acids give approximately neutral solutions in water. The empirical formula is

$C_{21}H_{37-39}N_7O_{12}$. It consists of a basic substance streptidine ($C_8H_{18}O_4N_6$) which is joined to a nitrogen-containing disaccharide called streptobisamine, $C_{13}H_{21-23}O_9N$, by a glucoside linkage.

Streptomycin is readily soluble in water, but it is poorly soluble in organic solvents. It is stable in the dry state at room temperature for a year, and aqueous solutions keep for two months at a temperature of 38° C.

Streptomycin is poorly absorbed from the intestinal tract even in large doses, and most of the drug can be recovered from the fæces. It can only be used by mouth therefore in the treatment of intestinal infections.

The method of choice for administration is by intermittent intramuscular injection. A dose of 1 g. gives a maximum blood level of 20–50 μg. per ml., falling to 4–10 μg. per ml., and less than 1 μg. per ml. at twenty-four hours. When streptomycin is given intramuscularly it diffuses into pleural and peritoneal fluids, but poorly into the cerebro-spinal fluid, except when there is inflammation of the meninges. Streptomycin is mainly excreted unchanged in the urine, most of the dose being excreted within twenty-four hours.

Dosage. Streptomycin is supplied in the dry state in rubber-capped vials each containing 1 g. of streptomycin hydrochloride, streptomycin sulphate, or streptomycin calcium chloride complex. The powder is dissolved by injecting 5 ml. of pyrogen-free distilled water into the vial with a syringe and needle. When the streptomycin has completely dissolved it is sucked up again into the syringe and injected into the upper and outer quadrant of the buttock, the upper third of the lateral aspect of the thigh, or into the deltoid muscle. For adult infections (excluding tuberculosis) 1 g. should be injected intramuscularly every six hours. This dose should be continued for three to four days or until there is a satisfactory clinical response, when the dose may be reduced to 0·5 g. six-hourly for two to four days. In children 10–20 mg. per pound body weight are given daily in divided doses.

Streptomycin may be given intrathecally in doses of 20–100 mg. dissolved in 5–10 ml. of pyrogen-free physiological saline. It should be injected into the subarachnoid space slowly. For injection into the pleural space 0·5 g. may be dissolved in 10 ml. of pyrogen-free distilled water. Streptomycin may be given by inhalation by means of a suitable nebuliser, 0·5 g. being dissolved in 10 ml. of sterile physiological saline, and 1 ml. is inhaled every two hours. Streptomycin (0·01 g. in 1 ml. of sterile physiological saline) may be used as eye drops. Hourly instillations should be used.

Toxicity. Toxic reactions to streptomycin appear most frequently when it is used for long periods, as in the treatment of tuberculous infections. As the commercial preparations have become purer, toxic reactions have become less frequent. The most important toxic effect of streptomycin is its effect on the vestibular apparatus, which is manifest by giddiness and may be accompanied by nystagmus. This effect occurs usually between the third and seventh weeks of treatment but it seldom persists for long after the drug is discontinued, except in older patients when it may last for months or even indefinitely. Bignall et al. (95) reported that some success was achieved by giving antihistamines in preventing the vestibular toxic effects, but their results were not conclusive. Other toxic effects which may occur are skin rashes, nausea, vomiting, drug fever, albuminuria and paraesthesiæ. Antihistamines are of value in treating skin rashes, and possibly in preventing nausea and vomiting. Skin sensitisation may develop through repeated local contact. This can be avoided by appropriate precautions, such as the wearing of rubber gloves by the nurse.

Dihydrostreptomycin is produced from streptomycin by reduction of the streptose aldehyde group to an alcohol group by means of hydrogen in the presence of platinum as a catalyst (96). Dihydrostreptomycin is said to have less effect on vestibular function than streptomycin, and to be therapeutically as effective. The dose is the same as for streptomycin.

Antibiotic Activity. Streptomycin is active against gram-negative bacilli and gram-negative cocci, and to a lesser extent against gram-positive cocci. It is often effective against penicillin-resistant organisms.

Bacterial Resistance. Bacteria acquire a high degree of resistance to streptomycin, sometimes very quickly. To achieve rapid control of the infection, it is advantageous to know the actual degree of sensitivity of the causative organism and to select the dosage accordingly. The dosage should be sufficient to attain a concentration of streptomycin in the tissues at least four times as great as that needed to inhibit their growth *in vitro*. The combination of para-amino salicylic acid with streptomycin in the treatment of tuberculosis is said to prevent or retard the development of streptomycin resistance.

Clinical Applications

H. Influenzæ Meningitis. Although this is a rare form of meningitis, the prognosis before the use of streptomycin was very grave. Early diagnosis is imperative and Allibone et al. (97) stress the importance of doing a lumbar puncture on children with fever and any evidence of meningeal irritation. Streptomycin is given by intermittent intramuscular injection, and this may be combined with intrathecal therapy. Treatment should be continued for at least seven days after the cerebro-spinal fluid has become sterile.

K. Pneumoniæ Pneumonia. Infection with K. pneumoniæ (Bact. friedländeri) may occur in three ways : as an acute primary infection, as a secondary invader in pneumonia which is primarily due to some other organism, or as a chronic pneumonia. Gill (98) has drawn attention to the improvement in prognosis which has resulted from the treatment of these infections of the lungs by streptomycin with or without sulphonamides.

H. Influenzæ Pneumonia. Streptomycin is of value in treating bacterial pneumonia when this organism is playing a part in the infection. It may be combined with penicillin therapy with advantage.

Urinary Tract Infections. Streptomycin is excreted in the urine when given by intramuscular injection. It is more active in an alkaline urine, so that alkalinisation of the urine by giving pot. citrate or sod. citrate, gr. 15 four-hourly, is advisable. Streptomycin is of value in treating acute and chronic urinary infections due to Bact. coli, Staph. pyogenes, Str. fæcalis, or K. pneumoniæ (Bact. friedländeri). It is often of value in treating infections with Proteus vulgaris and Pseudomonas pyocyanea, but these organisms may rapidly become streptomycin resistant. The dose is 1–3 g. at six-hourly intervals for five to seven days, or longer if the organism is still sensitive (99, 100, 101).

Septicæmia. Streptomycin is of value in treating septicæmic conditions due to gram-negative bacilli. Daily intramuscular injections of 2 g. of streptomycin for twelve days are recommended.

Streptomycin finds a place in treating sub-acute bacterial endocarditis due to penicillin resistant organisms. Treatment must be intensive and prolonged, and a constant check must be kept on the sensitivity of the causative organism to streptomycin (102, 103).

Tularæmia. This disease responds well to streptomycin in doses of 2 g. daily. Treatment is seldom needed for longer than a week (104).

Plague. Streptomycin has been reported of value in treating plague. *In vitro* streptomycin in a concentration of 0·5–2·5 μg. per ml. inhibits the growth of Past. pestis (105, 106).

Local Sepsis. Streptomycin may be used in local sepsis due to organisms within its range and against such organisms if they are penicillin-resistant. It is used as a powder for insufflation, or as an ointment.

Infantile Gastro-Enteritis. Streptomycin is of value in treating gastro-enteritis in infants. The drug is given by mouth before each feed. A total dose of 2 g. over seven days is recommended (107).

Gonorrhœa. Streptomycin may be used with advantage in the treatment of gonorrhœa. A single dose of 0·5 g. may cure the disease in the acute stage, and it does not mask an accompanying syphilitic infection.

Chancroid. Hirsch and Taggart report streptomycin to be of value in chancroid (108).

Terramycin

Terramycin was first reported in America by Finlay et al. in 1950 (109). It is derived from a soil actinomycete, *Streptomyces rimosus.* Terramycin is a pure amphoteric compound which is yellow in colour, and has a bitter taste. It is sparingly soluble in water, but it is readily soluble in solutions of strong acids or alkalis, when a salt is formed. The acid solution is stable up to thirty days at 0° C.

Antibiotic Activity. Terramycin is in general highly active against gram-positive and gram-negative cocci and gram-negative bacilli. Proteus vulgaris is highly resistant, but many strains of Pseudomonas pyocyanea are sensitive. It has been reported as being effective against brucella and rickettsiæ, and its effect on viruses is similar to that of aureomycin.

Dosage and Administration. The drug is usually given by

mouth in capsules. For adult infections 4 g. are given daily, and the interval between the dose should not exceed six hours, for although the drug remains detectable in the blood for as long as twenty-four hours after a single dose, its concentration begins to fall off after six hours. Bacterial resistance to terramycin has been reported *in vitro*.

Toxic Effects. The drug may cause gastro-intestinal upset; nausea and loose stools being predominant. In view of its powerful action upon the intestinal flora of the gut, changes in the mucous membranes of the mouth as seen with aureomycin and chloramphenicol may be expected, but Linsell and Fletcher did not observe any in their series (110).

Clinical Usage. Clinically terramycin has been used successfully in pneumonia, septicæmia, urinary tract infections, amœbiasis, brucellosis, pertussis, Rickettsioses, primary atypical pneumonia and post-operative sepsis (111).

The following table gives an indication of the best antibiotics to be used in various diseases, and in infections with different types of organisms. 1 = first choice, 11 = second choice, 111 = third choice.

It should be emphasised that to get the best results the organisms responsible for the infection should be isolated, grown in pure culture, and the sensitivity of the particular organism to the various antibiotics estimated. The antibiotic to which the organism is most sensitive should then be given in full dosage at the intervals recommended. Therapeutic failure may be due to the organism becoming resistant, or the presence of a " feeding focus " of infection which is not being reached by the antibiotic. Such "feeding foci", *e.g.* collections of pus, dead tissue, or mechanical obstruction to the normal outflow of the body secretion should be treated surgically.

Type of Infection or Disease	Penicillin G	Streptomycin	Aureomycin	Chloramphenicol	Sulphonamides
1. Group A β-hæmolytic streptococcal infections .	1		11		
2. α-hæmolytic streptococcal infections . .	1	11	1	11	
3. Streptococcus fæcalis .	11		1		

Type of Infection or Disease	Penicillin G	Strepto-mycin	Aureo-mycin	Chloram-phenicol	Sulphon-amides
4. Pneumococcal infections	1		1	11	
5. Meningococcal infections	1				1
6. Gonococcal infections .	1	11	11	11	11
7. Staphylococcal infections	1		1		
8. Brucellosis . . .		11 + sulpha-diazine	1	1	
9. Whooping cough . .			1	1	
10. Tularæmia . . .		11	1	11	
11. Typhoid fever . .				1	
12. H. influenzæ infections .		1 + sulpha-diazine	1	1	
13. Urinary tract infection .					
(i) Bact. coli . . .	111	11	1	1	1
(ii) Bact. aerogenes . .		11	1	1	
(iii) Proteus vulgaris . .		11		1	
(iv) Pseudomonas pyocyanea		1	1	1	
(v) Str. fæcalis . .	11		1		
14. Tuberculosis . .		1 + P.A.S.			
15. Chancroid . . .		11	1	1	
16. K. pneumoniæ (Bact. friedländeri) infections		1	1	1	
17. Salmonellæ infections .				1	
18. Bacillary dysentery .					1
19. Plague . . .		1			
20. Sub-acute bacterial endocarditis					
(i) α-hæmolytic streptococci . . .	1		1		
(ii) Str. fæcalis . .	1	11	1		
(iii) Staphylococci . .	1		11		
(iv) Gram-negative bacilli .		1	1	1	
21. Trachoma . . .	11		1	1	
22. Rickettsial diseases .			1	1	

Type of Infection or Disease	Penicillin G	Strepto-mycin	Aureo-mycin	Chloram-phenicol	Sulphon-amides
23. Primary atypical (non-bacterial) pneumonia .			1	1	
24. Psittacosis . . .			1	1	
25. Anthrax . . .	1				
26. Syphilis . . .	1		11		
27. Lymphogranuloma venereum			1	11	
28. Granuloma inguinale .		11	1	11	
29. Gas gangrene . .	1				
30. Diphtheria . . .	1 + anti-serum				
31. Actinomycosis . .	1 + sulpha-diazine		11		

Table modified from Long et al. *Journ. Amer. Med. Assocn.*, 1949, **141**, 315

REFERENCES

(1) Fleming. *Brit. Journ. Exp. Path.*, 1929, **10**, 226.

(2) Sullivan, Symmes, Miller and Rhodehamel. *Science*, 1948, **107**, 169.

(3) Boger, Oritt, Israel and Flippin. *Amer. Journ. Med. Sci.*, 1948, **215**, 250.

(4) Seeler, Wilcox, Clare and Finland. *Journ. Lab. Clin. Med.*, 1947, **32**, 807.

(5) Strauss, Ricjburg, Saba and Alexander. *Journ. Lab. Clin. Med.*, 1947, **32**, 818.

(6) Anderson and Landsman. *Brit. Med. Journ.*, 1947, *ii*, 950.

(7) Suchett-Kaye and Latter. *Brit. Med. Journ.*, 1947, *ii*, 953.

(8) Peck, Siegal and Bergamini. *Journ. Amer. Med. Assocn.*, 1947, **134**, 1546.

(9) Christie. *Penicillin*, 1950. Edited by Fleming. Butterworths Medical Publications, London.

(10) Rosenberg and Arling. *Journ. Amer. Med. Assocn.*, 1944, **125**, 1011.

(11) Daniels, Solomon and Laquette. *Journ. Amer. Med. Assocn.*, 1943, **123**, 1.

(12) Smith, Duthie and Cairns. *Lancet*, 1946, *i.*, 185.

(13) Grace and Bryson. *Journ. Amer. Med. Assocn.*, 1946, **130**, 841.

(14) Kirby and Hepp. *Journ. Amer. Med. Assocn.*, 1944, **125**, 1019.

(15) Boland, Headley and Hench. *Journ. Amer. Med. Assocn.*, 1944, **126**, 820.

(16) Florey and Florey. *Lancet*, 1943, *i*, 387.

(17) Welch, Putman, Randall and Herwick. *Journ. Amer. Med. Assocn.*, 1944, **126**, 1024.
(18) Romansky and Rittman. *Science*, 1944, **100**, 196.
(19) Romansky, Murphy and Rittman. *Journ. Amer. Med. Assocn.*, 1945, **128**, 404.
(20) Mahoney, Arnold and Harris. *Amer. Journ. Publ. Health*, 1943, **33**, 1387.
(21) Moore, Mahoney, Schwartz, Sternberg and Wood. *Journ. Amer. Med. Assocn.*, 1944, **126**, 67.
(22) Norcross. *Med. Bull. North Afric. Theat. Oper.*, 1944, **2**, 110.
(23) Leifer. *Journ. Amer. Med. Assocn.*, 1945, **129**, 1247.
(24) Lourie, Collier, Ross, Robinson and Nelson. *Lancet*, 1945, *ii*, 696.
(25) Dolkart and Schwemlein. *Journ. Amer. Med. Assocn.*, 1945, **129**, 515.
(26) *Journ. Amer. Med. Assocn.*, 1946, **131**, 265.
(27) McElligott. *Penicillin*, 1950. Edited by Fleming. Butterworths Medical Publications, London.
(28) Cutler. *Lancet*, 1943, *ii*, 639.
(29) Altemeier. *Journ. Amer. Med. Assocn.*, 1946, **130**, 67.
(30) Boland, Headley and Hench. *Journ. Amer. Med. Assocn.*, 1946, **130**, 556.
(31) Hamilton and Kirkpatrick. *Brit. Med. Journ.*, 1945, *ii*, 728.
(32) Duggar. *Annal. New York Acad. Sci.* 1948, **51**, 177.
(33) Lepper, Dowling, Brickhouse and Caldwell. *Journ. Lab. and Clin. Med.*, 1949, **34**, 366.
(34) Woods, Manning, Patterson and Durham. *Journ. Amer. Med. Assocn.*, 1951, **145**, 4, 207.
(35) Colbech. *Canad. Med. Assocn. Journ.*, 1949, **61**, 557.
(36) Astler and Morgan. *Univ. Mich. Med. Bull.*, 1950, **16**, 127.
(37) Long. *Amer. Journ. Pharm.*, 1949, **121**, 64.
(38) Shwachman, Crocker, Foley and Patterson. *New Eng. Journ. Med.*, 1949, **241**, 185.
(39) Herrell. *Proc. Staff. Meet. Mayo Clinic*, 1949, **24**, 612.
(40) Kneeland, Rose and Gibson. *Amer. Journ. Med.*, 1949, **6**, 41.
(41) Finland, Collins and Wells. *New Eng. Journ. Med.*, 1949, **240**, 241.
(42) Meiklejohn. *California Med.*, 1949, **71**, 319.
(43) Schoenbach and Bryer. *Journ. Amer. Med. Assocn.*, 1949, **139**, 275.
(44) Wong and Cox. *Annal. New York Acad. Sci.*, 1948, **51**, 290.
(45) Woodward. *Annal. Int. Med.*, 1949, **31**, 53.
(46) Cutileiro, Maderia, Custiano and Samparo. *Soc. das Ciencias Medicas Journ. de Lisboa*, 1949, **113**, 1949.
(47) Ross, Schoenbach, Burke, Bryer, Rice and Washington. *Journ. Amer. Med. Assocn.*, 1948, **138**, 1213.
(48) Bower. *Arizona Med.*, 1949, **6**, 30.
(49) Carroll, Allen and Flynn. *Journ. Urol.*, 1949, **62**, 574.
(50) Collins and Finland. *Surg. Gynaec. and Obst.*, 1949, **89**, 43.
(51) Dowling, Lepper, Caldwell, Whelton and Sweet. *Med. Annal. Distr. Columbia*, 1949, **18**, 335.
(52) Harris. *Bull. New York Acad. Med.*, 1949, **25**, 458.
(53) Debono. *Lancet*, 1949, *ii*, 326.
(54) Herrell and Barber. *Proc. Staff. Meet. Mayo Clinic*, 1949, **24**, 138.
(55) Rosenbaum and Reveno. *Harper Hosp. Bull.*, 1950, **8**, 1.
(56) Bradford and Day. *Journ. Pediat.*, 1949, **35**, 330.

(57) Bell, Pittman and Olson. *Pub. Health Rep.*, 1949, **64**, 589.
(58) Knight. *Journ. Amer. Med. Assocn.*, 1949, **141**, 315.
(59) Shaffer, Farquhar, Stokes and Sbovov. *Amer. Journ. Med. Sci.* 1950, **220**, 1.
(60) Farquhar, Stokes, Whitlock, Bluemle and Gambescia, *Amer. Journ. Med. Sci.*, 1950, **220**, 166.
(61) Shaffer, Bluemle, Sbovov and Neefe. *Amer. Journ. Med. Sci.*, 1950, **220**, 173.
(62) Gyorgy, Stokes, Smith and Goldblatt. *Amer. Journ. Med. Sci.*, 1950, **220**, 6.
(63) McVay, Larid and Sprunt. *Science*, 1949, **109**, 590.
(64) Chen, Dienst and Greenblat. *Journ. Amer. Med. Assocn.*, 1950, **143**, 8, 724.
(65) Rodriguez, Plotke, Weinstein and Harris. *Journ. Amer. Med. Assocn.*, 1949, **141**, 771.
(66) Willcox. *Brit. Med. Journ.*, 1949, *ii*, 1076.
(67) Runyan, Kraft and Gordon. *Amer. Journ. Med.*, 1949, **7**, 419.
(68) Willcox. *Brit. Med. Journ.*, 1951, *i*, 509.
(69) Erhlich, Bartz, Smith, Joslyn and Burkholder. *Science*, 1947, **106**, 417.
(70) Ley, Smadel and Crocker. *Proc. Soc. exp. Biol. N.Y.*, 1948, **68**, 9.
(71) Ross, Burke, Rice, Washington and Stevens. *New Engl. Journ. Med.*, 1950, **242**, 173.
(72) Woodward, Smadel, Ley, Green and Mankikar. *Annal. Int. Med.*, 1948, **29**, 131.
(73) Curtin. *Brit. Med. Journ.*, 1949, *ii*, 1504.
(74) Smadel, Woodward, Ley, Philip, Traub, Lewthwaite and Savoor. *Science*, 1948, **108**, 160.
(75) Harman. *Lancet*, 1949, *ii*, 1028.
(76) Whittick. *Brit. Med. Journ.*, 1950, *i*, 979.
(77) Wood. *Lancet*, 1949, *ii*, 55.
(78) Ludholm. *Swed. Med. Journ.*, 1949, **44**, 2351.
(79) Hewitt and Williams. *New Engl. Journ. Med.*, 1949, **242**, 110.
(80) Gray. *Lancet*, 1950, *i*, 150.
(81) Macrae. *Lancet*, 1950, *i*, 400.
(82) Payne, Levy, Zamora, Velarroel and Carelas. *Journ. Amer. Med. Assocn.*, 1949, **141**, 1298.
(83) Khalil and Abdin. *Lancet*, 1950, *ii*, 307.
(84) Walley and Cooper. *Brit. Med. Journ.*, 1949, *ii*, 265.
(85) Woodward, Smadel, Holbrook and Raby. *Journ. Clin. Invest.*, 1949, **28**, 968.
(86) Ralston and Payne. *Journ. Amer. Med. Assocn.*, 1950, **142**, 159.
(87) Hewitt and Williams. *New Engl. Journ. Med.*, 1950, **242**, 119.
(88) Recinos, Ross, Olshaker and Twible. *New Engl. Journ. Med.*, 1949, **241**, 733.
(89) Chittenden, Sharp, Vonden Heide, Bratton, Glazko and Strimpeit. *Journ. Urol.*, 1949, **62**, 771.
(90) Romansky, Clausky, Taggart and Robin. *Science*, 1949, **110**, 639.
(91) Robinson, Fox and Durace. *Amer. Journ. Syph. Gon. and Ven. Dis.*, 1949, **33**, 509.
(92) Greenblatt, Wammoch, Dienst and West. *Journ. Med. Assocn. Georgia*, 1949, **38**, 206.

(93) Willcox. *Brit. Med. Journ.*, 1951, *i*, 509.
(94) Schatz, Bugie and Waksman. *Proc. Soc. exp. Biol. N.Y.*, 1944, **55**, 66.
(95) Bignall, Crofton and Thomas. *Brit. Med. Journ.*, 1951, *i*, 554.
(96) Peck, Hoffhine and Folkers. *Journ. Amer. Chem. Soc.*, 1946, **68**, 1390.
(97) Allibone, Pickup and Zimmermann. *Lancet*, 1951, *i*, 610.
(98) Gill. *Amer. Journ. Med. Sci.*, 1950, **221**, 5.
(99) Wilson. *Lancet*, 1948, *ii*, 445.
(100) Fleming. *Brit. Med. Journ.*, 1948, *ii*, 831.
(101) Riches. *Brit. Med. Journ.*, 1948, *ii*, 832.
(102) Committee on Chemotherapeutics. National Research Council. *Journ. Amer. Med. Assocn.*, 1946, **132**, 4, 70.
(103) Hunter. *Amer. Journ. Med.*, 1947, **2**, 436.
(104) Foshay. *Amer. Journ. Med.*, 1947, **2**, 467.
(105) Herbert. *Lancet*, 1947, *i*, 626.
(106) Haddad and Valero. *Brit. Med. Journ.*, 1948, *i*, 1026.
(107) James, Ursula and Kramer. *Lancet*, 1948, *ii*, 553.
(108) Hirsch and Taggart. *Journ. Ven. Dis. Inform.*, 1948, **29**, 47.
(109) Finlay, Hobby, Pan, Regua, Routien, Seeley, Sheele, Sobin, Solomons, Vinson and Kane. *Science*, 1950, **111**, 85.
(110) Linsell and Fletcher. *Brit. Med. Journ.*, 1950, *ii*, 1190.
(111) Annotation. *Brit. Med. Journ.*, 1950, *ii*, 1209.

CHAPTER III

THE ANTIHISTAMINES

In 1910–11 Dale and Laidlaw (1) demonstrated that the injection of histamine into animals caused symptoms similar to those occurring in anaphylaxis. In 1927 Lewis described the effects of intradermal histamine on the human skin and its blood-vessels, showing that a "triple response", consisting of capillary dilatation, arteriolar dilatation, and increased capillary permeability, occurred similar to that resulting from minor traumatic damage. In 1932 Dragstedt and Gebauer-Fuelnegg (2) detected the release of histamine into the circulation of an animal during an anaphylactic reaction; thereafter histamine has been identified as the "H-substance" originally postulated by Lewis as responsible for the characteristic anaphylaxis symptom-complex. When a specific antigen combines with an antibody linked to fixed tissue cells, preformed histamine is released from the cells and can be attached to adjacent cells or be carried throughout the body. The damage thus caused gives rise to the allergic symptoms in man, or to the anaphylactic reaction in experimental animals. Most, but not all, of the symptoms of allergy can be attributed to histamine release; for example heparin, not histamine, is responsible for the increased clotting time of the blood in the anaphylactic state.

Properties of Histamine. Histamine

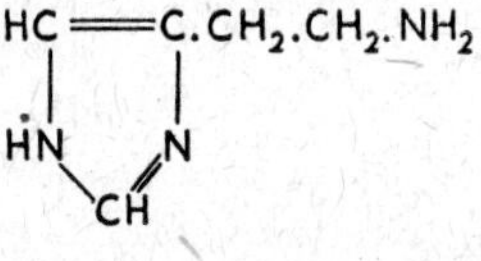

```
HC ===C.CH2.CH2.NH2
 |     |
 HN    N
   \  //
    CH
```

has been synthesised, and is a white water-soluble strongly basic compound. Its formation in the body may be by decarboxylation of histidine. When injected, it has powerful effects on many systems of the body, generally due to actions on smooth muscle. The more important are as follows :— *Skin.* When injected locally into the skin, marked capillary dilatation and an increase in capillary permeability occur, leading to œdema. Histamine release also causes itching and cutaneous pain. *Cardiovascular system.* If there is widespread cutaneous vasodilatation, due to circulating histamine, then a secondary fall of blood-pressure, tachycardia, and increase in cardiac output will result. *Gastro-intestinal tract.* Histamine is a powerful stimulant of the gastric and other secretory glands, and has some stimulatory action on the intestinal musculature. *Respiratory system.* Histamine has a local action on the bronchioles causing constriction by stimulation of smooth muscle, and it also causes an outpouring of mucus. In man such broncho-constriction does not occur in normals, but only in asthmatics (3).

To oppose the effects of an allergic response the following methods might theoretically be adopted :—

1. Prevent the original antigen-antibody reaction. 2. Prevent release of histamine from the antigen-antibody reaction (antigen desensitisation). 3. Prevent the formation of histamine (by inhibiting histidine decarboxylase, *e.g.* by the use of rutin). 4. Destroy histamine when released (by using a "histaminase"). 5. Desensitise the tissues to histamine (by repeated injection of small doses of histamine). 6. Use drugs which have actions opposed to that of histamine (*e.g.* adrenaline, which relaxes bronchiolar smooth muscle). 7. Peripherally block the actions of histamine by competitive action at the cell receptors, by using drugs which have no direct antagonistic effects. It is with this last class of "antihistamines" that we are further concerned.

Chemistry of the Antihistamines

In 1933 Bovet and his co-workers at the Pasteur Institute were studying the spasmolytic effects of a number of compounds including 929 F, of which the anti-anaphylactic properties were first described in 1937 (4): in the same year the anti-adrenaline compound 933 F (piperidino methyl 2 benzodioxane) was also found to be a histamine antagonist (5). Since that date an enormous number of antihistamine compounds have been manufactured and used for clinical or experimental purposes, compounds varying in potency and toxicity, but in general having the same range of action. Many of the antihistamines are derivatives of ethylenediamine.

$$\begin{matrix} H & & & & H \\ & \diagdown & & \diagup & \\ & N-CH_2-CH_2-N & & & \\ & \diagup & & \diagdown & \\ H & & & & H \end{matrix}$$

Ethylenediamine

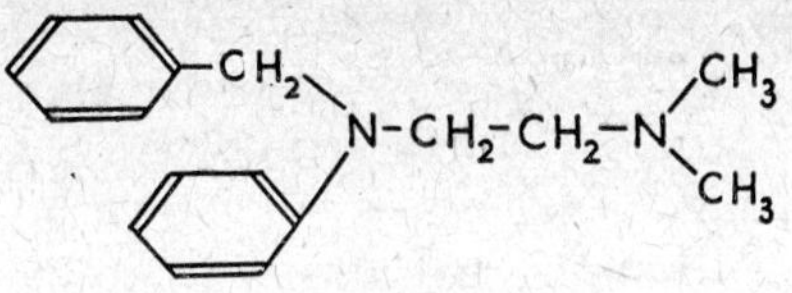

$C_6H_5-CH_2 \diagdown N-CH_2-CH_2-N(CH_3)_2$; $C_6H_5 \diagup$

Antergan

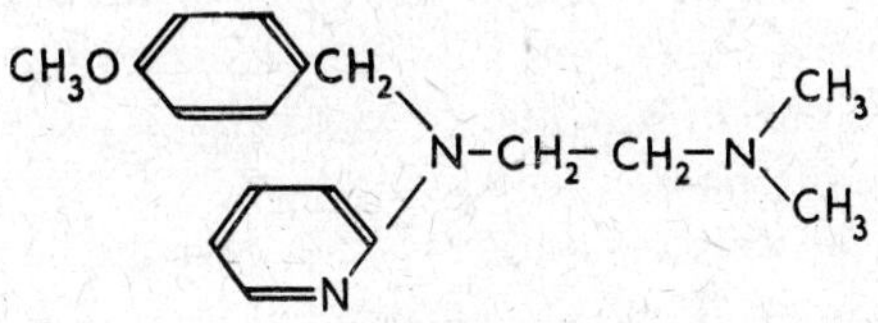

$CH_3O-C_6H_4-CH_2 \diagdown N-CH_2-CH_2-N(CH_3)_2$; $C_5H_4N \diagup$

Anthisan
(neoantergan)
mepyramine *

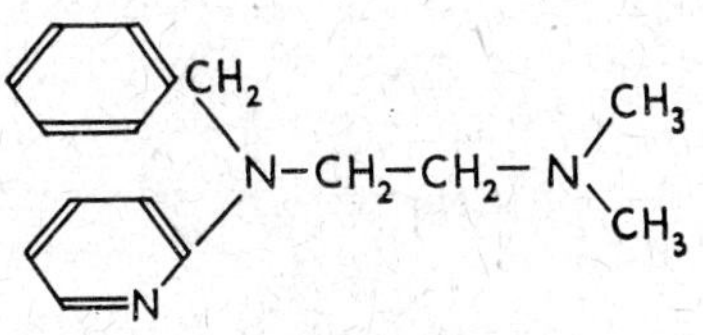

$C_6H_5-CH_2 \diagdown N-CH_2-CH_2-N(CH_3)_2$; $C_5H_4N \diagup$

Pyribenzamine
tripelennamine *

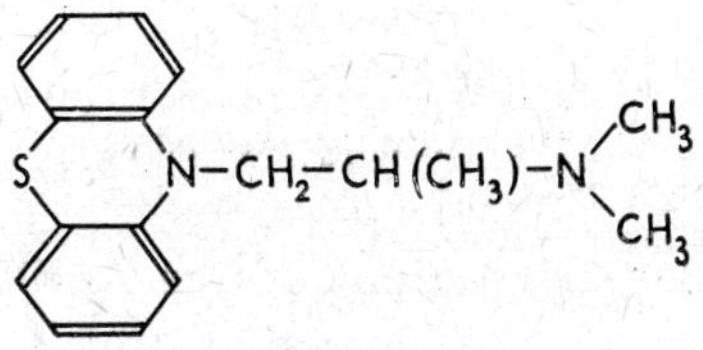

(Phenothiazine, S) $N-CH_2-CH(CH_3)-N(CH_3)_2$

Phenergan
promethazine *

Whilst the structures of some other of the important or commonly-used compounds are as follows :—

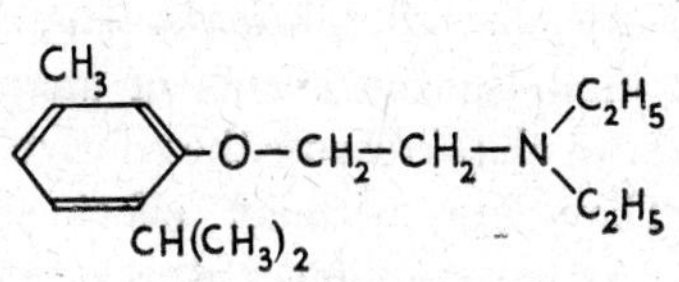

CH_3, $CH(CH_3)_2$ (on ring) $-O-CH_2-CH_2-N(C_2H_5)_2$

" 929 F."

* *G.M.C. approved name.*

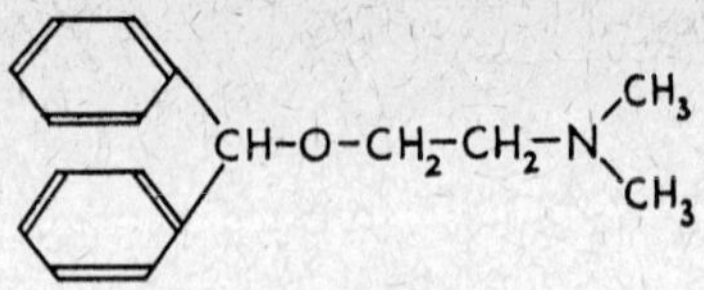

Benadryl
diphenhydramine *

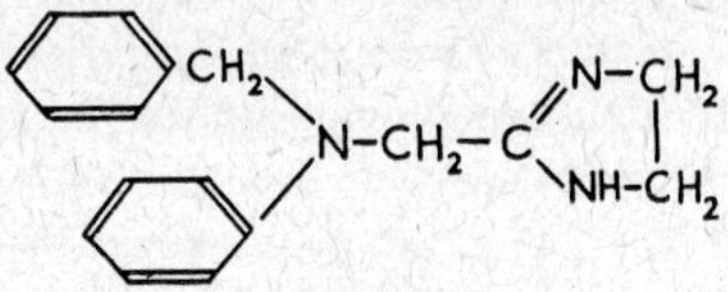

Antistin
antazoline *

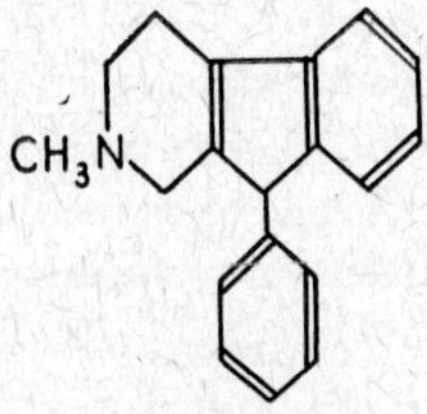

Thephorin
phenindamine *

* *G.M.C. approved name.*

Pharmacological Actions of the Antihistamines

These drugs are readily absorbed from the gut, and reach a peak blood level in a few hours (depending on the compound): degradation occurs mainly in the liver, and excretion in the urine.

Primary Actions. This series of drugs antagonises in man all the effects of histamine except the stimulation of hydrochloric acid formation in the stomach. *Anaphylaxis.* The antihistamines will both prevent and diminish the effects of anaphylactic shock in animals. Friedländer et al. (6) discuss the relative actions of different antihistamines. They are without effect, however, on the phenomenon of the Arthus reaction, as this is not due to histamine release, unless given in very large doses (7). *Skin Vessels.* The antihistamines abolish the "flare-wheal response" which results from damage to capillaries by histamine (dilatation—exudation); suitable control of this effect has been used for the bioassay of antihistamines in man (8). The effect of an antihistamine (promethazine) in inhibiting increases of capillary permeability due to drugs other than histamine (*e.g.* adrenaline, phosgene) has also been described (9). As well as the "antivasodilator" effect, the drugs also have a primary vasoconstrictor action; by these means they inhibit the hypotensive effects of histamine in anæsthetised animals. *Gastro-intestinal Tract.* The antihistamines effectively inhibit the spasmogenic effects of histamine on intestinal smooth muscle, but are not generally intrinsically anti-spasmodic. This action, on guinea-pig ileum, can be used for biological assay of antihistamines (10). *Lungs.* The antihistamines inhibit histamine-induced bronchospasm and mucosal œdema.

Actions not due to Histamine antagonism. *Nervous System.* Peripherally the antihistamines exert a local anæsthetic action. Centrally, in man, the vast majority of antihistamines have a depressant effect (Thephorin is a notable exception). In animals stimulation is the general result of moderate overdosage. *Miscellaneous Effects.* Certain antihistamines have been reported to have an anti-hyaluronidase action (11). Amongst other properties described are varying degrees of anti-acetylcholine, sympathomimetic or sympatholytic activity.

Therapeutic use of the Antihistamines

The antihistamines, like all other new drugs, have been tried for the treatment of most diseases known to medical science. In the following section only the more important therapeutic uses will be described.

The General Allergic Response. During therapeutic desensitisation with allergens the antihistamines have been found useful in the control of local and generalised reactions; such treatment should, however, only be used for patients in whom reactions frequently occur. If severe allergic reactions ("serum sickness"), due to abnormal sensitivity, occur during treatment with normally non-allergic drugs such as insulin, liver extract, or penicillin, then the use of the antihistamines is advised. They usually give considerable relief to the affected skin and mucous membranes, although the joint symptoms and pyrexia generally respond badly.

Allergic Affections of the Respiratory Tract. Hay fever and recurrent vasomotor rhinitis are the disorders most commonly treated with antihistamines. The response, though purely palliative, is generally good though long-standing vasomotor rhinitis may not improve so satisfactorily. The patient's distress is relieved, the sneezing and the itching of eyes and nose respond well, but the intranasal œdema may require treatment with ephedrine or similar vasoconstrictor drugs.

Although allergic cough also responds well, asthma—whether occurring independently or in association with hay fever—is little affected by the antihistamines, except possibly by their sedative effect.

Many exaggerated claims have been made for the efficacy of the antihistamines in the prevention and treatment of the common cold: use of these drugs was originally based on the theory that allergy plays a role in the ætiology of coryza. In the last few years, however, many carefully controlled clinical trials have been performed in which the efficacy of the antihistamines has been balanced against that of placebos, and present opinion is that the antihistamines are valueless in preventing or altering the duration of an attack of coryza (12, 13). In large doses they may give some symptomatic relief. The earlier fallacious reports omitted to consider two important factors: the differentiation of coryza from allergic rhinitis, and the value of any drug (albeit a placebo) in giving subjective symptomatic relief.

Affections of the Skin. The true characteristic allergic disorders of the skin, urticaria, angioneurotic œdema, and dermographia respond well to antihistamines. Itching is the symptom best relieved, œdema in the skin responds moderately well (though the associated serum sickness œdema, in *e.g.* the larynx, should be treated by ephedrine). The drugs are more effective in prevention and treatment of the acute condition than in treatment of chronic urticaria. Other allergic skin diseases respond variably. Atopic dermatitis responds inasmuch as the antihistamines reduce itching and have a sedative action; thus the patient scratches less and the lesions may improve on their own. When used for treating contact dermatitis, again the itching is greatly relieved: but cure of the condition depends on removal of the sensitising agent.

Affections of the Central Nervous System. The antihistamines have been found to possess a depressant action on the vomiting centre, and to be useful in the treatment of nausea and vomiting due to a variety of causes—streptomycin therapy, pregnancy, motion sickness. Much publicity has been given to the successful use of " Dramamine " (a derivative of benadryl) in 100 mg. doses in the prevention and treatment of sea and air sickness (14). The final status of the antihistamines, as compared with hyoscine derivatives, in the prevention of motion sickness is not yet established. Antihistamines have been used with moderate success in the treatment of Parkinson's disease (15). A beneficial palliative reduction in rigidity and muscular cramp is reported, with little action, however, on the tremor and akinesia.

Differential Action, Dosage and Administration of the Antihistamines

The principal actions of the different antihistamines are the same. For practical purposes the drugs may be divided into three groups :—

(*a*) Less potent, no sedative action, *e.g.* antistin (thephorin).
(*b*) Potent, moderately sedative, *e.g.* anthisan, pyribenzamine.
(*c*) Very potent, highly sedative, *e.g.* benadryl, phenergan.

Important exceptions to the general properties are that thephorin has a stimulant, not a sedative action ; and that phenergan is long-acting and has a maximum action at four to twenty hours after oral administration, as against the maximum action at one to four hours of the vast majority of the antihistamines.

It is impossible for the clinician to remember the actions and properties of the innumerable antihistamines at present on the market ; and he is advised to become familiar with one member of each group, to be used as the clinical condition warrants, remembering that individual patients may vary greatly in their responses.

The drugs are generally given orally in capsular form or as tablets or pills (which should be swallowed whole) : parenteral injection is rarely needed. Other methods of administration occasionally used and recommended for particular cases are as an ointment (*e.g.* 2% pyribenzamine) for atopic dermatitis, or as nasal drops or aerosol spray (*e.g.* 0·5% pyribenzamine) for hay fever. The usual single dose of compounds in groups (*a*) and (*b*) is 100–200 mg. (here thephorin is an exception : because of its stimulant action the maximum dose advised is 50 mg.); the usual single dose of the more potent compounds of group (*c*) is 10–50 mg. When using an antihistamine for the first time, the practitioner is strongly advised to consult the leaflet issued by the manufacturers before administering the drug to the patient.

The choice of drug to be used in a particular case depends to a large extent on the individual preferences of the physician, and should depend on the degree of sedation required and on the individual response of the patient. The size and frequency of the dose should depend on the severity of the symptoms, the sensitivity of the patient and also on the patient's size and age—to infants give 1/20–1/4 of the adult dose (depending on the weight), to children aged 2–5 give 1/3 of the adult dose, to children aged 5–12 give 1/2 of the adult dose. Potable " Elixirs " are available.

Some examples of suitable dosage may be suggested :—

Mild hay fever : 100 mg. of antistin twice daily. Serum sickness : 100 mg. of pyribenzamine four times daily. Urticaria with itching : 25 mg. of phenergan every night. Parkinsonism : 50 mg. of benadryl four times daily.

Further reference to doses which have been employed in various diseases may be found in the reviews cited at the end of this chapter. It must not be forgotten that the antihistamines exert a palliative effect only ; they do not affect the original lesion which is causing the release of histamine.

Toxic Effects of the Antihistamines

Despite the claims of the manufacturers, the perfect antihistamine has never been produced, and probably never will be—that is a drug which combines the maximum action in opposition to histamine with the minimum of side-effects. In general the more potent the drug, the higher its toxicity. Toxic side-effects, so severe that administration of the antihistamine must be stopped, occur in about 5% of cases.

The principle side-effect of the antihistamines is sedation. As already described, this sedation may be of value therapeutically, but in the majority of cases, in the ambulant patient, at best an unpleasant lassitude is produced, and at worst there is a marked degree of diminished alertness, drowsiness, and detachment from the surroundings. With average therapeutic doses, 25%–50% of patients show some symptoms of sedation. Benadryl is the most sedative of the common antihistamines and to avoid its soporific effect 5 mg. of amphetamine may be given with the benadryl each morning.

Conversely, excitation, convulsions and delirium may occur after very large doses of an antihistamine, but need not be feared with the normal therapeutic doses. Symptoms due to action on the gastro-intestinal tract are not uncommon; epigastric distress, nausea or mild colic may occur, especially in patients who already have some organic gastro-intestinal disorder. Other side-actions are dryness of the mouth, or palpitation and tachycardia; very occasionally skin rashes (occurring with systemic (16) or local (17) administration), and rare cases of agranulocytosis have been reported (18).

Deaths may occur from accidental overdosage: this has occurred especially in children, and fatalities have been reported (19) of infants or children, who ate 500 to 1,500 mg. of various antihistamine tablets (presumably thinking that they were sweets (20)) and who died in convulsions within the hour. Deaths may occur indirectly, usually in adults, from motor car or similar accidents which result from the common side-effects of drowsiness causing loss of alertness.

So it can be seen that the antihistamines are a valuable addition to the therapeutic armamentarium, but in a limited field; and that their dosage and distribution need to be carefully controlled. More detailed reference to the properties and uses of the antihistamines than has been possible in this brief survey may be found in the reviews of Loew (21), pharmacology; Huttrer (22), chemistry; Hunter and Dunlop (23), general survey; Lovelass and Dworin (24), allergy; and Feinberg et al. (25), general survey.

REFERENCES

(1) Dale and Laidlaw. *Journ. Physiol.*, 1910–11, **41**, 318.
(2) Dragstedt and Gebauer-Fuelnegg. *Amer. Journ. Physiol.*, 1932, **102**, 512.
(3) Curry. *Journ. Clin. Invest.*, 1946, **25**, 785.
(4) Staub and Bovet. *Compt. rend. Soc. de biol.*, 1937, **125**, 818.
(5) Ungar, Parrot and Bovet. *Compt. rend. Soc. de biol.*, 1937, **124**, 445.
(6) Friedländer, Feinberg and Feinberg. *Journ. Lab. Clin. Med.*, 1947, **32**, 47.
(7) Benacerraf and Fischel. *Proc. Soc. Exp. Biol. and Med.*, 1949, **71**, 349.
(8) Bain. *Proc. Roy. Soc. Med.*, 1949, **42**, 615.
(9) Halpern. *Bull. N.Y. Acad. Med.*, 1949, **25**, 323.

(10) Schild. *Brit. Journ. Pharmacol.*, 1947, **2**, 189.
(11) Elster, Freeman and Lowry. *Journ. Pharmacol. and Exp. Therap.*, 1949, **96**, 332.
(12) Council on Pharmacy and Chemistry, American Medical Assocn., *Journ. Amer. Med. Assocn.*, 1950, **142**, 566.
(13) Medical Research Council Special Committee. *Brit. Med. Journ.*, 1950, *ii*, 425.
(14) Gay and Carliner. *Science*, 1949, **109**, 359.
(15) Ryan and Wood. *Lancet*, 1949, *i*, 258.
(16) Ellis and Bundick. *Journ. Invest. Dermat.*, 1949, **13**, 25.
(17) Sherman and Cooke. *Journ. Allergy*, 1950, **21**, 63.
(18) Cahan, Meilman and Jacobson. *New England Journ. Med.*, 1949, **241**, 865.
(19) Tobias. *Brit. Med. Journ.*, 1949, *i*, 1098.
(20) Editorial. *Lancet*, 1950, *i*, 28.
(21) Loew. *Physiol. Rev.*, 1947, **27**, 542.
(22) Huttrer. *Enzymologia*, 1948, **12**, 277.
(23) Hunter and Dunlop. *Quart. Journ. Med.*, 1948, **17**, 271.
(24) Loveless and Dworin. *Bull. N.Y. Acad. Med.*, 1949, **25**, 473.
(25) Feinberg, Malkiel and Feinberg. *The Antihistamines : their clinical application*, 1950. The Year Book Publishers, Chicago.

CHAPTER IV

THE USE OF ISOTOPES IN MEDICINE

ALTHOUGH radioactive isotopes were used in biological investigations by Hevesy (1), Hamilton (2) and Hertz (3), and in therapy by Lawrence (4) before 1940, their extensive use in medicine and related subjects commenced in 1945. Since that time, certain nuclear reactors have become available for the cheap production of radioactive isotopes, and simple mass spectrometers have been developed for the measurement of stable isotopes. Their use in fundamental metabolic studies is now established, but their therapeutic application has proved disappointing. At the present time only in one disease, polycythæmia vera, is therapy with a radioactive isotope the treatment of choice.

Isotopes of the same element have the same atomic extra-nuclear structure and therefore possess similar chemical properties. Their nuclear structure and atomic weights differ however and they can be distinguished by physical methods, *e.g.* their atomic weights can be compared by means of a mass spectrometer. If the nuclear structure is unstable the isotope is radioactive and a certain proportion of the atoms disintegrate per second emitting particles and radiations which can be detected by such instruments as the Geiger counter, or less sensitively by using photographic emulsion. The radioactive isotopes can be detected with greater sensitivity than the stable variety and hence can be used at greater dilution in biological experiments. They can also be detected *in situ* in the human body and these two advantages have led to their more extensive use in medical research than the stable isotopes. However, for two important biochemical elements, nitrogen and oxygen, the only suitable isotopes are stable.

An important unit for the measurement of amount of radioactivity is the curie which represents $3{\cdot}700 \times 10^{10}$ atoms disintegrating per second. Smaller units, which are usually encountered in tracer work, are the milli- and micro-curie, which are 1/1,000 and 1/1,000,000 of a curie respectively. The activity of any particular radioactive isotope decays with time, and a measure of this rate of decay is its half-life, which is the constant time interval during which the amount of radioactivity halves in value. This may range from fractions of a second to millions of years for different isotopes. If the half-life is too short, then the isotope may be unsuitable for most investigations, *e.g.* the oxygen isotope of atomic weight 15 which has a half life of one hundred and twenty-six seconds.

Most naturally occurring elements consist of a mixture of stable isotopes, *e.g.* oxygen consists of 99·757% O^{16}, 0·039% O^{17} and 0·204% O^{18}. Labelling a group of atoms by means of stable isotopes, therefore, involves the preparation of material which contains an abnormal proportion of isotopes, *e.g.* 2% O^{18}, 98% O^{16}. This abnormal ratio, or the degree of dilution of this ratio by the oxygen normally present in the organism or system, is detected by the mass spectrometer. The use of radioactive isotopes is simpler in principle as only one commonly occurring element, potassium, contains an isotope which is radioactive. Thus it is possible to introduce a group of radioactive atoms, all of which are labelled, into a system which previously contained no such atoms. In practice, the group of introduced atoms is not always "carrier-free" but consists of a mixture of radioactive and normally occurring atoms of an element.

Use of Isotopes in Metabolic Studies

The technique of an isotope experiment consists in the introduction of labelled atoms, which may or may not be incorporated into molecules, into the system under investigation. Although the system may contain the same element or compound as the introduced material, the labelled atoms are distinguishable because of their physical properties and the movement of these particular atoms can be followed. Thus, the dynamic properties of a system may be revealed, although the chemical state remains in equilibrium.

It is not proposed to review in detail here the application of tracers to fundamental metabolic investigations. The development of the technique has reached such a stage that it is now best considered in its true place as an invaluable and unique method to be used and considered in conjunction with other methods for the investigation of any particular problem. A bibliography of general reference sources for the more recent work is presented at the end of this chapter. However, it may be of value to state some general considerations which are vital to such applications:—

(*a*) The chemical properties of the labelled atoms must be indistinguishable from those occurring naturally. That this is approximately the case is shown by determinations of the natural ratio of isotopes in various body compartments. Lasnitzki and Brewer (5) have investigated the ratio of K^{41}/K^{39} in biological tissue and found it to be constant, except for bone marrow and blood plasma where the ratio is about 3% higher than in other tissue. The chemical properties of the isotopes of hydrogen, however, cannot be regarded as identical. The atoms of the isotopes H^3 (tritium) and H^2 (deuterium) have twice and three times the mass of the most abundant naturally occurring atom, H^1. This produces differences in their chemical behaviour which particularly affect certain enzyme reactions (6).

(*b*) The radiation from the radioactive atoms must not disturb the normal metabolic processes. Ionising radiation may, of course, even be lethal to living organisms. Thus it is advisable to use as small a dose of radioactivity as possible, but in general it is not considered that tracer doses cause any short term physiological effect (7).

(*c*) If molecules are to be labelled by the incorporation of tracer atoms, then the unambiguous following of such molecules in a chemical process precludes any exchange of the tracer atoms with the corresponding constituents of other molecules. That this is generally true has been shown by many workers (8, 9, 10). However, it has been shown that hydrogen atoms bound to oxygen and nitrogen are easily exchangeable with those of water (11). The possibilities of such exchange mechanisms can be explored by multi-labelling of a molecule. Thus more than one atom of a molecule may be labelled in various positions by different isotopes and the proportion of the isotopes measured by utilising their dissimilar physical properties, *e.g.* by using stable H^2 and radioactive H^3.

(*d*) If all the atoms of a labelled element are radioactive then it is generally necessary to introduce only about 10^{-12} g. of the element in a tracer experiment. However, it is possible that greater amounts of the element may be necessary because of dilution of the radioactive atoms with inert atoms of the same element in the physical production process. In the case of compounds the position is less satisfactory because the chemical synthesis will again lower the specific activity (ratio of radioactive to inert atoms). Tracer experiments demand compounds of high specific activity and negligible mass, or the experiment may be carried out under pharmacological rather then physiological conditions. Thus the fate of 10 mg. of œstradiol in a 100 g. rat is of little interest compared with that of 10μg. The metabolism of 14 mg. of labelled iodine in humans has been shown to differ very greatly from that of 0·1 μg. (12) and Pochin (13) has shown that the metabolism of labelled thyroxine differs with the amount of hormone injected. As many isotopes are now available carrier-free, and detection methods are very efficient, the onus for increase in overall efficiency lies with the methods of chemical synthesis.

Although these considerations and limitations must be carefully considered in isotopic investigations, their use in the field of fundamental metabolic studies in conjunction with other methods has brought revolutionary progress in the understanding of the dynamic state of body constitutents. This is brought out in the following extract :—"Components of an animal are rapidly degraded into specific molecular groups which may wander from one place to another. The chemical reactions must be balanced so delicately that, through regeneration, the body components remain constant in total amount and in structure. This constancy is not to be taken as an indication that the structural matter of the living organism is inactive and takes little part in metabolism" (14, 15).

The Use of Isotopes in Clinical Diagnosis

Radioactive isotopes are much more generally used than stable isotopes for clinical diagnosis. Even so the number of radio-isotopes which can be used is restricted to those with suitable half-lives and radiation properties and which can be economically produced (preferably in an atomic pile). The half-life must not be inconveniently short and yet must not be so long as to be potentially dangerous to patient and investigators.

The isotopes most generally used emit β rays and sometimes also γ rays in addition. Even the most energetic β rays, which are actually high velocity electrons, do not penetrate more than 1 cm. of tissue, whereas γ rays, which could be described as very hard X-rays, penetrate tissue with very little absorption. Thus, those isotopes which emit γ rays can be detected *in situ* by Geiger counters but those, such as P^{32}, Ca^{45} and C^{14}, which emit β rays only cannot be located in any but the most superficial positions. It is possible to measure quantitatively the amount of a γ ray emitting isotope in almost any position in the body, but even though a pure β ray emitter may be superficially located it is generally impossible to obtain any quantitative results other than a comparative distribution survey. The ideal isotope for diagnostic purposes should have a half-life of one to fourteen days, should emit γ rays of about 0·5 Mev and should be produced economically, if possible in a carrier-free state, by the atomic pile. Such an isotope is radioactive iodine, I^{131}, which has a half-life of eight days, emits a γ ray of 0·36 Mev as well as β rays and is available at the time of writing in Great Britain carrier-free at 10s. per 0·5 millicurie from the Harwell pile.

The use of isotopes for diagnosis can be divided into two types :—static and dynamic investigations.

Static Investigations

These investigations are concerned with the distribution of a radioactive isotope with position in a patient at a particular fixed time. The survey is usually carried out at a definite time (often

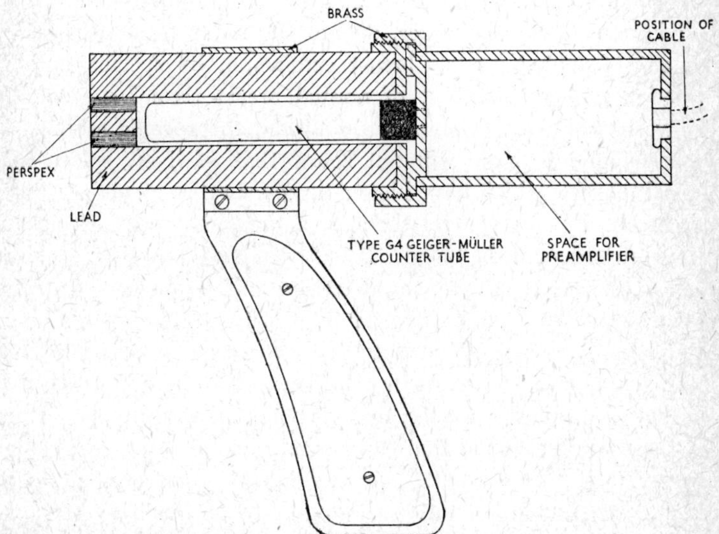

FIG. 1. A sectional view of a typical directional Geiger-Müller counter. The collimating property depends on the lead shielding.

twenty-four hours) after the administration of the isotope and its distribution localised by means of a specially shielded directional Geiger counter such as is shown in Fig. 1.

Tumour Localisation. The uptake of an isotope or labelled compound by neoplastic tissue may differ from that of the surrounding tissue. This may yield useful diagnostic information although the differential uptake may not be great enough for therapeutic application. This property of neoplastic tissue is thought to be due to the following causes :—

(*a*) *Increased Metabolic Activity of the Tumour Tissue.* The specific uptake (per cent of isotope administered per g. of tissue) of a particular tissue depends on :—

(i) The amount of the chemically identical element or compound present in the tissue.

(ii) The rate of turnover of the element or compound.

In the case of rapidly growing tissue, such as tumours, the second of these factors is increased ; and, the first factor being the same, tumours will show a higher uptake of radioisotope than most normal tissue when specific uptakes are measured shortly after administration of the tracer. Thus Kenney et al. (16) found that osteogenic sarcoma had four times the specific uptake of P^{32} than had normal bone. However, due to the lower total phosphorus content of such tissue as breast carcinoma, its specific uptake, although higher than that of normal breast tissue, is generally below that of normal bone. In addition, the specific activity of such malignant tissue will fall below that of liver, spleen and sternal marrow which have higher turnover rates. This precludes the use of P^{32} for general therapy of malignant cells except for certain disorders of the blood. It has been used, however, by Low-Beer et al. (17, 18, 19) for the detection and estimation of malignancy of breast tumours. Investigation was made, forty-eight hours after administration of the isotope, by *in situ* measurements, but as P^{32} emits β rays only, its distribution could only be measured in superficial neoplastic tissues, and then not quantitatively. Even so, these workers found that carcinomata had at least, and benign lesions at the most, a 25% greater uptake than normal breast tissue. There was an increased uptake of as much as 150% in acute inflammations because of increased vascularisation. They claim that, using these criteria as a basis for diagnosis, the method was reliable for 89% of carcinomata, 91% of benign lesions and 100% of inflammations.

Radiostrontium and radiocalcium are also taken up at high specific activities by osteogenic sarcomata, but this property is of little use for diagnostic purposes as both these isotopes are pure β ray emitters. It has recently been reported that radiogallium (20), which is selectively absorbed by bone, is concentrated to a greater extent by bone tumours. This may be especially valuable for diagnosis as radiogallium is a γ ray emitter, and is safe because of its short half-life.

(*b*) *Differential Membrane Permeability of Tumours.* Most ions with a negative charge pass more slowly from the plasma into the central nervous system than do other ions. This selective barrier is broken down in vessels supplying such abnormal regions as brain tumours, abscesses, granulomata and traumatised tissues. Thus the fluorescein radicle penetrates into such areas more readily than into normal brain tissue and may be detected there during neuro-surgical operations by its fluorescence under ultraviolet light irradiation. Radioactive di-iodofluorescein, in which I^{131} is incorporated, also exhibits this property; and a survey of the skull after administration of this compound to a patient can reveal the presence and location of regions in which the blood-brain barrier has been broken down. Moore et al. (21) report that, except for very small tumours, with little associated œdematous tissue, the method is reliable for the diagnosis and location of glioblastomata, ependymomata, meningiomata, ependymoblastomata and metastatic tumour (in that order of dependability), but is unreliable for acoustic neuromata and astrocytomata. It is generally about 95% efficient for diagnosis of the gliomata. Ashkenzaky et al. (22) who have also done extensive work in this field agree with this figure.

(*c*) *Specific Differentiation by Tumour Tissue.* It is very desirable that some radioactive compound or element be found that is selectively localised by neoplastic tissue, perhaps to be retained there as a synthesised metabolite. Such a compound has not yet been discovered, which is hardly surprising. However, the normal thyroid has the ability to absorb one particular element, iodine, and it also absorbs the radioactive isotope I^{131} very efficiently. Thus twenty-four hours after oral administration of a carrier-free drink containing I^{131}, 30% of the dose is taken up by the normal thyroid. A survey of the thyroid after such a tracer drink will show the position of the lobes and isthmus in a normal gland. Results of such an investigation are best presented in the form of projection contour maps with lines of equal activity as shown in Fig. 2. These maps may indicate to the surgeon areas of high functional activity before thyroidectomy and regions of residual activity after the operation. Any disturbance of the normal function of such tissue affects the specific uptake. Most thyroid carcinomata have a reduced ability to concentrate radioactive iodine, and this may be shown in thyroid surveys (Fig. 2). As about 5% of cases of well differentiated adenocarcinomata retain this characteristic of I^{131} retention, this test can only supply a positive answer regarding the possible presence of cyst or tumour. Metastases of thyroid primary tumour of a differentiated type may also have I^{131} retaining ability and particularly after thyroidectomy, these may be detected and treated by the use of this radioisotope.

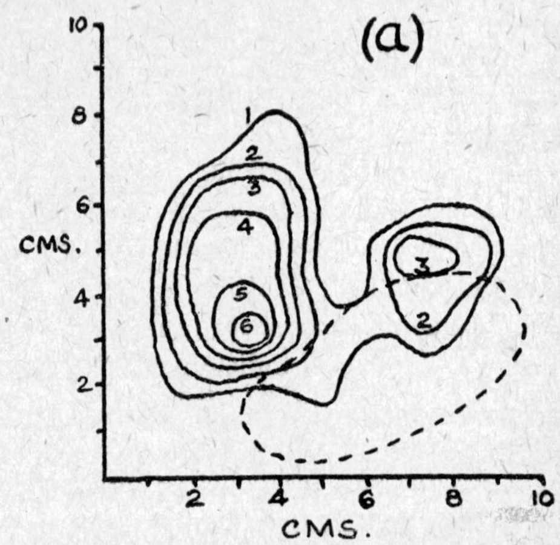

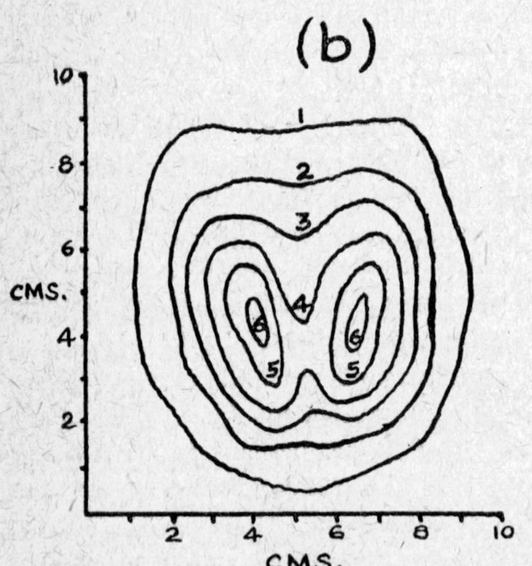

FIG. 2. Diagrams of distribution of I^{131} in the thyroid obtained by using a directional counter of the type shown in Fig. 1. Figures represent activity. (a) Shows the distribution diagram obtained in a particular case of thyroid adenoma. The position of the palpable mass is shown by the dotted line. It can be seen that this is not composed of functional tissue. (b) Shows the type of distribution obtained for a normal gland.

Technique of Autoradiography. Autoradiography consists in the placing of a tissue section of about 10 μ thickness in contact with a photographic emulsion. The presence and location of radioactive material is indicated by blackening of the emulsion, *e.g.* the presence of I^{131} in thyroid colloid can be demonstrated. Thus a biopsy followed by autoradiography can be very informative in static investigations. A resolution of about 2 μ can be obtained by this method at the present time but it is likely that further advances in technique will lead to its extension from histological to cytological studies.

Dynamic Investigations

These studies are concerned with the variation of the quantity of radioistope with time at a particular position.

Determination of Distribution Characteristics. When a tracer is injected intravenously and its subsequent plasma concentration followed, a graph of concentration against time generally shows a multiple exponential decay curve. Thus the concentration of radiosodium, Na^{24}, in plasma shows a rapid decay, followed after about four hours by a much more gradual decrease. This has been interpreted as a rapid diffusion of the isotope into the extracellular space followed by a more gradual exchange with sodium in such tissue as bone apatite crystal layers, and in nervous tissue. A similar curve is obtained using radioactive potassium or heavy water (water labelled with deuterium), but for these substances the exponential curve is simple and single. The concentration of plasma I^{131} also shows a decay curve but, after about twenty-four hours, the concentration begins to increase. This is due to the output of protein bound I^{131} by the thyroid gland, which is significant at this time particularly for thyrotoxic patients (23). However, in the case of many tracers (Na^{24}, K^{42}, D_2O) the concentration in the plasma is very nearly constant after about twelve hours when allowance is made for excretion. Then if it is assumed that the tracer atoms have completely exchanged with the body constituents, the total body content of the introduced compound or element can be found. Moore (24) and many others have used D_2O to estimate the total body water of humans. He has carried out the same measurement in rabbits and then estimated the water directly, finding that the results agree very closely. Also, just as inulin is used to estimate extracellular space so tracers can be used to estimate sodium and potassium spaces. It should be emphasised that these space values are useful physiological concepts only and represent the effective space occupied by the tracer at the same concentration as in the plasma. As many elements are present in intracellular tissue at much greater concentration than in blood plasma, the space values do not represent actual space occupied by the element although in the case of sodium this may nearly be so.

If R represents the amount of tracer introduced, r represents the amount of tracer per ml. plasma after equilibrium has been attained, and i represents the amount of substance chemically identical with the tracer in 1 ml. plasma after equilibriation then,

$$R/r \times i = \text{total body content of the substance and}$$

$$R/r = \text{distribution space of substance.}$$

The information which can be obtained by the simultaneous use of heavy water, K^{42} and Na^{24}, and inulin measurements includes the values for the average intracellular cation concentration. Thus heavy water measurements give values of total body water and inulin measures extracellular space. Subtraction of these two values gives the intracellular water. Use of K^{42} and Na^{24} together with flame photometer measurements of plasma potassium and sodium concentrations gives values for total body sodium and potassium, and subtraction of the total extracellular sodium and potassium values (obtained from inulin space $\times$ plasma concentration of sodium and potassium) gives the total intracellular potassium and sodium. Thus intracellular water, potassium and sodium are known and the average intracellular cation concentrations can be calculated. Corrections must be made for the amount of tracers excreted.

By similar methods, total red cell volume and plasma volume can be estimated by the use of tracers. Total red cell volume has been estimated by the use of tagged red cells in which radioactive iron (25) or P^{32} (26) or Cr^{51} (27) are incorporated into the erythrocyte. Storaasli, Friedell et al. (28) have used I^{131} tagged human serum albumin to estimate total plasma volume. They report that the method has decided advantages over the T 1824 dye method which has previously been used for this estimation, a determination which is becoming increasingly important in clinical medicine.

THE USE OF I^{131} IN DIAGNOSIS OF THYROID FUNCTION

The most frequent application of radioactive isotopes to clinical diagnosis is the study of I^{131} metabolism in selected patients suspected of suffering from disorders of the thyroid gland.

I^{131} is a γ and β ray emitter and by the use of suitably designed calibrated Geiger counters (29) the amount of the tracer in the thyroid gland can be estimated *in situ* by external measurements. The amount of I^{131} in plasma and urine is usually measured by a β ray counter.

If the content of I^{131} in the thyroid, expressed as percentage of administered tracer, is plotted against time of measurement, curves such as Fig. 3 are obtained. The carrier-free I^{131} may be given

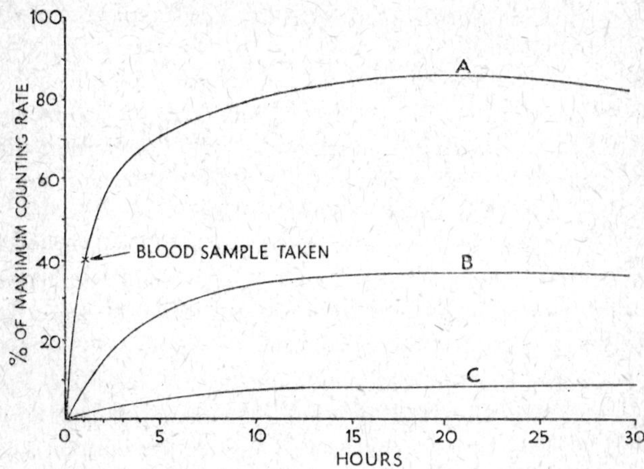

FIG. 3. Typical I^{131} uptake curves. Curve A was obtained with a thyrotoxic patient. A blood sample was taken sixty-five minutes after the administration of approximately 15 μc. of I^{131}. The slope of the curve at this point showed an uptake rate of 0·27% per minute. Assay of the plasma sample showed the I^{131} content to be 0·000415% per ml., thus the clearance rate of the gland was 650 ml. per minute. Curve B shows a typical normal uptake curve, and curve C the type of curve obtained with a myxœdematous patient.

orally or intravenously, for apart from a slight initial delay in uptake after oral administration, the results are similar. As can be seen from Fig. 3, thyroid glands of different activity show differences in the slope of their uptake curves and certain characteristics of such graphs may be chosen as an index for diagnosis of thyroid function. The curves can be described by three characteristics :— Initial rate of uptake, maximum value of uptake and shape of curve after twenty-four hours. Both initial rate of uptake and maximum value of uptake increase as the functional activity of the gland increases. For patients with thyroid glands of low or normal activity, and with normal renal iodide clearance values, the uptake remains constant or increases slowly after twenty-four hours, but for hyperactive glands the uptake decreases after this time. This is due to a high rate of output of protein-bound I^{131} by such glands. Diagnosis may be based on these three characteristics as follows :—

Twenty-four hour Thyroid Uptake. This index is the value of thyroid uptake expressed as per cent of given oral dose measured twenty-four hours after administration. It has the virtue of great simplicity but has two main disadvantages :— (*a*) The measurement may be made during the downward trend of the curve and so may be much less than the maximum value of thyroid uptake, (*b*) It is dependent on renal iodide clearance values and may give false results for patients with renal disorders.

Werner, Quimby and Schmidt (30) have published observations on 269 patients using this method. They found that euthyroid states give values of 10–40% for the twenty-four hour thyroid uptake value, hyperthyroid conditions values over 35% (mostly over 50%) and hypothyroid conditions low values of less than 10%. There was a small overlap of values for euthyroidism and hyperthyroidism and they found lack of correlation between uptake and B.M.R. values in Hashimoto's disease, malignant exophthalmos and general hypometabolic states such as Simmonds' disease, Addison's disease and anorexia nervosa.

Thyroid Clearance. This index is based on the initial rate of uptake and corresponds in concept to the renal clearance value. It is the minimum volume of plasma cleared of I^{131} by the thyroid per minute and is determined by the rate of uptake (per cent per minute) one to two hours after administration of tracer, divided by the plasma concentration (per cent per ml.) at that time. Hence it is expressed in ml./min. This index was first shown to be of value by Pochin, Mayant and Goldie (31). It has the advantage of being a direct measure of thyroid function independent of renal functions, and is probably the best of the numerous suggested methods based on the radioiodine accumulating ability of the gland. Measurements of thyroid clearance should be made after equilibrium has been approximately attained in body tissues other than the thyroid and before the thyroid commences to secrete I^{131} in organic form. As Pochin (13) has suggested, intravenous injection may be of advantage to ensure rapid equilibration, but measurements made one hour after oral administration of the isotope are usually satisfactory. Iodine medication must not be given in the three weeks before the test and the diet must be reasonably normal in iodine content (fish have a high iodine content).

The following values have been found by various British workers:—

Thyroid condition	Workers and reference	No. of cases	Range of values of thyroid clearances ml/min.	Mean value of thyroid clearance	Method of administration
Hyperthyroidism	Pochin (13)*	12	84–350	240	Intravenous
	Pochin (31)	11	198–1390	486	oral
	Macgregor (23)	31	30–560	163	oral
Non-toxic goitre	Pochin (13)	12	7–42	25	Intravenous
	Pochin (31)	4	28–100	62	oral
	Macgregor (23)	16	15–59	32	oral
Normal . .	Pochin (13)	12	9–37	25	Intravenous
	Pochin (31)	8	9–38	16	oral
	Macgregor (23)	12	15–37	19	oral
Hypothyroidism	Macgregor (23)	4	0·4–34	13	oral

* Hyperthyroid cases quoted in (13) are clinically more doubtful than those in (31).

There is no doubt that thyroid clearance rates are a reliable measure of thyroid activity and this index is becoming of general use in Great Britain. The use of this test is of value for examining thyroid function in such conditions as anxiety states, essential hypertension, cardiac disease and chronic alcoholism in which B.M.R. values are nearly always raised, independently of the condition of the thyroid. However, as stated by Keating et al. (32), diagnosis based on radioiodine-accumulating function of the thyroid gland is as liable to give false results as relying on B.M.R. values, so that these two tests are supplementary. It should be noted that these results are false only from the standpoint of diagnosis of toxicity and not necessarily from certain other aspects of thyroid activity.

Protein-bound I^{131} values. The estimation of protein-bound non-radioactive iodine in plasma as a reliable index of toxicity is now realised but the technique of measurement is extremely difficult. The concentration of protein-bound I^{131} in plasma measured forty-eight hours after administration of the tracer is a similar index but the measurement is much easier technically. Clark et al. (33), McConahey, Keating and Power (34), McGregor (23) and Freedberg et al. (35) have discussed its value in diagnosis.

The relationship of B.M.R., thyroid clearance and protein-bound iodine values is not clear at present. It seems, however, that the B.M.R. is a non-specific measurement of the rate of body metabolism, whereas the thyroid clearance and protein-bound iodine values are specifically related to thyroid function. Perlmuter, Martin and Riggs (36) have shown that although radioiodine accumulating function decreases with age, protein-bound iodine values remain constant. They suggest that this is due to a decreasing rate of utilisation of thyroxine by the peripheral tissues. Thus, protein-bound iodine and thyroid clearance values also represent different aspects of thyroid function. Stanbury and Hedge (37) have shown that in certain cases of goitrous cretins, the I^{131} accumulating properties may be normal but the protein-bound iodine values are very nearly zero. Thus there is a blocking of the synthesis of thyroxine in such glands. The evidence suggests that I^{131} accumulating function represents the ability of the gland to synthesise iodine to an intermediate compound and is not necessarily a measure of the rate of secretion of thyroxine.

Use of Isotopes in Circulatory Studies

The flow of blood may be followed *in situ* by the injection of a γ ray emitting isotope into the blood stream. Radioactive sodium (Na^{24}, half-life 14·9 hours) has been extensively used for this purpose (38). It is not the perfect isotope for the purpose as it rapidly diffuses into the whole extracellular space and it emits a penetrating γ ray which is very difficult to locate directionally. However, radiosodium can be used without chemical processing, it is easily produced and is very safe because of its short half-life and general distribution in the body. Quimby and Smith (39) have measured arm to foot circulation times by this method. Radiosodium was injected into the antecubital vein and a shielded Geiger counter, placed against the sole of the foot, recorded the delayed pulse of radiation. No valuable correlation was established between circulation time and clinical condition. Prinzmetal (40) has also applied this method in a procedure which he terms " radio-cardiography ". Na^{24} was injected very rapidly into the raised arm and a directional γ ray counter, placed over the heart, recorded the pulses of radioactivity as can be seen in Fig. 4. Prinzmetal claims that diagnosis of certain cardiac conditions can be quickly and surely made by this simple procedure. A comparison of the method with electrocardiography, ballistocardiography and angio-cardiography would be useful.

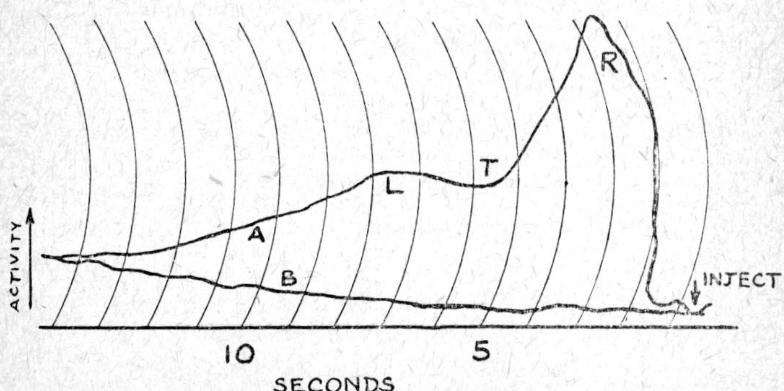

FIG. 4. Typical cardiograms obtained by Prinzmetal et al. (*Journ. Amer. Med. Assocn.*, 1949, **139**, 617). Curve A was obtained with a normal patient, the R wave represented blood entering and leaving the right side of the heart, whilst the L wave represented blood entering and leaving the left side, the transition point T being the point where most of the blood was in the lungs. Curve B was obtained after injecting radiosodium into the antecubital vein of a patient having a superior vena caval obstruction. The delayed and ill-defined R wave denoted blocking of venous return.

An application of isotopes to circulatory conditions, which is rather different in principle, is the study of " build-up " or " rate of disappearance curves ". Quimby and Smith have observed the increase in radioactivity in a particular site after the injection of radiosodium in another part of the body. Fig 5 shows such a curve. These workers claim that various disorders can be diagnosed by this test and sites of amputation can be decided upon. Veall (41) states that this test is very dependent on external conditions such as temperature and humidity. It would seem that variation between individuals is so great that this test is of the greatest use in the comparative study of the progress of the individual patient with treatment. This also applies to a similar method proposed by Kety and Cooper (42) in which the rate of disappearance of radio-sodium from an injected site is followed.

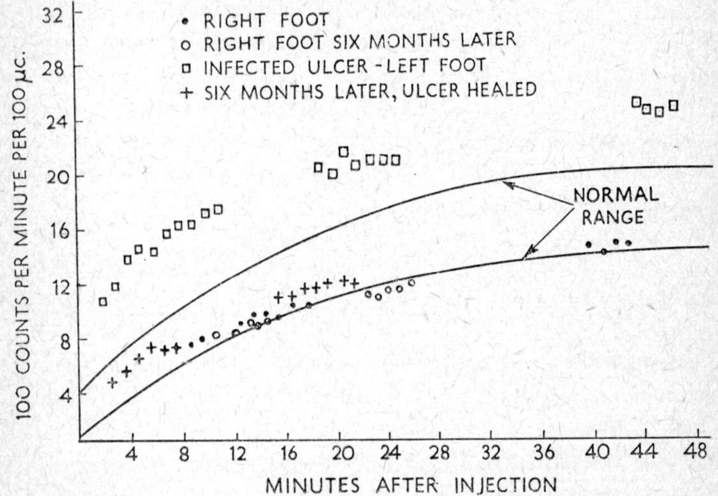

FIG. 5. Radiosodium " build-up " curves in a diabetic arteriosclerotic patient with an infected ulcer in the sole of the left foot. The upper curve (□) indicates the " build-up " in the left foot in its original condition, and the points (•) the " build-up " in the unaffected right foot. Six months later the ulcer had healed, as a result of local therapy, the " build-up " being represented by (+). The right foot " build-up " is unaltered (o). (E. H. Quimby. *Amer. Journ. Roentgenol.*, 1947, 58, 746.)

MISCELLANEOUS APPLICATION OF TRACERS IN CLINICAL DIAGNOSIS

Further applications of isotopes to clinical diagnosis which are merely in an experimental stage are the diagnosis of cartilagenous tumours by investigation with S^{35} labelled sodium sulphate (43), and the use of S^{35} labelled methionine for the study of protein metabolism. Kinsel et al. (44) state that patients with chronic liver disease, idiopathic hypoproteinæmia and Cushing's syndrome showed a significant deviation of protein metabolism from the normal metabolic pattern.

Isotopes have also been used for mechanically tracing the rate of absorption of compounds from various ointments and the extent of the penetration through the skin of injurious compounds such as the nitrogen mustards.

Radioactive Isotopes in Therapy

Radium or X-ray therapy involves the localised irradiation of neoplastic tissue. This localisation is carried out by mechanical methods which must necessarily be inefficient, and generally if therapy is to be successful the malignant tissue must be more radio-sensitive than normal tissue. The possibility of selective irradiation of tumours by radioactive isotopes promised, in principle, a much more efficient method of therapy. However, because of the reasons outlined in the section "Tumour Localisation" only four diseases are now regularly treated by isotopes. These are chronic myeloid leukæmia, polycythæmia vera, functioning metastases of thyroid carcinoma and a non-malignant condition, thyrotoxicosis. The former two are treated with P^{32} and the latter two with I^{131}.

Chronic Myeloid Leukæmia. P^{32} treatment of this condition results in slightly longer remissions than does X-ray therapy. An effective dose of 6 millicuries maintained over six weeks will generally result in a remission of over a year (45). Splenomegaly, lymphadenopathy, hepatomegaly, erythrocytopenia and thrombocytopenia are rapidly improved. The advantages over X-ray therapy are ease of treatment and lack of radiation sickness.

Polycythæmia Vera. P^{32} therapy is now the treatment of choice in this condition. Six millicuries are generally given intravenously, followed one to two months later by a second dose whose magnitude is determined by the individual response. Response to treatment is delayed by a time interval corresponding to the mean life of an erythrocyte. Complete remission is induced in some patients by a single dose. In certain other neoplastic diseases of the hæmopoietic system, particularly chronic lymphatic leukæmia, P^{32} therapy may be of value. Brues and Jacobson (46) have reviewed the comparative therapeutic effects of radioactive and chemo-therapeutic methods for such conditions.

Thyroid Carcinoma. Differentiated metastases of adenocarcinoma of the thyroid may retain I^{131} concentrating ability.

They may then be treated, after thyroidectomy, by the oral administration of large doses of I^{131} (a single dose may be as large as 200 mc.). Very dramatic results have been obtained by such therapy (Fig. 6). However, the proportion of metastases with this ability is small (approximately 10%) and the value of this method is as a demonstration of principle.

Thyrotoxicosis. The highly selective uptake of I^{131} by the thyroid gland provides a method of diagnosis and treatment of thyrotoxicosis. Radiation of the thyroid by I^{131} is mainly accomplished by the emitted β rays, which have a range of only 1 mm. in tissue. Thus the radiation is very local and even the parathyroids are not greatly damaged. Many workers (47) have treated Graves' disease by this method, which is regarded by a few as the treatment of choice. The required dose of 1–5 millicuries I^{131} is determined by the size of the gland, the severity of the condition and by the uptake of a preliminary tracer dose of the isotope. A possible disadvantage of the method is the theoretical likelihood of a delayed carcinogenic effect but this has yet to be proved, although the method is now ten years old. However, because of this risk, most clinicians restrict I^{131} treatment to carefully selected patients.

Therapy with radioactive isotopes has not fulfilled its earlier theoretical promise but the work of biochemists in this field may alter the picture. The most promising line of investigation seems to be that carried out by Pressman (48). He has been preparing tagged tissue anti-sera, such as kidney anti-serum, which, on injection is selectively concentrated in kidney tissue. The preparation of tagged tumour anti-sera is a possible development.

Future Development. In this field it is safe to prophesy only on future technical developments. The most important of these will be the preparation of large numbers of labelled compounds of high specific activity and the development of the scintillation counter. This counter has twenty times the efficiency of a Geiger counter for the detection of γ rays and will probably revolutionise *in situ* work.

It is to be hoped that the more fundamental metabolic studies with isotopes will be applied in clinical diagnosis, not as an interesting novelty, but as a unique method of clinical pathology to be used in conjunction with other biochemical procedures.

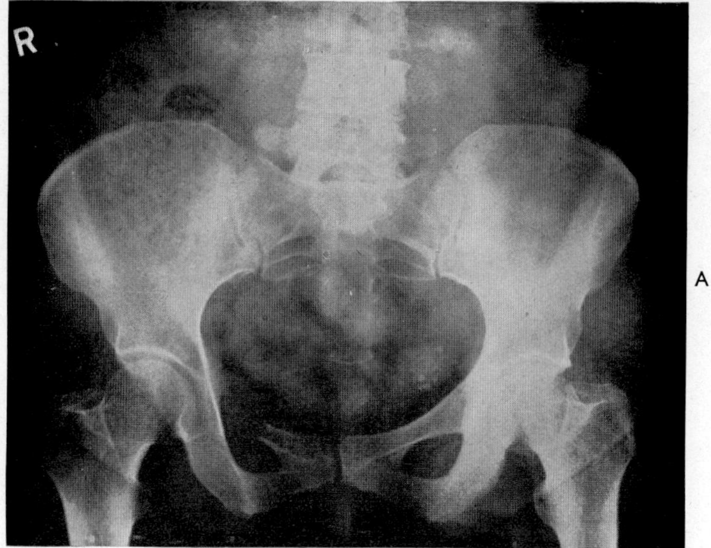

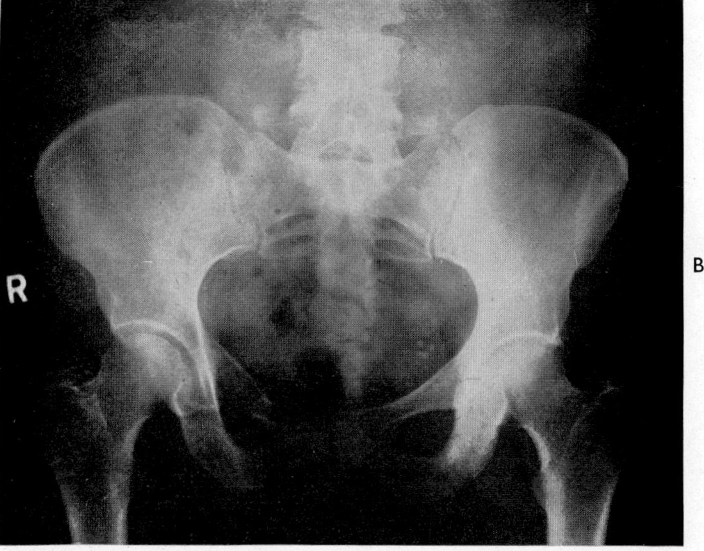

FIG. 6. X-ray films of the pelvis showing a differentiated metastasis of adenocarcinoma of the thyroid in the right os pubis. A was taken in June, 1949 before treatment and B in January, 1950 six months after beginning treatment with 100 mc. I^{131}. (Green, Tait and Worsnop, *Brit. Journ. Radiol.*, 1951, **24**, 148.)

[*To face p.* 72.

REFERENCES

GENERAL

"*Radioactive Indicators.*" George Hevesy. Interscience Publishers. 1948.

"*Isotopic Carbon.*" Calvin, Heidelberger, Reid, Talbot and Yankerwich. John Wiley and Sons. 1949.

"*Radioactive Tracers in Biology.*" Kamen. Academic Press, New York. 1947, new Edition 1951.

"*Nucleonics. Biological Synthesis of Radioisotope Labelled Compounds.*" 1950, **7**, No. 2, 26.

"*Nucleonics. Radioisotopes in Pharmaceutical and Medical Studies.*" 1950, **7**, Nos. 5 and 6; 1951, **8**, 1.

"*Advances in Biological and Medical Physics.* Lawrence and Hamilton. Vol. 1. Academic Press Inc., New York. 1948.
Also Vol. II, 1950. Vol. III to be published.

"*Symposium in the Use of Isotopes in Biology and Medicine.*" University of Wisconsin Press.

"*Clinical Use of Radioactive Isotopes.*" Low-Beer. Charles C. Thomas, Publishers, Springfield, Illinois. 1950.

TEXT

(1) Chievitz and Hevesy. *Nature*, 1935, **136**, 754.
(2) Hamilton and Soley. *Amer. Journ. Physiol.*, 1939, **127**, 557.
(3) Hertz, Roberts and Evans. *Proc. Soc. Exper. Biol. and Med.*, 1938, **38**, 510.
(4) Lawrence, Scott and Tuttle. *Internat. Clin.*, 1939, **3**, 33.
(5) Lasnitzki and Brewer. *Biochem. Journ.*, 1941, **35**, 144.
(6) Norris, Ruben and Allen. *Journ. Amer. Chem. Soc.*, 1947, **64**, 3037.
(7) Evans and Quimby. *Amer. Journ. Roentgenol.*, 1946, **55**, 55.
(8) Wilson. *Journ. Amer. Chem. Soc.*, 1938, **60**, 2697.
(9) Tuck. *Journ. Chem. Soc.*, 1939, 1292.
(10) Voge and Libby. *Journ. Amer. Chem. Soc.*, 1937, **59**, 2474.
(11) Taylor. "*Advances in Nuclear Chemistry and Theoretical Organic Chemistry.*" Interscience, New York, 1945.
(12) Hamilton. *Radiology*, 1942, **39**, 541.
(13) Pochin. *Clin. Sci.*, 1950, **9**, 405.
(14) Tabern, Taylor and Gleason. *Nucleonics*, 1950, **7**, No. 6, 46.
(15) Schoenheimer. Monograph "*Dynamic State of Body Constituents,*" pp. 63–64 rev. Rittenberg et al. 1942. Harvard Univ. Press, Cambridge, Mass.
(16) Kenney, Marinelli and Woodard. *Radiology*, 1941, **37**, 683.
(17) Low-Beer. *Science*, 1946, **104**, 339.
(18) Low-Beer, Bell, McCorkle, Stone, Steinbach and Hill. *Radiology*, 1946, **47**, 492.
(19) McCorkle, Low-Beer, Bell and Stone. *Surgery*, 1948, **24**, 409.
(20) Dudley and Mulrey. *Journ. Lab. and Clin. Med.*, 1951, **37**, 239.
(21) Moore, Kahl, Marvin, Wang and Caudill. *Radiology*, 1950, **55**, 344.
(22) Ashkenazy, Davis, Martin, LeRoy and Fields. *Journ. Lab. and Clin. Med.*, 1949, **34**, 1580.
(23) MacGregor. *Brit. Journ. Radiology*, 1950, **23**, 550.
(24) Moore. *Science*, 1946, **104**, 157.
(25) Hahn, Balfour, Ross, Bale and Whipple. *Science*, 1941, **93**, 87.

(26) Hahn and Hevesy. *Acta. Physiol. Scand.*, 1940, **1**, 3.
Hevesy and Rebbe. *Acta. Physiol. Scand.*, 1940, **1**, 171.
(27) Gray and Sterling. *Science*, 1950, **112**, 179.
(28) Krieger, Storaasli, Friedell and Holder. *Proc. Soc. Exper. Biol. and Med.*, 1948, **68**, 511.
Storaasli. *Surg. Gynecol. and Obstet.*, 1950, **91**, 458.
(29) Tait, Worsnop and Cook. *Brit. Journ. Radiology*, 1951, **24**, 14.
(30) Warner, Quimby and Schmidt. *Journ. Clin. Endocrinol.*, 1949, **9**, 342.
(31) Pochin, Myant and Goldie. *Clin. Sci.*, 1949, **8**, 109.
(32) Keating, Haines, Power and Williams. *Journ. Clin. Endocrinol.*, 1950 **10**, 1425.
(33) Clark, Moe and Adams. *Surgery*, 1949, **26**, 331.
(34) McConahey, Keating and Power. *Journ. Clin. Invest.*, 1949, **28**, 191.
(35) Freedberg, Hertz and Vreks. *Proc. Soc. Exper. Biol. and Med.*, 1949, **70**, 679.
(36) Perlmuter, Martin and Riggs. *Journ. Clin. Endocrinol.*, 1949, **9**, 430.
(37) Stanbury and Hedge. *Journ. Clin. Endocrinol.*, 1950, **10**, 1471.
(38) Quimby. *Amer. Journ. Roentgenol.*, 1947, **58**, 741.
(39) Smith and Quimby. *Surg. Gynaec. and Obst.*, 1949, **79**, 142.
(40) Prinzmetal, Corday, Spritzler and Flieg. *Journ. Amer. Med. Assocn.* 1949, **139**, 617.
(41) Veall. *Brit. Journ. Radiol.*, 1950, **23**, 527.
(42) Kety. *Amer. Heart Journ.*, 1949, **38**, 321.
Cooper. *Southern Med. Journ.*, 1949, **42**, 870.
(43) Layton and Frankel. *Cancer*, 1949, **2**, 1089.
(44) Kinsel, Margen, Tarver, Frantz, Flanagan, Hutchin and McCallie. *Journ. Clin Invest.*, 1950, **29**, 238.
(45) Low-Beer. " *Clinical Use of Radioactive Isotopes.*" p. 295.
(46) Brues and Jacobson. *Amer. Journ. Roentgenol.*, 1947, **58**, 774.
(47) Soley and Miler. *Med. Clin. North America*, 1948. *Amer. Journ. Roentgenol.*, 1948, **60**, 45. *Journ. Clin. Endocrinol.*, 1949, **9**, 29.
Werner, Quimby and Schmidt. *Radiology*, 1948, **51**, 564.
Trunnell. *New York Acad. Sci.*, 1949, **2**, 195.
Prinzmetal. *California Med.*, 1949, **70**, 236.
Blomfield. *Brit. Journ. Radiology*, 1950, **23**, 566.
(48) Pressman. *Trans. New York Acad. Sci.*, 1949, **11**, 203. *Journ. Amer, Chem. Soc.*, 1950, **72**, 2226. *Journ Immunol.*, 1949, **63**, 375.

CHAPTER V

THE VITAMINS

THE actual date of discovery of the vitamins is difficult to place, since early travellers, even as far back as the Middle Ages, were aware that scurvy and similar diseases could be prevented only by feeding with fresh food, and more particularly fresh fruit. The matter received its first scientific establishment through the work of Sir Frederick Gowland Hopkins and Casimir Funk, who proved experimentally that animals could not exist on a diet composed of pure protein, fat, and carbohydrate. Hopkins showed that animals fed on such a diet not only failed to grow, but rapidly lost weight, and that this state of affairs could be immediately rectified by the addition of small quantities of milk to the diet, the quantity added being so small as to make no appreciable difference to the calorie intake. Since that time a great deal of work has been done on these accessory food factors, as Hopkins originally called them, and they have now been separated into a number of groups; in all, there are to-day some thirty-one vitamins and provitamins which have either been definitely isolated or their presence proved by pharmacological experimentation. It is proposed now to describe those which are concerned with human nutrition :—

Vitamin A. This vitamin is present in fats and is soluble in fat solvents. It was discovered simultaneously in 1912 by McCollum and Osborn and Mendel. These observers showed that the liver of certain fishes such as the cod, and animal fats such as butter, contained a substance necessary for the growth of young animals. If animals are fed on a diet lacking this vitamin they suffer from a series of degenerative conditions, such as xerophthalmia, and succumb to intercurrent infections. Mellanby has maintained that this vitamin is responsible for raising the general level of resistance against infection, and so it has been termed by him the anti-infective vitamin. It has been shown that a certain chemical test gives a rough indication of the amount of the vitamin which is present in a fat or oil. This test consists in treating the oil with a solution of antimony trichloride or arsenic trichloride, when a blue colour will develop. The amount of vitamin may be judged by the intensity of the blue colour. A quantitative estimation may be performed by estimating the colour by means of a Lovibond tintometer. The result is expressed as an arbitrary unit, which is known as the Lovibond unit if a 20 % dilution of the oil in chloroform is used. The vitamin may also be estimated by a feeding test in which young rats are given a diet containing the optimum of protein, fat, carbohydrate and mineral salts and the other vitamins. The test is run on a series of animals, and as soon as they are losing weight steadily or are ceasing to grow, the unknown preparation is administered in varying quantities and the effect noted. The relationship between the chemical test and the physiological test is difficult to express, since it is highly probable that the efficacy of the vitamin in feeding tests is dependent upon a number of other factors which are at present uncontrolled.

As the administration of carotene to animals fed on a diet deficient in vitamin A confers all the benefits they would have received had the vitamin been present, it is now generally accepted that carotene is the main precursor of vitamin A, being converted in the body into vitamin A, and the international unit of vitamin A is taken as 0·6 γ of β carotene. From the chemical point of view the relationship is interesting, since carotene is a highly unsaturated hydrocarbon with the formula :—

β-Carotene (Karrer).

```
CH3  CH3
  \  /
   C                  CH3                    CH3
  / \                  |                      |
CH2  C - CH = CH - C = CH - CH = CH - C = CH - CH =
 |   ||
CH2  C - CH3                                                       CH3  CH3
  \  /                                                               \  /
   CH2                  CH3                 CH3                        C
                         |                   |                        / \
          CH - CH = C - CH = CH - CH = C - CH = CH - C  CH2
                                                           ||  |
                                                   CH3 - C  CH2
                                                            \  /
                                                             CH2
```

whilst vitamin A has the following formula :—

```
CH3  CH3
  \  /
   C                  CH3                    CH3
  / \                  |                      |
CH2  C - CH = CH - C = CH - CH = CH - C = CH - CH2OH
 |   ||
CH2  C - CH3
  \  /
   CH2
```

The vitamin has been synthesised and has a potency of 3 to 3·3 million international units per g. Vitamin A_2, which occurs in freshwater fish, differs only slightly from vitamin A in constitution.

Clinical Applications. Coward and Morgan (1) give the vitamin A content of foods in international units per g. or ml. as follows: Butter, average 60, egg yolk 30, carrots 19, cabbage 9, runner beans 6, milk 3 to 5. In 1937 a technical commission of the League of Nations decided that an adult requires about 3,000 international units of vitamin A daily. Children require about 4,000 international units and pregnant and nursing mothers 6,000 to 8,000 international units daily. A pint of milk, 1 egg, 1 oz. of butter and a helping of green vegetables will supply about 2,000 international units of vitamin A, and 1,000 international units of carotene. In war time the average adult only received about 500 to 800 international units of preformed vitamin A daily. Carotene is less well absorbed from the alimentary tract in man than is vitamin A; probably only 25% of carotene is absorbed. Carrots, spinach and broccoli tops are good sources of carotene, and with the war-time allowance of milk and vitaminised margarine (which has only about half the vitamin A content of butter), ½ lb. of carrots should be eaten weekly. They are best eaten cooked, as they are more easily digested and the carotene is not destroyed by cooking. It would appear that the diet of ordinary middle or lower class workers was deficient in vitamin A, and to this fact has been attributed the frequency of common ailments such as colds, bronchitis and septic complications, etc. The work of Mellanby has also indicated that lack of vitamin A may play a big part in the ætiology of puerperal sepsis. A severe degree of deficiency of vitamin A in the diet leads to xerophthalmia, which was prevalent in Denmark in 1917, and is a common cause of blindness in India and China to-day. Further, striking evidence of relative hypovitaminosis A in apparently normal subjects is found by a study of the adaptation of the retina to light. It is now known that vitamin A is concerned in the regeneration of visual purple, the photo-sensitive substance of the retina which is responsible for rod vision. Investigations have shown that a large number of apparently healthy persons are affected with night-blindness in varying degrees, which may be tested by a special photometer. Thus Jeghers (2) testing 162 medical students at Boston found 55 deficient in vitamin A, as shown by this test. Harris and

Abassy (3) reported similar results in school children attending elementary schools in London and Cambridge; 40 to 50% were normal, 20 to 30% slightly below normal, and 20 to 30% definitely deficient. A correlation was found between the diet and the dark-adaptation tests. "Among children having ⅔ pint of milk at school 67% were normal on test, whereas of those having ⅓ pint or less, only 37% were normal." Under war conditions in England, Yudkin (4) "found low adaptation in 9% of children at an urban institution, 15% among urban children from poor homes and 18% among some village children." It has been shown that the sensitivity to dim light may be greatly increased in these individuals by the administration of vitamin A. Yudkin (4) has shown that large doses are necessary to effect prolonged improvement, as much as 100,000 international units daily. A total dosage of 300,000 to 2,000,000 international units may be required, and the beneficial effect may last for weeks or months. It is usually given by the mouth in the form of one or other of the fish oils. At present the most concentrated form of natural oil is obtained from halibut liver. This may be administered either in the form of drops or in capsules. An alternative method of administration is to give the various concentrates, but it is stated by competent authorities that these are not so stable as the halibut liver oil. The preparation, Liq. vit. A. Conc. (B.P. Add.), contains 2,500 international units in 1 minim. Cod liver oil contains on an average 2,000 international units per g., and halibut liver oil 160,000 units per g. Thus a teaspoonful of cod liver oil contains 6,400 units, and a drop of halibut liver oil 3,200 units. When administered subcutaneously the preparation is said to be not so active as when given orally. Although clinically the risk of hypervitaminosis A seems remote, Moore and Wang (5) have produced an experimental condition in rats which they attribute to massive oral doses of vitamin A. The symptoms, which include tenderness of the limbs and bone fractures, are absent if the vitamin is oxidised prior to administration. Post-mortem examination confirmed the presence of subcutaneous and intra-muscular hæmorrhage, whilst X-ray photographs showed that the majority of the fractures occurred at the centre region of the long bones. Although the symptoms in many ways resembled those of scurvy, they did not respond to treatment with l-ascorbic acid or calciferol.

The Vitamin B Complex. Vitamin B was originally regarded as a single substance which was necessary for the maintenance of normal health in animals. It is now known to be a very complex mixture, the following constituents of which have been isolated and synthesised: aneurin, riboflavin, nicotinic acid, pyridoxin, biotin, folic acid, *p*-amino-benzoic acid and pantothenic acid. The last two compounds have not yet been proved to play an essential part in human nutrition.

Vitamin B_1. The absence of the B_1 factor is responsible for the peripheral neuritis of beri-beri, which is often accompanied by heart failure and gastro-intestinal disturbances. The first observations on this interesting substance were made by Eijkman in 1897. He showed, whilst working in a prison in Java, that fowls suffered from a type of polyneuritis similar to beri-beri, which at that time affected the prisoners with considerable severity. The fowls were fed on polished rice of the same variety as was given to the prisoners, and Eijkman showed that when the fowls were fed on unpolished rice the symptoms disappeared. A large scale experiment was carried out on the prisoners, and feeding a carefully controlled group on unpolished rice proved that the disease could be stamped out.

Vitamin B_1 is soluble in water. In 1932 Windaus (6) determined its composition to be $C_{12}H_{17}N_4OS$, and Windaus (7) and Williams (8), working independently, finally established the structure. The formula given below is that of aneurin, thiamine or vitamin B_1 chloride hydrochloride :—

```
                                         CH3
       N—C—NH2.HCl                        |
       |   |                             C===C—CH2CH2OH
 CH3—C   C—CH2————————N<          |
       ||  ||                       |   \CH—S
       N—CH                        Cl
```

The naturally occurring vitamin is identical with the synthetic substance, both chemically and physiologically. The international unit of vitamin B_1 is defined as the anti-neuritic potency possessed by 3 γ of vitamin B_1 hydrochloride.

The assay of vitamin B_1 has been the subject of a number of publications which are summarised by Williams and Spies (9). The two main methods are the rat bradycardia test and a chemical test, known as the thiochrome method, whereby the vitamin may be estimated by measuring the intensity of fluorescence of one of its derivatives.

Considerable insight into the physiological function of aneurin has resulted from the discovery by Peters (10) that the oxygen uptake of brain tissue from avitaminose pigeons on a substrate of lactic acid or pyruvic acid is subnormal. When aneurin or aneurin pyrophosphate is added the respiration returns to normal and lactic and pyruvic acids disappear. The suggestion of Lohman and Schuster (11) that aneurin pyrophosphate is identical with co-carboxylase, the co-enzyme responsible for the metabolism of pyruvic acid, is now generally accepted.

Clinical Applications. The Scientific Adviser's Division, Ministry of Food (12) found that of 322 samples of National Wheatmeal Flour 81% of the samples contained more than 1·0 international unit per gram.

Harris and Wang (13) give the vitamin B_1 content of certain foods as follows, expressed in international units per gram: yeast extract 4·6 to 8·0, bacon 4, wheat germ 9·5, whole meal 0·87 to 1·7, oats 1·8, egg yolk 0·5, fresh milk 0·10 to 0·15. An adult requires about 700 international units daily, and 3 mg. of synthetic vitamin B_1 hydrochloride are equivalent to 1,000 international units. National Wheatmeal bread, made from 85% extraction flour, should supply sufficient vitamin B_1, and also nicotinamide.

For purposes of treatment vitamin B_1 can be administered by mouth in the form of Benerva tablets (3 mg.) t.i.d. or by intramuscular or intravenous injections of 5 to 25 mg. daily for 12 doses.

Children, pregnant and nursing women require a specially high vitamin B_1 intake, as do patients suffering from diabetes mellitus, increased thyroid activity and febrile diseases, and individuals undergoing prolonged muscular activity.

Alcoholic peripheral neuritis and other cases of neuritis of unknown origin may be due to deficient intake or absorption of the vitamin, and treatment in such cases with vitamin B_1 is worthy of trial.

Severe vitamin B_1 deficiency leading to beri-beri is rare in this country, but various complex and ill-defined conditions can be traced to partial deficiency. Early symptoms have been summarised by Williams and Spies (9) as follows: "Loss of appetite, weight, and strength; muscle cramps; diarrhœa, abdominal pain;

palpitation; dyspnœa; œdema; burning sensations in various parts of the body; vertigo; headache; cessation of menstruation; numbness and tingling; nervousness; depression; irritability; distractibility; apprehension and forgetfulness." We have found that in some cases in adults anorexia and flatulent dyspepsia have been improved by the administration of vitamin B_1. Sub-clinical deficiency in infants and children may be evidenced by constipation and a subnormal weight.

Heart failure, associated with chronic alcoholic poisoning, is in some cases due to vitamin B_1 deficiency. In these cases œdema may precede the onset of dyspnœa, and the face may be swollen as well as the legs. The vitamin deficiency may be demonstrated chemically by examination of the blood or the urine. The usual treatment for heart failure is not successful unless supplemented by injections of vitamin B_1. Attention was drawn to the condition by Aalsmeer and Wenckebach (14), and subsequently by Jones and Bramwell (15), by Bowe (16), and by Stannus (17).

Williams, Shapiro and Bartelot (18), Forsyth (19) and Gretton-Watson (20) have reported on the treatment of acrodynia, or pink disease, by the administration of vitamin B_1. Very little is known of the causes of this condition, and the course varies widely, but it is well known that spontaneous and sudden recovery frequently occurs. Acrodynia in rats is associated with vitamin B_6 deficiency.

Wernicke (21) in 1881 described a syndrome characterised by oculomotor palsies, mental changes and ataxia, resulting from acute hæmorrhagic polioencephalitis superior. Small degenerative foci and varicosities are present in the periventricular grey matter. It is associated with chronic gastro-intestinal disorders, many cases being due to chronic alcoholic poisoning. It has subsequently been shown by Wortis et al. (22) that there is a disturbance of pyruvic acid metabolism, and in many cases improvement rapidly follows the administration of vitamin B_1, although it is not thought to represent a simple aneurin deficiency. A similar disease, known as chastek paralysis, can be produced in silver foxes by feeding them largely on raw fish. This can be prevented by adding aneurin to the diet, and it is possible that an anti-vitamin is present in raw fish, which inactivates aneurin.

Vitamin B_2 (Riboflavin). This is no longer regarded as the anti-pellagra vitamin, though its deficiency is considered to be responsible for some of the symptoms often associated with pellagra. Its constitution has been revealed through the work on the flavins. It has been known for many years that all plant and animal tissues contain a water-soluble yellow pigment known as riboflavin (lactoflavin) which exhibits blue fluorescence. This substance has been crystallised by many workers from various sources such as whey, egg-albumen, egg-yolk, liver, urine, etc.

Györgyi, Kuhn and Wagner-Jauregg (23) suggested in 1933 that vitamin B_2, an essential growth-factor for rats, was a flavin. They were able to show that for finely crystalline lactoflavin a dose of 7 to 10 γ constituted a rat unit. The Heidelberg group of workers proved that the synthetic riboflavin is both biologically and chemically identical with the naturally occurring vitamin B_2. The formula of riboflavin is shown here. In rats the absence of vitamin B_2 from the diet causes cataract, stunting of growth, loss of hair and general lowering of condition.

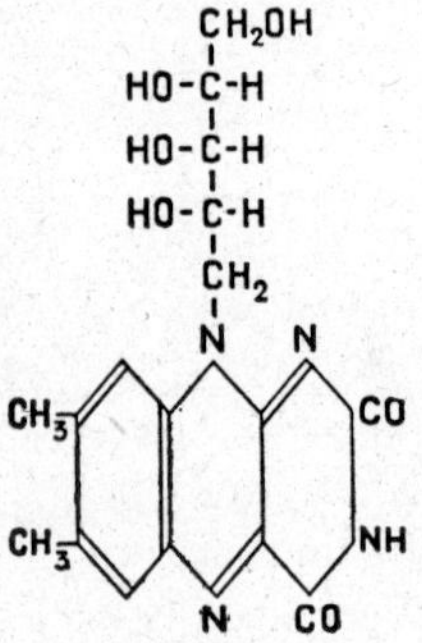

Riboflavin

The physiological function of riboflavin, like that of aneurin, is enzymic in character and is intimately associated with cell respiration. As a phosphoric acid ester, in association with a protein carrier, riboflavin has been identified with Warburg's "Yellow enzyme". The connection between this important respiratory function and the symptoms of ariboflavinosis are not yet understood.

Clinical Applications. The chief source of vitamin B_2 is plant tissue, particularly young green leaves, but milk is a stable and dependable source containing 1 to 2 γ per ml. National flour contains 1·3 to 1·9 γ per g. and dried yeast 0·1 to 0·2 mg. per g.

Stannus (24) first described the chief clinical features of riboflavin deficiency twenty years before the discovery of riboflavin. Sebrell, Butler, Wooley and Isbell (25) found, by study of the riboflavin balance in ten women, that the requirement of this vitamin is approximately 3 mg. per day. Lack of this vitamin in man produces a condition described by Sebrell and Butler (26) as ariboflavinosis. Eighteen women were given a diet with a low riboflavin content, and thirteen developed ariboflavinosis.

The lips become red along the line of closure, and the mucous membrane is thin, shiny and denuded. This is known as cheilosis. Maceration and fissuring occur at the angles of the mouth, resembling the lesions known as perlèche, so-called from the verb *lécher*, as the patient licks the sore with the tip of the tongue. Seborrhœic accumulations are also noted at the naso-labial folds, on the alæ nasi, in the vestibule of the nose, and occasionally on the ears and eyelids. These lesions disappeared with the administration of 0·025 mg. riboflavin per kg. of body weight, and reappeared on discontinuing the vitamin. The tongue may also be affected, being purplish-red or magenta in colour, clean, with flattened or mushroom-shaped papillæ, and a burning sensation may be complained of. Further, Kruse and his co-workers (27) have found that vitamin B_2 deficiency leads to keratitis and that the condition can be cured both in animals and in human subjects by the administration of the vitamin. Johnson and Eckardt (28) treated thirty-six patients suffering from rosacea keratitis with the vitamin, giving 3 mg. daily, and found that it will correct the condition when it arises from vitamin B_2 deficiency in the diet, but not when it arises in patients whose diet is not deficient but who show hypochlorhydria. Engorged limbic vessels are not a definite indication of ariboflavinosis. In order to diagnose the condition on ocular signs, new capillaries should be seen by slit-lamp microscopy, arising from the apices of the limbal loops and spreading on to the cornea, around the whole circumference and in each eye. Mann (29) has described a further corneal manifestation of ariboflavinosis, with marginal vascularities and opacities in the substantia propria. These changes disappear when riboflavin is administered. Jones et al. (30) described an outbreak of stomatitis due to riboflavin deficiency in a camp in North Africa when the daily riboflavin intake was reduced from 1·61 mg. to 1 mg. per head. It was quickly cured by giving 100 mg. riboflavin in five days, or by ½ oz. of fresh yeast daily. Partial syndromes of ariboflavinosis, without eye signs or tongue changes, have also been described by Duckworth (31), and in one case under our observation a patient complained of a sore hard palate ; the mucous membrane over the affected part was pale, and the symptoms were promptly relieved by the administration of 3 to 5 mg. of riboflavin daily, nicotinic acid and other remedies having failed. Relapse occurred when the treatment was omitted. Scarborough (32), describing some cases of circumcorneal injection as a sign of riboflavin deficiency, comments on this tendency to relapse in certain patients in whom an abnormally large amount of riboflavin appears to be required. Manson-Bahr (33) has suggested that vitamin B_2 deficiency (riboflavin and nicotinic acid) may be responsible for the glossitis found in pellagra, sprue, pernicious anæmia, the nutritional anæmias and idiopathic steatorrhœa. Stannus (34) suggests that the first tissue to feel the evil effect of riboflavin deficiency is the capillary endothelium.

Nicotinic Acid (Niacin). This is also known as the pellagra-preventing (P-P) factor. Pellagra is a deficiency disease prevalent in districts where maize is one of the staple foodstuffs, such as the southern states of the U.S.A., Rumania, Italy, Egypt and Southern Russia. Its symptoms are severe gastro-intestinal disturbances and wasting, associated with characteristic dermatitis; in addition many subjects develop chronic dementia.

Experiments on dogs and rats, and later on human subjects, have shown that pellagra is essentially a deficiency disease which can be cured by the administration of nicotinic acid or its amide. Their formulæ are given below :—

CO.OH — N — Nicotinic Acid

$CO.NH_2$ — N — Nicotinamide

Nicotinic acid, like several other members of the vitamin B complex, is known as a widespread and important constituent of carbohydrogenase systems. Coenzyme I (adenosine-ribose diphosphoric-ribose nicotinic amide) plays the part of hydrogen carrier to enzyme systems which oxidise such substrates as alcohol, lactic acid and malic acid, whilst Coenzyme II (adenosine-ribose triphosphoric-ribose nicotinic amide) plays a similar rôle in the dehydrogenation of glucose, hexose monophosphate and glutamic acid. The reduced coenzymes are subsequently reoxidised by transferring their acquired hydrogen to Warburg's "yellow enzyme". This important function has not yet been related to the clinical symptoms which characterise pellagra.

Clinical Applications. The distribution of nicotinic acid in foodstuffs has been determined by chemical and microbiological methods. Liver, kidney, pork flesh and yeast are good sources, whereas milk contains only small amounts. The daily requirement is 15 to 40 mg. From 30 to 50% of the ingested nicotinic acid is normally excreted in the urine as derivatives of nicotinic acid or as trigonelline. The blood level and urinary excretion of nicotinic acid in pellagrins does not differ markedly from the normal, using chemical methods of assay. It has been shown by Kark and Meiklejohn (35) that, contrary to the general view, porphyrins are not necessarily present in the highly pigmented urine of pellagrins. The blue fluorescence of the urine in these cases is attributed to the presence of a substance F_1 of unknown chemical composition. A second bluish fluorescent substance F_2, which is possibly thiochrome, is a normal constituent of urine and is diminished in quantity in the urine of pellagrins. Najjar and co-workers (36) found that the administration of nicotinic acid to pellagrins decreased the output of F_1, while raising the quantity of F_2. The minimum effective dosage is still not yet worked out either for the cure or prevention of pellagra, but Spies, Cooper and Blankenhorn (37) recommend 0·5 g. daily, given in five doses of 100 mg., as safe and effective in the usual case of pellagra. For parenteral injection they found that 50 to 80 mg. a day, in sterile physiologic solution of sodium chloride, were effective when injected intravenously. Sebrell (38) has emphasised that the best method of prevention is to bring about a permanent change in diet by adding as much green vegetables, milk and lean meat as possible. Since it seems likely that vitamin B_1 plays some part in the development of the pellagra syndrome, the diet must provide for an adequate intake of this factor also.

King (39) suggests that Vincent's disease in man, in which there is ulceration of the mouth accompanied by the presence of fusiform bacilli and spirochætes, may be a pre-pellagrous condition. He records good results from the administration of nicotinic acid, 250 mg. by mouth in water, given daily for ten days. In glossitis and stomatitis due to nicotinic acid deficiency the tip and sides of the tongue are fiery red and swollen, and ulcers form on the tongue and buccal mucous membrane. Vincent's organisms may be found in the greyish exudate. On account of its vasodilator action intravenous injections of nicotinic acid (5 to 10 mg.) have been given in cases of cerebral thrombosis by Furtado (40), and in angina pectoris by Neuwahl (41), and in Ménière's syndrome by Atkinson (42), with promising results. Nicotinic acid may also be given by mouth in doses of 25 to 150 mg. daily, according to the flushing effect produced, in cases of intermittent claudication. In some cases the walking capacity of the patient is considerably improved. Gottlieb (43) described 5 cases of acute nicotinic acid deficiency, characterised by mental confusion or excitement, which were relieved by the administration of nicotinic acid in doses of 400 to 600 mg.

Vitamin B_6 (Pyridoxin). In 1934 Gyorgy (44), investigating the condition of acrodynia in rats, showed that, although the symptoms were associated with a dietary factor, none of the known members of the vitamin B complex afforded relief. In 1938 five independent groups of workers succeeded in crystallising the essential factor, for which the name "pyridoxin" was finally adopted. In the same year degradation and synthesis (45, 46) showed that pyridoxin was a pyridine derivative with the constitution shown:

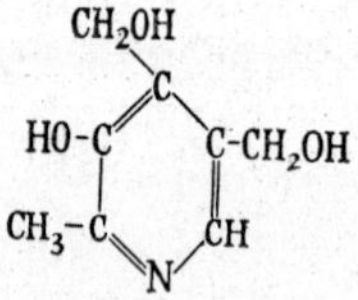

```
          CH2OH
           \
            C
          //  \
     HO-C      C-CH2OH
        |      ||
    CH3-C      CH
         \\   /
            N
```

Pyridoxin appears to be widespread in the animal and vegetable kingdoms. Good sources are to be found in yeast, rice polishings and wheat germ, and although found in many other foodstuffs it is frequently associated with protein or starch, and, as such, is only assimilated after hydrolysis by cooking.

Whilst rats on being deprived of pyridoxin show loss of weight, œdema and dermatitis of the extremities, the corresponding condition in dogs and pigs is associated amongst other things with a disturbance of erythropoiesis. Independent workers (Chick et al. (47), Wintrobe et al. (48) and Borson and Mettier (49)) working variously on pigs and dogs, agree that the condition is one of hypochromic microcytic anæmia. The condition, although having elements of similarity with pernicious anæmia, does not respond to iron or liver extract therapy. On the contrary, as the symptoms intensify, there is a rise in serum iron which runs parallel to the anæmia. There is marked hypoplasia of the bone marrow and hæmosiderosis of the liver and spleen. Neurological disturbances of an epileptiform character also occur. At least in experimental animals, all these symptoms are relieved by the administration of pyridoxin. There is little doubt that much of the experimental work in the past has been complicated by the failure to recognise the part played by nicotinic acid and folic acid in related conditions.

Our clinical knowledge of pyridoxin is far from complete. The synthetic compound has been used in substantial quantities in the treatment of anæmias (Vilter, Schiro and Spies (50)), muscular atrophy and dystrophy (McBryde and Baker (51)), and Parkinsonism (Spies, Hightower and Hubbard (52)). The reports are conflicting and no well-defined clinical condition has yet been clearly associated with deficiency. The new information regarding the function of folic acid in macrocytic anæmia may help to resolve this problem.

Biotin. In 1927 Boas (53), showed that rats maintained on a raw egg-white diet developed symptoms of an eczema-like dermatitis which was associated with a loss of hair. Factors which protect rats from "egg-white injury" were isolated independently by Kogl and Tonnis (54) from egg-yolk, α-biotin, and by Du Vigneaud et al. (55) from liver concentrate, β-biotin, formerly known as vitamin H. Despite former assurances that these two compounds were identical, it now seems likely that they are indeed distinct (56). The factor responsible for the symptoms of biotin deficiency has been isolated by Eakin, Snell and Williams and named Avidin (57). Avidin, which has been crystallised (58), is a protein-carbohydrate complex of molecular weight about 70,000. It forms a complex with biotin which renders the latter inactive.

The constitution of β-biotin has been elucidated and confirmed by the synthesis by Du Vigneaud and colleagues (59, 60) as:

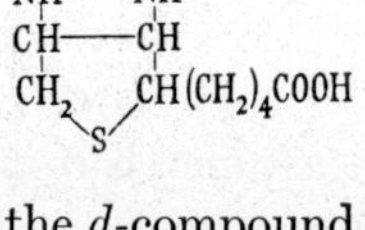

```
      CO
     /  \
   NH    NH
   |     |
   CH----CH
   |     |
   CH2   CH(CH2)4COOH
     \  /
      S
```

The natural vitamin is the *d*-compound and as the racemic form, tested on rats, has only half of the activity of the naturally occurring material, it is questionable whether the *l*-form has any activity (Emmerson (61), Ott (62)). According to Kogl et al. (63), the constitution of α-biotin differs significantly from that put forward by the American school, but as the compound has not yet been synthesised, no clinical significance is yet attached to it.

Biotin is found in close association with other members of the vitamin B complex, the chief sources being yeast, liver, eggs, peas and cereals. According to Sydenstricker et al. (64), the daily requirement of adult humans is about 150 μg.

The symptoms of biotin deficiency are not limited to rats. As an essential growth factor for many bacteria and moulds (Bios IIB), biotin has been known for over two decades, yet the recognition of its clinical importance is of very recent development. Experimental deficiency in monkeys may be induced by limiting the biotin intake, by adding raw egg-white to the diet, or by suppressing the synthesis of biotin by the intestinal flora by the administration of sulphonamides (Waisman et al. (65)). The syndrome in monkeys is characterised by a thinning of the fur, a loss of hair colour and by a conspicuous dermatitis of the face, legs and arms, all of which symptoms are relieved by the administration of 20 μg. of synthetic biotin daily. Symptoms of biotin deficiency in man described by Sydenstricker (64) include a scaly dermatitis, a greyish pallor of the skin, atrophy of the lingual papillæ and disturbed erythropoiesis. A very remarkable case of clinical biotin deficiency has been quoted by Williams (66).

Folic Acid. The subdivision of the vitamin B complex is apparently so endless that it is a pleasant task to be able to report some simplification. With the purification of the various reported essential factors, it becomes increasingly probable that three factors hitherto treated as separate entities are, in fact, identical. These are (*a*) folic acid, the acid factor isolated by Williams et al. (67) from spinach, and found by him to be a growth-stimulant of the organism streptococcus lactis, (*b*) the " norit eluate factor " reported by Snell and Peterson (68) in yeast and liver, and found to be an essential factor for the growth of lactobacillus helveticus, and (*c*) vitamin B_C, a dietary factor described by Hogan and Parrott (69), the absence of which is responsible for the symptoms of macrocytic hypochromic anæmia in chicks. The earlier claim of Mitchell and Williams (70) that folic acid bore a close resemblance to xanthopterin, a pigment found in butterfly wings, seems to be inconsistent with the inability of this compound to relieve the characteristic symptoms of vitamin B_C deficiency in chicks. Notwithstanding this fact, the close similarity in physical and chemical properties, together with the stimulatory effect upon lactic acid organisms, held in common by these three factors, support the claim to identity (Pfiffner et al. (71)). Some clarification of this problem may be anticipated following the recent characterisation of the liver factor. Angier et al. (72) have shown by degradation and synthesis that this factor possesses the following structure :

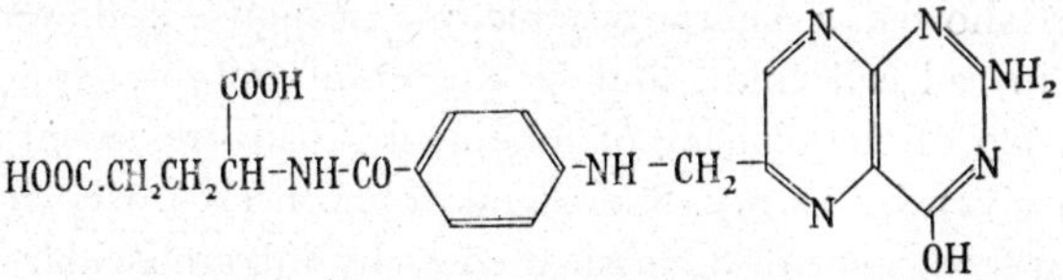

COOH
HOOC.CH$_2$CH$_2$CH–NH–CO–⟨benzene ring⟩–NH–CH$_2$–⟨pteridine ring: N, N, NH$_2$, N, N, OH⟩

N-[4-{[(2-amino-4-hydroxy-6-pteridyl) methyl]amino}benzoyl]glutamic acid.

The presence of glutamic acid and *p*-aminobenzoic acid residues in the molecule is interesting. Hitherto the pteridyl ring has not been encountered as such in the biological field.

The synthetic compound stimulates the growth of L. Helveticus (casei) and is active against anæmia in chicks. An analogous synthetic compound prepared by omitting the glutamic acid residue fails to do either, but stimulates the growth of Streptococcus fæcalis R. Angier and co-workers also describe a second factor isolated from a fermentation mixture which, as it can be readily converted into the above compound, must be closely related to it.

Folic acid, as its name implies, is found in green leaves. Concentrates of the vitamin are usually obtained from spinach tops, yeast, or, if an animal source is preferred, from liver extracts. As this factor is almost certainly synthesised by the intestinal flora, it is difficult to estimate the daily requirements. Established deficiency in adults has been cured by the administration of 5 mg. per day for ten days.

Rats maintained on a diet supplemented with aneurin, riboflavin, pantothenic acid, pyridoxin, nicotinic acid, choline and biotin, but containing 1% sulphaguanidine, developed symptoms of agranulocytosis and leucopenia which responded promptly to the administration of crystalline folic acid (Daft and Sebrell (73)).

Within four days, the white cell counts rose from 2,700 to 14,400 per cubic millimetre, with a simultaneous increase in the percentage of granulocytes from 1 to 40.

That folic acid not only stimulates the production of white cells but also exerts a profound effect upon erythropoiesis is apparent from the clinical reports of Spies (74, 75) on the treatment of nutritional macrocytic anæmia. Out of 42 cases of macrocytic anæmia treated, 26 responded immediately to treatment with 20 mg. of synthetic crystalline folic acid administered either parenterally or orally. The cases, which included five of Addisonian pernicious anæmia as well as macrocytic anæmia of pregnancy and of sprue, showed a sharp reticulocyte response followed by an increase in red cell count and hæmoglobin content. Independent confirmation of the efficacy of folic acid in the treatment of sprue has been given by Darby, Jones and Johnson (76), who report the successful treatment of 3 classical cases by intramuscular injection of 15 mg. of folic acid.

The use of folic acid or of synthetic pteroylglutamic acid in the treatment of pernicious anæmia is now universally condemned. It is true that the initial response is good. Thus Wilkinson (77) showed there is a prompt reticulocytosis, with a rapid rise in the red cell count, hæmoglobin percentage, and, in some cases, the white cell and platelet counts. Later, increasing amounts of folic acid are necessary to prevent relapse in some cases, and finally there may be no response at all. Most serious of all is the fact that neurological changes are not relieved by folic acid, and in some cases which were originally free from nervous lesions, subacute degeneration of the cord may rapidly appear, despite a good hæmatological response. It seems even that folic acid may precipitate spinal cord degeneration.

Wilkinson and Israëls (78) treated 13 patients suffering from pernicious anæmia with synthetic folic acid conjugates, pteroyl-γ-triglutamic acid (teropterin) and pteroyl-α-diglutamic acid (diopterin). The hæmatological response was satisfactory, indicating that the sufferers from pernicious anæmia can hydrolyse and utilise these folic acid conjugates, if given in adequate doses.

Para-aminobenzoic Acid. This substance was first recognised as a vitamin by Ansbacher (79). He fed black and piebald rats on a diet which produced greying of the fur, a condition known as achromotrichia. When this diet was supplemented daily by 3 mg. of *p*-aminobenzoic acid, the animals grew normally pigmented fur within a month. Ansbacher (79) also showed that the vitamin improved the condition of chicks reared on a heated vitamin K-deficient diet, while Sure (80) found that *p*-aminobenzoic acid was an essential dietary factor for lactation and reproduction in the rat. It is evident that the above results require further confirmation, since some workers have failed to substantiate the claims of Ansbacher. The formula of *p*-aminobenzoic acid, which is one of the B-complex vitamins, is as follows :

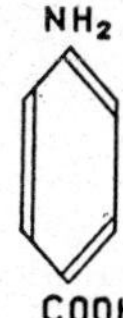

The substance has aroused considerable interest in recent years because of its inhibitory effect on the activity of sulphanilamide. This inhibition, which was demonstrated by Woods and Fildes (81) *in vitro* and by Selbie (82) in mice infected with streptococcus hæmolyticus, led Fildes (83) to conclude that *p*-aminobenzoic acid is an essential metabolite for bacteria. The vitamin appears to be widespread in plants and animals and has been isolated from yeast, which has been found to contain 0·5 mg. per 100 g. Little is known of the effect of a deficiency of the vitamin in human subjects or of the normal daily requirement. Sieve (84), however, claimed that *p*-aminobenzoic acid caused darkening of the hair in 30 cases of human achromotrichia.

Microbiological Assay of Members of the Vitamin B Complex. In no single sphere of biochemistry have the methods of microbiological assay been more successful than in the estimation of vitamin B factors. As with more complex animals, selected strains of bacteria are apparently very discriminating in regard to the composition of the medium upon which they grow. Although organisms will fail to grow on a medium lacking in one essential factor, yet, over a limited range of concentration, they respond in an almost linear manner to addition of micro-quantities of the missing factor. It is upon this principle that the method of microbiological assay rests. Factors essential to bacteria include most members of the vitamin B complex and an impressive list of amino acids, including all of those essential to man. By using pure solutions to produce standard graphs of growth against added factor, it has been possible to estimate, with a greater degree of accuracy than is possible by chemical methods, the concentration of these factors in foodstuffs.

The method will doubtless lend itself to the assay of these factors in biological materials. In most assays it has been possible to circumvent the technical difficulty of measuring the growth of bacterial cultures by using lactic acid producing organisms, and the linear relation between lactic acid production and the concentration of the missing factor has been demonstrated in many cases.

Phycomyces Blakesleanus has been used for a number of years in the determination of aneurin (Schopfer and Jung (85)). Less well known, but not less accurate, is the use of Lactobacillus Helveticus (L. casei ϵ) for the estimation of riboflavin (Snell and Strong (86)), pyridoxin (Carpenter and Strong (87)), biotin (Snell, Hutchings and Peterson (88)) and folic acid (Snell and Peterson (68)). For the estimation of nicotinic acid Lactobacillus Arabinosus is the organism of choice (Barton-Wright (89), Kent-Jones and Meiklejohn (90)). Other organisms which have been employed in similar assays include Neurospora Sitophila (Stokes et al. (91)), Streptococcus lactis (Snell, Guirard and Williams (92)) and Leuconostoc Mesenteroides (Barton-Wright et al. (93)). The latter is also recommended for amino acid assays.

Vitamin B_{12}. The isolation from liver of the highly potent anti-anæmic factor, known as vitamin B_{12}, was accomplished independently, and almost simultaneously in 1948 by Rickes et al. (94) in America, and by Lester Smith (95) in England. Rickes et al. (94), by successive purifications of clinically active liver fractions, isolated in minute amounts a crystalline substance highly active for the growth of the Lactobacillus lactis Dorner, and they called this substance vitamin B_{12}. Short (96) had shown that the Lactobacillus lactis requires for its growth two unidentified factors, one of which (LLD factor) appeared to be related to the activity of commercial liver preparations used in the treatment of pernicious anæmia. It was found that vitamin B_{12} was either wholly or partially responsible for the LLD growth activity observed for liver extracts. Rickes et al. were therefore able to use this microbiological method of assay of the various liver fractions isolated, instead of the more tedious and somewhat uncertain clinical trials employed by Ungley (97) on material supplied by Lester Smith.

Method of Isolation from Liver. Lester Smith and his colleagues have given details of their methods of isolation of vitamin B_{12} in a series of publications (95, 98, 99, 100). They used the method of partition chromatography invented by Martin and Synge (101). Smith (100) outlines the process as follows : " The method employs a tube packed with an inert porous powder capable of soaking up a considerable proportion of water without appearing damp ; the material to be separated is applied to this column dissolved in an organic solvent not completely miscible with water, and development is combined with the same solvent. These columns do not differ in appearance from the familiar adsorption chromatograms using alumina, for example, but the mechanism of separation is different ; it depends on differences in the partition of the various substances present between water (held in the pores of the solid) and the solvent, instead of upon differences in adsorbability." Purified liver extracts separated into 3 coloured zones, yellow below, brown above and pink in between. Nearly colourless material was present between the pink and yellow zones.

Smith (102) says that the method is very complicated involving " at least 6 chromatographic procedures in succession, interspersed with other steps of purification, such as salting out with ammonium sulphate, proteolysis, precipitation with phosphotungstic acid and partition between aqueous solution and solvent mixtures. The chromatographic steps included adsorption in alumina, silica and charcoal." The active principle was present in two red bands in the chromatogram column. Eventually 20 mg. of vitamin B_{12} were obtained from a ton of liver. Both Rickes et al. (103) and Smith (104) showed that the red crystalline B_{12} contained cobalt to the extent of 4%, each molecule probably containing one atom of cobalt and three atoms of phosphorus.

Cobalt had been shown by Martin (105) to prevent or cure anæmia in ruminants resulting from feeding on pastures deficient in cobalt. The use of the cobalt ion alone is ineffective in the treatment of pernicious anæmia.

A further advance was made in the preparation of vitamin B_{12} when it was shown by Rickes et al. (106) that the streptomyces griseus, from which streptomycin is prepared, forms in its metabolism fluid vitamin B_{12} identical with that obtained from liver, and producing a similar clinical response in pernicious anæmia. It appears probable that there are four or more active forms of B_{12}, these have been called B_{12a}, B_{12b}, B_{12c} and B_{12d}. Articles on these forms of vitamin B_{12} have been published by Smith (107), Ungley and Campbell (108) and Chalmers (109).

Clinical Applications. Vitamin B_{12} is active in very small doses. West (110) tested the crystalline substance, isolated by Rickes et al., in the clinical treatment of pernicious anæmia in relapse. He found that in two patients doses of 3 and 6 micrograms respectively produced a rapid increase in the reticulocytes, red cells and hæmoglobin. Ungley (97) tested clinically the crystalline vitamin B_{12}, prepared by Smith, on 53 patients suffering from pernicious anæmia, most of whom had received no previous treatment, and a few who were in a stage of relapse after discontinuing treatment. The vitamin was injected intramuscularly as a single dose. The doses were graded logarithmically from 1·25 to 160 micrograms. The reticulocytes usually began to rise on the second or third day and reached a peak on the fifth or sixth day. A good reticulocytosis was not always a precursor of a correspondingly good rise in the red cell count. It was found that the increase of red cells in fifteen days was the best criterion of hæmatological response to the vitamin. The amount of vitamin B_{12} required to raise the red cell count to over 4,500,000 per c.mm. varied from 15 to 140 micrograms. The bone marrow showed changes from a megaloblastic to a normoblastic picture. Soreness of the tongue disappeared within a few days of the injection, and allergic reactions were not met with. Ungley has also reported on the favourable effects produced by vitamin B_{12} on the neurological manifestations of pernicious anæmia.

For an uncomplicated case of pernicious anæmia he recommended an initial dose of 40 to 80 micrograms, followed by 20 micrograms weekly for three months, and 30 micrograms every three weeks subsequently.

In cases showing neurological changes, such as peripheral neuritis or subacute combined degeneration, larger doses are required, such as 40 micrograms every week for six months, and 20 micrograms weekly afterwards. Berk et al. (111) reported rapid regression of neurological manifestations and absence of allergic reactions in a patient sensitive to injectable liver extracts. The patient was a forty-one-year-old mulatto woman, who had previously been treated with injections of purified liver extracts and folic acid. Eight daily injections of 5 micrograms of B_{12} were given. On the tenth day of treatment remarkable changes in the neurological signs were noted. The numbness and clumsiness of the fingers vanished, the plantar responses became flexor, the patient could walk without support, and vibration sense returned. It is clearly essential that the neurological changes in pernicious anæmia should be adequately treated before structural damage in the cord renders them irreversible. Ungley (112) has also compared the efficacy of vitamin B_{12} with that of more crude liver extracts in the treatment of subacute degeneration of the cord. He found that it was equally effective and stated that " the existence of a separate neuropoietic factor need no longer be postulated ". Weekly doses of 40 micrograms of B_{12} are usually effective in the first six months, with half this dose for the subsequent maintenance treatment. At the least sign of relapse, or if there is an intercurrent infection, the dosage should be increased.

Vitamin B_{12} is available in Great Britain as Cytamen in ampoules containing 20 and 50 micrograms equivalent per ml., or Anacobin, in ampoules containing 10 micrograms in 1 ml. Vitamin B_{12} has also been effective in the treatment of tropical macrocytic anæmia, nutritional macrocytic anæmia and sprue. It is ineffective in secondary anæmias and in aplastic anæmia.

Jacobson and Bishop (113) have brought forward evidence to show that the hæmopoietic effect of vitamin B_{12} is inferior to a comparable dose of commercial liver extract. It is suggested that in addition to the primary factor, B_{12}, accessory factors are required. These accessory factors include l-tyrosine, a peptide, xanthopterin, tryptophane and guanosine. If this is so, then a liver extract, such as Anahæmin is preferable to B_{12} in the routine treatment of pernicious anæmia.

Vitamin C. This substance, which is water-soluble, is responsible for protection against scurvy. It is found distributed fairly widely in animal tissues and also in the juice of fresh fruit, particularly citrus fruits. It has been shown to be *l*-ascorbic acid which has the constitution shown below :—

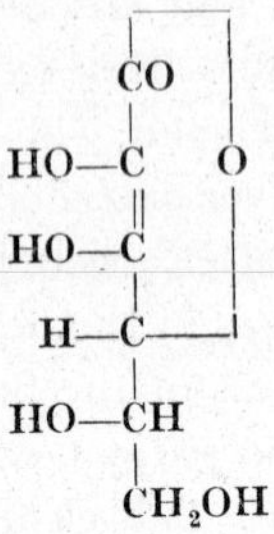

```
         ┌─────┐
         CO    │
         │     │
    HO—C      O
        ‖      │
    HO—C      │
         │     │
     H—C─────┘
         │
    HO—CH
         │
        CH2OH
```

The compound is a powerful reducing agent and is unstable in alkaline solution. It is estimated biologically by its ability to protect guinea-pigs from scurvy, and chemically by titration with phenol-indo-2 : 6-dichloro-phenol.

Clinical Applications. The vitamin is administered in the prophylactic and curative treatment of scurvy, usually in the form of fresh orange juice. Orange juice contains 0·2 to 0·9 mg. per ml., rose-hip syrup 0·4 to 2·2 mg. per ml., blackcurrant purée 0·66 to 1 mg. per ml., blackcurrant syrup 0·63 mg. per ml., spinach 0·9 mg. per g., human milk 0·06 mg., and cow's milk 0·02 mg. per ml. The vitamin C content of cow's milk is lowered by pasteurisation, by standing, by further heating and by dilution.

Vegetables should be cut up only just before cooking, and dropped in small quantities into boiling water, care being taken that the water does not go " off the boil ". Further, if vegetables are not eaten as soon as cooked, the ascorbic acid gradually deteriorates. The daily requirement of vitamin C for an adult is 50 to 100 mg., for a child 50 to 150 mg., and for an infant 15 to 50 mg. Alternatively it may be given as tablets of ascorbic acid each containing 50 mg. of crystalline vitamin C, 1 to 3, t.d.s., or in adult scurvy, ascorbic acid mg. 100 to 300 may be administered subcutaneously, t.i.d. There is no danger of hypervitaminosis. It has been suggested that many chronic illnesses may be due to a degree of vitamin C subnutrition (latent scurvy). Abbasy, Hill and Harris (114) have shown that in active rheumatism the ascorbic acid excretion in the urine is below normal, and they conclude that in the infection which underlies rheumatic fever there is a greatly increased metabolic use of, and need for, vitamin C, and a correspondingly lower degree of saturation of the body reserves. Kaiser (115), however, determining the vitamin C content of the blood in normal and rheumatic children, found no striking difference and considered that vitamin C is probably not a significant ætiological factor in rheumatic infections. Thus children may show a fragility of capillaries, especially in the early spring. Campbell and Cook (116) found that gingivitis, characterised by painful and bleeding gums, rapidly healed if ascorbic acid was given in doses of 300 mg. daily for four days. Glazebrook and Thomson (117) made observations on youths between the age of fifteen and twenty years who were having a diet in which the vitamin C was largely destroyed by the methods of cooking and distribution ; 335 had ascorbic acid administered daily for several months. None of them developed pneumonia or rheumatic fever, whereas in a group of 1,100 controls there were 17 cases of pneumonia and 16 of acute rheumatism. Lack of healing of wounds (Bourne (118)) and of gastric ulcers in patients undergoing treatment has been ascribed to deficiency of vitamin C in the diet. In some cases of pernicious anæmia a satisfactory response to liver therapy is not obtained until ascorbic acid is also administered. Harris (119) concluded that the addition of extra vitamin C to wartime diets increased resistance to infections, promoted healing of wounds, and improved weight and height gains in children.

The diagnosis of vitamin C subnutrition may be carried out as follows : Harris and his co-workers (120) have studied the concentration of ascorbic acid in the urine both before and after the administration of test doses of ascorbic acid to human subjects. They found that normal individuals excrete significant amounts of ascorbic acid in their urine, usually over 13 mg. daily. The vitamin is derived from the diet. If the ascorbic acid is withheld from the diet, ascorbic acid is excreted at a steady rate for a time, indicating the existence of appreciable reserve stores of the vitamin. In general, the urinary excretion reaches an equilibrium level proportional to the dietary intake of the vitamin. Harris regards a daily excretion below 13 mg. as suggestive of vitamin C deficiency. The effect of a test dose of 700 mg. of ascorbic acid per 10 stones of body-weight depends on the state of nutrition of the subject with respect to vitamin C. In normal individuals there is a sharp increase in the excretion of ascorbic acid, usually on the first day following the test dose. A patient is regarded as " unsaturated " if the excretion rate does not show a rapid increase above the resting level. When dealing with patients with a low reserve of ascorbic acid a better idea of the degree of unsaturation may be obtained if the test dose is administered for several consecutive days and the daily output of vitamin recorded.

The chief difficulty of the test is due to the instability of ascorbic acid, which oxidises rapidly in air. For this reason, the urine should be collected in dark stoppered bottles and treated with one-tenth of its volume of glacial acetic acid. Analysis should be performed at once. The night urine should be collected in the same way and despatched to the laboratory for analysis early in the morning. The whole of the urine passed in twenty-four hours must be collected. Unless these precautions are taken, loss of ascorbic acid will occur and may lead to an erroneous conclusion. If the output is under 13 mg. per day a deficiency of vitamin C may exist. For the test dose, about 700 mg. of ascorbic acid should be given for every 10 stones of body-weight, and the urine collected for the following two or three days. If a small response results, the dose should be repeated on one or two further days in order to distinguish between the milder degrees of deprivation and more severe hypovitaminosis.

Harris and Abbasy (121) have proposed a modified test over a shorter period, suitable when the collection of full twenty-four-hourly specimens may be inconvenient. At 9 a.m. the patient is instructed to urinate. This specimen is discarded. The patient is then instructed not to urinate until 12 noon if possible, when the test specimen representing one-eighth of the total day's excretion is obtained and analysed. The same programme is repeated on a second and third day in order to establish the resting level. After this, the test dose of 700 mg. of ascorbic acid per 10 stones of body-weight is administered on one or more further days. In these cases the urine samples are collected during the same afternoon over a three-hourly period, *e.g.* 2 to 5 p.m., and analysed at once.

Investigation of the ascorbic acid content of the blood has indicated the existence of a threshold valuc of about 1 mg. per 100 ml. of plasma. Lower thresholds are sometimes observed. Normally, the effect of a test dose is to increase the plasma ascorbic acid over the threshold value, with the appearance of the vitamin in the urine. Ungley (122) showed that with deficiency of vitamin C the resting level of ascorbic acid in the plasma is low, and is only slightly increased by the dose. However, the plasma value, although dependent on the intake of ascorbic acid in the diet, is not a good index of a significant deficiency of the vitamin. Thus, Lund and Crandon (123) in a study of a human volunteer found that the plasma level of ascorbic acid dropped to zero in six weeks, whereas clinical scurvy took five months to develop in a subject placed on a diet free from ascorbic acid. It was also found that the reducing substance in the " buffy coat " of centrifuged blood, presumably consisting of ascorbic acid, took four months to drop to zero and thus provided a more reliable index to the danger of clinical scurvy.

Vitamin D. This anti-rachitic vitamin is found in fish liver oils, but can also be prepared by the irradiation of inactive sterols found in nature. Thus, the irradiation of ergosterol leads to the formation of calciferol which was formerly thought to be the naturally-occurring vitamin. The constitution of the naturally-occurring vitamin is not certain, since many sterols on irradiation produce active compounds. At least 10 provitamins D are known, the 4 listed below having been isolated in the pure state :—

Vitamin D	*Provitamin D*
D_2 . . .	Ergosterol
D_3 . . .	7-dehydrocholesterol
D_4 . . .	22-dehydroergosterol
D_5 . . .	7-dehydro-sitosterol

The compound D_3, which has been isolated from tunny fish oil, has a high activity when tested in chickens and it is suggested that this is the naturally-occurring vitamin D. The formulæ for ergosterol, calciferol and vitamin D_3 are as follows :—

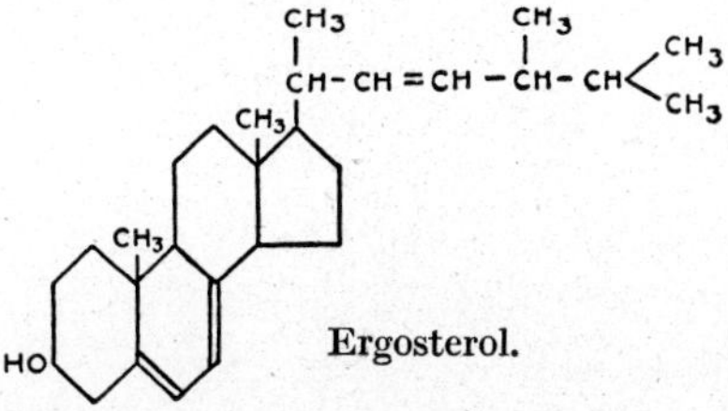

Ergosterol.

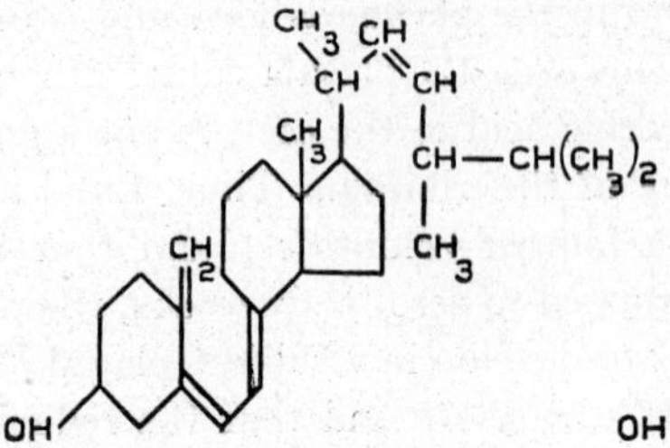

Calciferol (vitamin D_2).

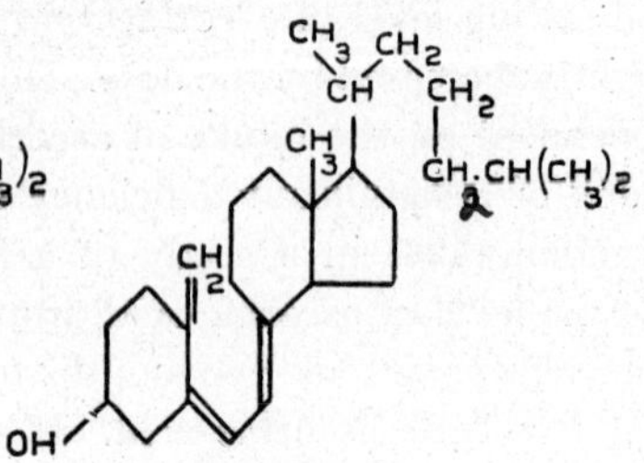

Vitamin D_3.

The method of standardising vitamin D consists in employing the same type of method as already recounted for the other vitamins. There is, however, considerable difference in that the great importance of the presence of this vitamin has succeeded in producing a definite quantitative method of estimation. Rats are fed on a special diet containing no vitamin D until rickets develops. The stock is then divided into groups, and to each group graded doses of the preparation are given by mouth. To another series a standard preparation of vitamin D is given, and by carefully grading the doses attempts are made to produce the same effect as with the standard preparation, and by this means a definition of the activity of the unknown in terms of the standard may be arrived at. The actual technique of determining the degree of healing of the rickets varies considerably. For example, X-ray photographs may be taken of the leg bones, when uncalcified areas can readily be seen. An alternative method is that known as the " line test ". In this, animals are killed and sections of the long bones are made and the epiphyses are stained with silver nitrate. The preparation is then exposed to the light, with the result that at the epiphyseal line a black area is produced. By this means the degree of healing may be studied. It is thus possible to obtain the potency of the unknown in terms of the standard. The international unit is $\frac{1}{10000}$ mg. of irradiated ergosterol. The D vitamins are stable to cooking.

Clinical Applications. The vitamin D content of certain foods, according to Coward and Morgan (1), is as follows, expressed as international units per g. : Egg yolk 1·5 to 5, cream 0·5, butter 0·4 to 4, milk 0 to 0·1, cod liver oil 480 units per teaspoonful, and halibut liver oil 48 units per drop. Fresh herrings contain 250 international units per oz. The use of vitamin D is very wide, and it is usually given either in the form of cod liver oil, halibut liver oil, or some similar preparation, or, alternatively, as irradiated ergosterol. As a prophylactic against rickets, most foods given to children are reinforced either by the addition of irradiated ergosterol or by the irradiation of the actual product ; infants usually require 700 to 1,500 international units daily, and as a curative dose 3,000 to 5,000 international units daily. The British Pædiatric Association recommends 700 international units daily for a baby during the first year. This is contained in 8 drops of Radiostoleum, 10 drops of halibut liver oil, 12 drops of Adexolin, 280 drops of cod liver oil compound, and 560 drops of 50% emulsion of cod liver oil (2 drops = 1 minim). Liq. vit. D Conc. (B.P. Add.) contains 1,500 international units in 3 minims. Ten thousand units daily would constitute an overdosage, resulting in increased density of bone, fever, etc. Massive doses of vitamin D, in the form of irradiated ergosterol (300,000 international units or more daily) have been used to raise the blood calcium in tetany, and in the treatment of lupus vulgaris, rheumatoid arthritis and hay fever. Such doses are not devoid of danger. Tumulty and Howard (124) record the case of a man given 750,000 international units daily for twelve days to aid the union of a fracture. His blood calcium rose to 15 mg. per 100 ml., the serum phosphorus not falling below 3·8 mg. per 100 ml. He was seized with nausea, abdominal pains and severe vomiting, associated with renal failure. The vitamin D had been administered in milk, in which vehicle it is ten times more potent than in oil.

Dihydrotachysterol (A.T. 10), although possessing only slight antirachitic potency, has also been employed to raise the level of blood calcium in idiopathic and post-operative (hypoparathyroid) tetany. It appears to possess no special advantage over calciferol for this purpose. Albright (125) recommends that the urine of patients under treatment with massive doses of calciferol or A.T. 10 should be regularly tested for calcium by the Sulkowitch reagent. This reagent consists of 2·5 g. oxalic acid, 2·5 g. ammonium oxalate and 5 ml. of glacial acetic acid dissolved in water to make 150 ml. One volume of urine is treated with 1 volume of reagent. If no precipitate of calcium oxalate is obtained there is little calcium present in the urine and the serum calcium level is probably from 5 to 7·5 mg. per 100 ml. If there is a fine white cloud the level of the calcium in the serum is in the satisfactory range. If the mixture looks like milk, the danger of hypercalcæmia is present. No method has been worked out for the actual isolation of vitamin D from the urine, and therefore we have no definite evidence of a sub-rickets condition.

Vitamin E. It has been shown that animals fed on diets deficient in certain vegetable substances can no longer reproduce. The fœtus becomes resorbed following placental changes after the twelfth day. In the male this deficiency leads to destruction and atrophy of the testes. The distribution of vitamin E in nature is widespread, cereal grain, green leaves, legumes and nuts being good plant sources of the material. As far as is known, wheat germ oil is the richest source, and most workers attempting to obtain the pure vitamin from natural sources have used this as a starting material. Vitamin E is classified among the fat-soluble vitamins, and is destroyed by atmospheric oxygen in the presence of alkali.

Three substances, α-, β- and γ-tocopherol have been isolated and found to possess vitamin E activity. α-tocopherol has been synthesised by Karrer et al. (126) and Todd et al. (127), and is as active as the most potent vitamin E concentrates. The formula of α-tocopherol is shown below :

```
        CH3    CH3         CH3        CH3        CH3
         |   O  /           |          |          |
   CH3 /\  /\  C—(CH2)3.CH(CH2)3 CH(CH2)3 CH.CH3
       |   ||   |
    HO  \/  \/ CH2
       CH3 CH2
```

β- and γ-tocopherol possess one methyl group less than α-tocopherol and exhibit only half the activity of α-tocopherol when tested on rats.

Clinical Applications. Vitamin E is put up in 3 m. capsules (Viteolin), each containing the unsaponifiable matter of 5 g. wheat germ oil, or as α-tocopherol tablets, 3 mg. (Ephynal). Fresh dried whole-wheat germ may also be given by mouth, $\frac{1}{2}$ oz. twice daily. One international unit corresponds with 1 mg. of the acetate.

Sterility. Good results have been claimed by some authors such as Currie (128) in the treatment of habitual and threatened abortion by the administration of vitamin E in the form of wheat germ oil extract 3 m. capsules, one capsule daily for three to six months up to the onset of labour. It is difficult, however, to obtain adequate controls, and some authorities are sceptical of the results claimed. Drummond (129) says that in human beings the process of normal pregnancy, like that in the goat and unlike that in the rat, may not be dependent on vitamin E.

Nervous and Muscular Lesions. Bicknell (130) suggests that vitamin E may be deficient in the normal diet of man and that the nervous and muscular systems may suffer in cases of hereditary disposition or from toxic influences such as syphilis. He also suggests that the anti-sterility factor, α-tocopherol, is not identical with the myotropic and neurotropic factors, although all are present in wheat germ oil. He treated cases of muscular dystrophy in children, and amyotrophic lateral sclerosis and tabes dorsalis in adults with fresh dried whole-wheat germ, $\frac{1}{2}$ oz. twice daily for a period up to eighteen months. He obtained good results with the myopathies and came to the conclusion that they are deficiency diseases and curable. Demole (131) considers that only one factor, α-tocopherol, is needed to prevent paralysis in experimental animals deficient in vitamin E. Wechsler (132) obtained good results in two cases of amyotrophic lateral sclerosis treated with pure synthetic α-tocopherol in the form of Ephynal tablets, 3 mg., 2 to 3 t.d.s. Subsequent work by various investigators, such as Sheldon et al. (133), Doyle and Merritt (134), Denker and Scheinman (135), Ferrebee et al. (136), and Fitzgerald and McArdle (137) indicate that vitamin E lack does not cause muscular dystrophies or motor-neurone disorders in man. Further, administration of vitamin E, either in the crude form or as the synthetic preparation, alone or combined with vitamin B_6, does not cure such disorders. This opinion is based both on clinical observations, and on the estimation of urinary creatine. The excretion of the latter results from nutritional muscular disturbances, and, if the patient is on a creatine-free diet, its excretion should diminish as the muscular disease improves. Bicknell and Prescott (138) criticise these adverse findings on the efficacy of vitamin E, and say that in many cases enormous doses were administered which may act adversely by actually causing a fall in the vitamin E content of the blood. They further say that in many of the unsuccessful cases the disease had lasted for many years, when recovery of muscular function could hardly be expected.

Vitamin K. The history of vitamin K, the " Koagulations-vitamin ", dates back to the suggestion of Dam (139) made in 1934, that the spontaneous hæmorrhages found in newly-born chicks were the result of the absence of a fat-soluble factor from the diet. These hæmorrhages, although closely resembling those of scurvy, did not respond to the administration of 1-ascorbic acid, and, furthermore, differed from those of avitaminosis C in that they were associated with hypoprothrombinæmia and a prolonged blood clotting time (Schonheyder (140), Dam et al. (141). The analogous clinical conditions in man were recognised by Brinkhous et al. (142) in 1937 as hæmorrhagic disease of the newborn and as a hæmorrhagic tendency in cases of biliary obstruction.

Although fat-soluble, vitamin K differs from vitamins A and D in that it predominates in plant sources. Doisy and his co-workers (143) isolated two crystalline compounds, vitamin K_1 (alfalfa) and vitamin K_2 (putrefied fish meal) which, although similar in physiological activity, differed in detail in their chemical composition.

Vitamin K_1 has been shown to be 2-methyl-3-phytyl-1 : 4-naphthoquinone and is represented by the following formula :—

$$\text{(naphthoquinone ring, O at 1 and 4)}\ \begin{array}{l} -CH_3 \\ -CH_2-CH=\underset{\displaystyle CH_3}{\underset{|}{C}}-(CH_2)_3-\underset{\displaystyle CH_3}{\underset{|}{CH}}(CH_2)_3\underset{\displaystyle CH_3}{\underset{|}{CH}}-(CH_2)_3\,\underset{\displaystyle CH_3}{\underset{|}{CH}}-CH_3 \end{array}$$

2-methyl-3-phytyl-1 : 4-naphthoquinone (vitamin K_1).

Vitamin K_2 (144), the second of the naturally-occurring vitamins, differs in that the phytyl group in the 3-position is replaced by

$$=CH(CH=\underset{\displaystyle CH_3}{\underset{|}{C}}.CH_2.CH_2)_5CH=C\begin{array}{l} \diagup CH_3 \\ \diagdown CH_3 \end{array}$$

The molecular structure is not very specific and many synthetic 1 : 4 naphthoquinone derivatives display activity. An intact benzene ring and methyl group in the 2-position have been found in all active compounds to date. Not only can the group in the 3-position be replaced by hydrogen without loss of activity, but the quinonoid oxygens may also be replaced by a variety of groups. Phthiocol (2-methyl-3-hydroxy-1 : 4-naphthoquinone) was the forerunner of a series of compounds in which lyophilic groups (—OH, SO_3H, etc.) were deliberately introduced to endow the synthetic drugs with water-solubility. Typical water-soluble vitamin K substitutes such as sodium 2-methyl-1 : 4-naphthoquinone-3 sulphonic acid, and 2-methyl-1 : 4-naphthoquinone bisulphite (Stewart (145)) are readily absorbed even in the absence of bile secretion and are suitable for oral administration (Smith and Owen (146)). The fat-soluble analogues are usually administered intramuscularly in an oily medium or orally accompanied by bile salts to aid absorption.

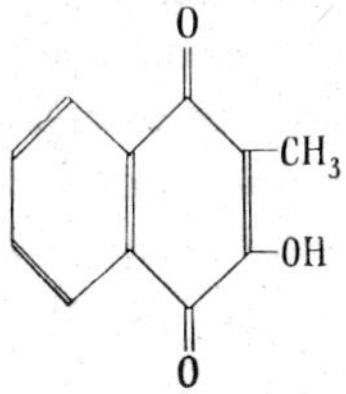

O O O
$-CH_3$ $-CH_3$ $-CH_3$
$-OH$ $-SO_3Na$
O O O

Phthiocol 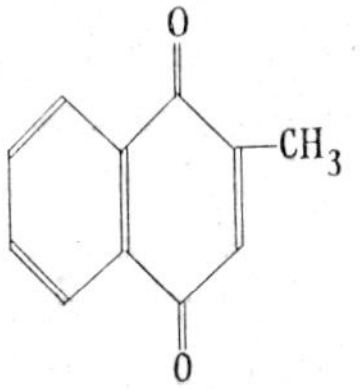 Menaphthone 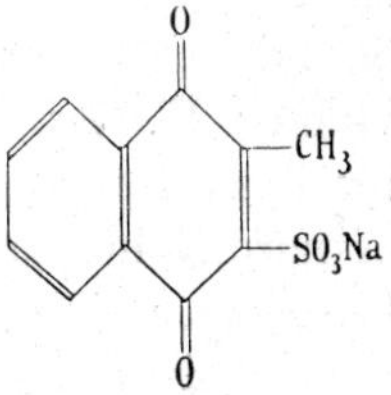 Sodium 2-methyl-1 : 4-naphthoquinone-3-sulphonic acid.

Some doubt exists as to the site and mode of action of vitamin K. The older school of thought maintained that the " Koagulations-vitamin " played no direct part in the coagulation of blood, but was only associated with prothrombin formation. Ample evidence is forthcoming (Fitzgerald and Webster (147), Kark and Souter (148)) that some four hours after the administration of vitamin K to patients suffering from hypoprothrombinæmia there is a distinct rise in the blood prothrombin concentration and a corresponding fall in prothrombin time, but as to whether vitamin K is an essential unit in prothrombin, or whether it stimulates the formation of prothrombin in the liver, no opinion was expressed. Lyons (149) has produced definite evidence which bears on this problem. According to the classical theory of Morawitz, supported by Mellanby (150), thrombin reacts with, or combines with, fibrinogen to form the insoluble fibrin clot. Lyons succeeded in dividing thrombin into two active components, Thrombin A and B, neither of which alone will convert fibrinogen into fibrin, although a combination of both will do so. Thrombin A reacts with fibrinogen to form an intermediate compound, fibrinogen B, between fibrinogen and fibrin. Fibrinogen B can be converted into a normal fibrin clot by the addition of Thrombin B or a minute quantity of 2-methyl-1 : 4-naphthoquinone (vitamin K).

Lyons suggests, therefore, that either vitamin K is the prosthetic group of the enzyme thrombin, or that vitamin K along with a protein carrier acts as an oxido-reductase system. Support to the former theory is given by the fact that the products of tryptic digest of thrombin give colour reactions characteristic of 1 : 4-naphthoquinones.

Within a few days of birth, the danger of hæmorrhagic disease of the newborn recedes and with the establishment of an intestinal flora the child becomes less dependent upon an exogenous source of vitamin K. As this synthesis and absorption from the intestine persists throughout adult life, it is difficult to get an accurate idea of normal human requirements. Sells, Walker and Owen (151) place the requirements of the newborn at 1 to 2 μg. per day. Figures given by other workers are substantially the same.

In vitamin K therapy synthetic substitutes have largely replaced concentrates from natural sources. Phthiocol (2-methyl-3-hydroxy-1 : 4-naphthoquinone), the first synthetic analogue, no longer finds as widespread use as Menaphthone (2-methyl-1 : 4-naphthoquinone) which is put up in capsules of 1 to 10 mg. for oral administration and in oil for intramuscular injection. For more rapid control of hæmorrhage, intravenous injection of water-soluble derivatives is recommended (Almquist and Klose (152)). The prompt response in these circumstances, however, is not maintained, and a prolonged rise in prothrombin level is best achieved by intramuscular injection of an oil-soluble derivative.

Clinical Applications. Various preparations are available for clinical use. Klotogen is an oily concentrate of the naturally-occurring vitamin. It is put in capsules for oral administration. Kapilon is an oily solution of a synthetic analogue of vitamin K. It is put up in 1 ml. ampoules containing 5 mg. of the pure substance, for intramuscular injection, and in tablets of 10 mg., and in " liquid " containing 10 mg. in 1 ml. for oral administration. Prokayvit is a similar synthetic substance put up in 1 ml. ampoules each containing 5 mg. for intramuscular injection. The synthetic substances have the advantage of being considerably cheaper than the naturally-occurring vitamin. Bilein capsules each contain gr. 5 bile salts.

The chief indications for the use of vitamin K are :—

1. *Spontaneous subcutaneous and internal hæmorrhages, or the liability to bleeding during and after operation.* The predisposing condition here is the absence of bile from the intestinal tract, resulting in deficient absorption of the vitamin. The most important causes are obstructive jaundice, biliary fistula, and less often acute hepatosis and yellow fever. Investigations have shown that vitamin K is a fat-soluble vitamin which cannot be absorbed from the intestine in the absence of bile-salts. The hæmorrhagic tendency which results is due to a low plasma prothrombin level. The method for estimating this is described on p. 371, and this appears to be the best guide to the need for vitamin K therapy. If vitamin K is given by mouth in the absence of bile from the intestinal tract, bile-salts must also be administered in order to ensure its absorption from the intestine. This is not necessary if the vitamin is injected. In some cases, however, absorption appears to be slow after intramuscular injection. In cases of operation for obstructive jaundice, Klotogen, 1 capsule, or Kapilon, 1 tablet, and Bilein, 2 gr. 5 capsules, are given t.i.d. with meals for at least four days before operation and for three to four days subsequently. Successful results have been obtained by Macfie et al. (153) in cases of obstructive jaundice using intramuscular injections of the synthetic vitamin K. Thus Kapilon or Prokayvit, 1 to 2 ml., may be given daily by intramuscular injection for two to three days prior to the operation, and 1 ml. subsequently for two to three days. In many cases of obstructive jaundice in which the prothrombin level of the blood is low, there is a failure of response to vitamin K. This is probably due to extensive liver damage. In such cases, as shown by Kark and Souter (154), if the vitamin fails to raise the prothrombin level, the only alternative method of treatment is blood transfusion.

2. *Hæmorrhagic disease of the newborn.* In newborn infants it is common to find slight hæmorrhagic tendencies during the first week, but occasionally the hæmorrhages are so severe as to cause death. The investigations of Dam et al. (155) indicated that the cause of the hæmorrhage is vitamin K deficiency developing a few

days after birth, and ceasing usually after the eighth day. They have found that in one case the administration of the vitamin together with bile-salts through a stomach tube raised the prothrombin level to normal within forty-one hours. A low prothrombin level, however, is probably not the sole cause of the hæmorrhage, as the level may be low without bleeding occurring. Subsequent investigations in America by Sandford et al. (156) have thrown some doubt on the matter. Although the administration of vitamin K to newborn babies lessened the normal fall in the prothrombin level during the first three days of life, hæmorrhagic manifestations occurred as frequently in the babies thus treated as in the untreated. These, however, were all minor hæmorrhages, and not those characteristic of hæmorrhagic disease of the newborn. They further showed that the administration of vitamin K to the mother before delivery will raise the plasma prothrombin value of the infant. Norris and Bennett (157) determined the prothrombin value of the mother and of the newborn child, and showed that as there appears to be no relationship between the two, it is unlikely that the prothrombin passes directly from the mother to the fœtus, and it may be formed in the placenta. It does not seem possible to decide by an examination of the maternal blood, whether or not vitamin K should be given to the mother before the birth of the child. In addition to the pathological hypoprothrombinæmia, the clotting time of the blood is prolonged in the hæmorrhagic disease of the newborn. The hypoprothrombinæmia occurring in icterus gravis neonatorum, anæmia neonatorum and hydrops congenitus also responds to the administration of vitamin K.

The prophylactic treatment of neonatal hæmorrhage consists in giving the mother Kapilon 5 tablets or 1½ drams liquid by mouth twelve to four hours before the baby is born, and the baby is given 36 drops (18 m.) by mouth on the first day of its life. Lehmann (158), in Sweden, using a vitamin-K analogue, sodium-2-methyl-1, 4-naphthohydroquinone disulphate, which is completely soluble in water and absorbed without the presence of bile salts, treated 13,250 full term infants with doses of 1 mg. (20 drops of a 0·1% solution) by mouth within an hour of birth, the results being controlled by prothrombin estimations. In comparison with 17,740 untreated cases, Lehmann concluded that death from bleeding was reduced by 1·6 per 1,000 in the treated infants, and recommends the method for general prophylaxis. The curative treatment consists in the intramuscular injection of a preparation such as Kapilon, 1 ml., repeated daily. In severe cases blood transfusions should be given.

The question as to whether vitamin K deficiency may arise through some dietary lack in otherwise normal subjects cannot yet be answered. A study by Kark and Lozner (159) of four non-jaundiced subjects with diminished prothrombin levels suggests that there may be a dietary deficiency of vitamin K in man, but it seems likely that such a condition can only arise under abnormal circumstances and in conjunction with other nutritional deficiencies. A low plasma prothrombin level may occasionally be responsible for hæmoptysis in pulmonary tuberculosis. We have had one such case under our care, and Sheely (160) reports four cases of hæmoptysis associated with prothrombin deficiency in which the administration of vitamin K appeared to be a likely factor in controlling the bleeding.

Readers are referred for further consideration of this subject to the monograph by Butt and Snell (161).

Dicoumarol. No account of the relationship of vitamin K deficiency to hypoprothrombinæmia would be complete without reference to the hæmorrhagic symptoms which characterise sweet clover disease in cattle, as described by Roderick (162) and Quick (163). The cause of this condition has been shown by the Wisconsin school to be due to the action of a substance present in the sweet clover diet. The active principle, isolated and synthesised by Link et al. in 1941 (164), is Dicoumarol (3 : 3-methylene-bis-4-hydroxycoumarin):

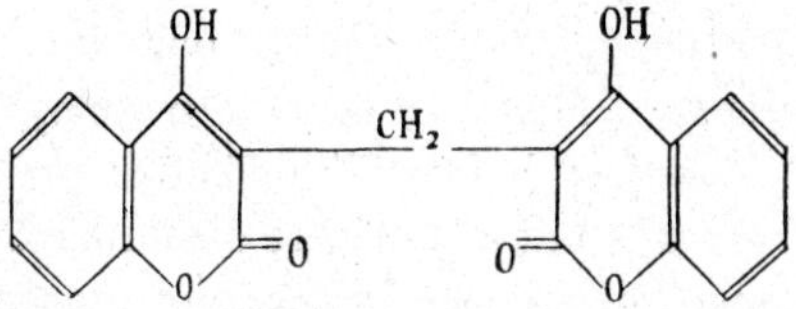

Dicoumarol.

Krumer and Barker (165) and Lucia and Aggeler (166) showed that, administered orally, this compound induces hypoprothrombinæmia inside seventy-two hours unless considerable amounts of vitamin K analogue are administered simultaneously. The fact that the prolonged clotting time in hæmorrhagic disease is always associated with a fall in blood prothrombin level, together with the relatively slow recovery following protection by vitamin K therapy, suggests that dicoumarol inhibits the production of prothrombin by the liver. Link et al. (167) have shown that in rats with pronounced hepatic disorder, recovery is very slow even when ample vitamin K is administered.

Clinical Applications. For the prevention of post-operative thrombosis, pulmonary embolism, and as a prophylactic in thrombophlebitis, dicoumarol has advantages over heparin. Apart from considerations of cheapness, it is effective orally and exercises a more prolonged action. The dangers of spontaneous hæmorrhage are never absent, however, and the course of treatment with dicoumarol must always be controlled by daily determinations of the prothrombin time.

The drug is put up in mg. 50 tablets, called Dicoumarin. Allen, Barker and Waugh (168) gave to their patients 200 to 300 mg. by mouth on the first day and 200 mg. on the second day, and subsequently it was administered in doses sufficient to keep the prothrombin time between thirty-five and sixty seconds (normal fifteen to twenty seconds). This effect should be maintained for about ten days after pulmonary embolism, or after the onset of acute thrombophlebitis. It should not be used for patients who are bleeding and it is particularly dangerous in subacute bacterial endocarditis. Further, it should not be used in cases in which there are ulcerating lesions, renal disease, obstructive jaundice, severe liver damage or high fever. Zucker (169) reported the successful use of dicoumarol in cavernous sinus thrombosis. Davis and Porter (170) recommend the daily administration of three separate doses of 100 mg. every eight hours in the treatment of puerperal thrombosis. There is usually a delay of twenty-four hours after the first dose before the effect is produced, and this may persist for two to ten days after the dicoumarol is discontinued. Signs of overdosage may occur if the prothrombin time is over sixty seconds. They include lassitude, aching in the costo-vertebral joints, bleeding into the skin, joints, brain, viscera or from the gums. A blood transfusion, using blood not more than four days old, will restore the prothrombin time to normal. Vitamin K is useless for this purpose.

Vitamin P. Szent-Györgyi and co-workers (171) isolated from paprika and lemon juice a substance which, whilst capable of controlling the petechial hæmorrhages which characterise certain diseases such as vascular purpura, was not l-ascorbic acid. Chemical investigation of the material showed that it was an equilibrium mixture of two flavanone glucosides, hesperidin and its chalcone, eriodictin, but, as concentrates of the vitamin have been produced by Bacharach and Coates (172) which, when tested by these workers, were many times more active than crystalline hesperidin, the identity of the essential factor is by no means established beyond doubt.

Clinical Applications. Scarborough (173) considered that Szent-Györgyi's cases were unsuitable for the demonstration of a new vitamin and that the only suitable cases for investigation are those of known low vitamin intake, many of which show capillary fragility unrelated to vitamin C deficiency. Scarborough (174) says that as the result of nutritional deficiency and vitamin P lack, petechial hæmorrhages occur in the skin with much decreased capillary resistance. The patient complains of lassitude with pains in the shoulders and legs, but there are no hæmatological changes. These symptoms are relieved by the administration of vitamin P but not by vitamin C. Scarborough (175) recorded two cases of purpura senilis in which the capillary resistance was low and associated with a tendency to bruise. Administration of Permidin apparently increased the capillary resistance and controlled the tendency to bleeding. Permidin is available in tablet form for clinical use. Each tablet contains the equivalent of 0·25 g. of hesperidin, the usual dose being 1 to 4 tablets daily. Kugelmass (176) treated successfully two cases of allergic purpura in girls, characterised by fever, abdominal pain, bloody stools and purpura. He prepared the vitamin P from orange peel. The solution contained 50 mg. per ml. of flavones consisting of eriodictyol glucoside and hesperidin and the dose was 150 mg. orally. Vitamin P does not appear to be efficacious in the treatment of purpura hæmorrhagica, or of mechanical purpura.

REFERENCES

(1) Coward and Morgan. *Brit. Med. Journ.*, 1935, *ii*, 1043.
(2) Jeghers. *Journ. Amer. Med. Assocn.*, 1937, **109**, 756.
(3) Harris and Abbasy. *Lancet*, 1939, *ii*, 1299, 1355.

(4) Yudkin. *Proc. Roy Soc. Med.*, 1942, **35**, 619.
(5) Moore and Wang. *Biochem. Journ.*, 1945, **39**, 222.
(6) Windaus. *Hoppe-Seyl. Zeits.*, 1932, **204**, 123.
(7) Windaus. *Hoppe-Seyl. Zeits.*, 1935, **237**, 98.
(8) Williams. *Journ. Amer. Chem. Soc.*, 1935, **57**, 229.
(9) Williams and Spies. "*Vitamin B_1 and Its Use in Medicine*," 1938, Macmillan, New York.
(10) Peters. *Biochem. Journ.*, 1937, **31**, 2240.
Banga, Ochoa and Peters. *Biochem. Journ.*, 1939, **33**, 1109.
(11) Lohman and Schuster. *Biochem. Zeitschr.*, 1937, **294**, 188.
(12) National Flour and Bread, Second Report. From the Scientific Adviser's Division, Ministry of Food. *Nature*, 1942, **150**, 538.
(13) Harris and Wang. *Biochem. Journ.*, 1941, **35**, 1050.
(14) Aalsmeer and Wenckebach. *Wien. Arch. Inn. Med.*, 1929, **16**, 193.
(15) Jones and Bramwell. *Brit. Heart Journ.*, 1939, *i*, 187.
(16) Bowe. *Lancet*, 1942, *i*, 586.
(17) Stannus. *Lancet*, 1942, *i*, 756.
(18) Williams, Shapiro and Bartelot. *Lancet*, 1940, *i*, 76.
(19) Forsyth. *Med. Journ. Aust.*, 1939, **2**, 751.
(20) Gretton-Watson. *Lancet*, 1940, *i*, 244.
(21) Wernicke. *Lehrbuch der Gehirnkrankheiten*, 1881, **2**, 229. Berlin.
(22) Wortis, Bueding, Stein and Jollife. *Arch. Neurol. and Psych.*, 1942, **47**, 215.
(23) Györgyi, Kuhn and Wagner-Jauregg. *Naturwissenschaften*, 1933, **21**, 560.
(24) Stannus. *Trans. Soc. Trop. Med. Hyg.*, 1912, **5**, 112.
(25) Sebrell, Butler, Wooley and Isbell. *Publ. Hlth. Rep., Wash.*, 1941, **56**, 510.
(26) Sebrell and Butler. *Publ. Hlth. Rep., Wash.*, 1939, **54**, 2121.
(27) Kruse, Sydenstricker, Sebrell and Cleckley. *Publ. Hlth. Rep., Wash.*, 1940, **55**, 157.
(28) Johnson and Eckardt. *Arch. Ophthal., Chicago*, 1940, **23**, 899.
(29) Mann. *Amer. Journ. Ophthal.*, 1945, **28**, 243.
(30) Jones, Armstrong, Green and Chadwick. *Lancet*, 1944, *i*, 720.
(31) Duckworth. *Brit. Med. Journ.*, 1942, *i*, 582.
(32) Scarborough. *Brit. Med. Journ.*, 1942, *ii*, 601.
(33) Manson-Bahr. *Lancet*, 1940, *ii*, 318, 356.
(34) Stannus. *Brit. Med. Journ.*, 1944, *ii*, 103, 140.
(35) Kark and Meiklejohn. *Amer. Journ. Med. Sci.*, 1941, **201**, 380.
(36) Najjar and Wood. *Proc. Soc. Exp. Biol. and Med.*, 1940, **44**, 386.
Najjar and Holt. *Proc. Soc. Exp. Biol. and Med.*, 1941, **48**, 413.
Najjar and Holt. *Science*, 1941, **93**, 20.
(37) Spies, Cooper and Blankenhorn. *Journ. Amer. Med. Assocn.*, 1938, **110**, 622.
(38) Sebrell. *Journ. Amer. Med. Assocn.*, 1938, **110**, 1665.
(39) King. *Lancet*, 1940, *ii*, 32.
(40) Furtado. *Lancet*, 1942, *i*, 602.
(41) Neuwahl. *Lancet*, 1942, *ii*, 419.
(42) Atkinson. *Journ. Amer. Med. Assocn.*, 1942, 119, 1194.
(43) Gottlieb. *Brit. Med. Journ.*, 1944, *i*, 392.
(44) Gyorgy. *Nature*, 1934, **133**, 498 ; *Biochem. Journ.*, 1935, **29**, 741, 760, 767.

(45) KUHN, WESTPHAL, WENDT and WESTPHAL. *Naturwissenschaften*, 1939, **27**, 469.
(46) HARRIS and FOLKERS. *Journ. Amer. Chem. Soc.*, 1939, **61**, 1245.
HARRIS, STILLER and FOLKERS. *Journ. Amer. Chem. Soc.*, 1939, **61**, 1242.
(47) CHICK, MACRAE, MARTIN and MARTIN. *Biochem. Journ.*, 1938, **32**, 2207.
(48) CARTWRIGHT, WINTROBE and HUMPHREYS. *Journ. Biol. Chem.*, 1944, **153**, 171.
(49) BORSON and METTIER. *Proc. Soc. Exp. Biol. and Med.*, 1940, **43**, 429.
(50) VILTER, SCHIRO and SPIES. *Nature*, 1940, **145**, 388.
(51) McBRYDE and BAKER. *Journ. Ped.*, 1941, **18**, 727.
(52) SPIES, HIGHTOWER and HUBBARD. *Journ. Amer. Med. Assocn.*, 1940, **115**, 292.
(53) BOAS. *Biochem. Journ.*, 1927, **21**, 712.
(54) KOGL and TONNIS. *Zeitschr. physiol. Chem.*, 1936, **242**, 43.
(55) DU VIGNEAUD, HOFMANN, MELVILLE, GYORGY and ROSE. *Science*, 1940, **92**, 62, 609.
(56) KOGL and TEN HAM. *Zeitschr. physiol. Chem.*, 1943, **279**, 140.
(57) EAKIN, SNELL and WILLIAMS. *Journ. Biol. Chem.*, 1940, **136**, 801; 1941, **140**, 535.
(58) PENNINGTON, SNELL and EAKIN. *Journ. Amer. Chem. Soc.*, 1942, **64**, 469.
(59) MELVILLE, MAYER, HOFMANN and DU VIGNEAUD. *Journ. Biol. Chem.* 1942, **146**, 487.
(60) DU VIGNEAUD, MELVILLE, FOLKERS, WOLF, MOZINGO, KERESZTESY and HARRIS. *Journ. Biol. Chem.*, 1942, **146**, 475.
(61) EMMERSON. *Journ. Biol. Chem.*, 1945, **157**, 127.
(62) OTT. *Journ Biol. Chem.*, 1945, **157**, 131.
(63) KOGL, VERBEEK, ERXLEBEN and BORG. *Zeitschr. physiol. Chem.*, 1943, **279**, 121.
(64) SYDENSTRICKER, SENGAL, BRIGGS, DE VAUGHN and ISBELL. *Journ. Amer. Med. Assocn.*, 1942, **118**, 1199.
(65) WAISMAN, McCALL and ELVEHJEM. *Journ. Nutrit.*, 1945, **29**, 1.
(66) WILLIAMS. *New England Journ. Med.*, 1943, **228**, 247.
(67) MITCHELL, SNELL and WILLIAMS. *Journ. Amer. Chem. Soc.*, 1941, **63**, 2284; 1944, **66**, 267.
(68) SNELL and PETERSON. *Journ. Bact.*, 1940, **39**, 273.
(69) HOGAN and PARROTT. *Journ. Biol. Chem.*, 1940, **132**, 507.
(70) MITCHELL and WILLIAMS. *Journ. Amer. Chem. Soc.*, 1944, **66**, 271, 274.
(71) PFIFFNER, BINKLEY, BLOOM, BROWN, BIRD, EMMETT, HOGAN and O'DELL. *Science*, 1943, **97**, 404.
(72) ANGIER, BOOTHE, HUTCHINGS, MOWAT, SEMB, STOKSTAD, SUBBAROW, WALLER, COSULICH, FARENBACH, HULTGUIST, KUH, NORTHEY, SEEGAR, SICHELS and SMITH. *Science*, 1945, **102**, 227; 1946, **103**, 667.
(73) DAFT and SEBRELL. *Publ. Health Rep. Wash.*, 1943, **58**, 1592.
(74) SPIES. *South Med. Journ.*, 1945, **38**, 781.
(75) SPIES. *Lancet*, 1946, *i*, 225.
(76) DARBY, JONES and JOHNSON. *Science*, 1945, **103**, 2665, 108.
(77) WILKINSON. *Brit. Med. Journ.*, 1948, *i*, 771, 822; *Lancet*, 1949, *i*, 249, 291, 336.
(78) WILKINSON and ISRAËLS. *Brit. Med. Journ.*, 1949, *ii*, 1072; *Lancet*, 1949, *ii*, 689.
(79) ANSBACHER. *Science*, 1941, **93**, 164.
(80) SURE. *Science*, 1941, **94**, 167.

(81) Woods and Fildes. *Journ. Soc. Chem. Ind.*, 1940, **59**, 133.
(82) Selbie. *Brit. Journ. Exp. Path.*, 1940, **21**, **90**.
(83) Fildes. *Lancet*, 1940, *i*, 955.
(84) Sieve. *Science*, 1941, **94**, 257.
(85) Schopfer and Jung. *Compt. Rend. Acad. d. Sc.*, 1937, **204**, 1500.
(86) Snell and Strong. *Ind. Eng. Chem. Anal.*, 1939, **11**, 346.
(87) Carpenter and Strong. *Arch. Biochem.*, 1944, **3**, 375.
(88) Snell, Hutchings and Peterson. *Journ. Biol. Chem.*, 1942, **142**, 913.
(89) Barton-Wright. *Biochem. Journ.*, 1944, **38**, 314.
(90) Kent-Jones and Meiklejohn. *Analyst*, 1944, **69**, 330.
(91) Stokes, Larsen, Woodward and Foster. *Journ. Biol. Chem.*, 1943, **150**, 17.
(92) Snell, Guirard and Williams. *Journ. Biol. Chem.*, 1942, **143**, 519.
(93) Barton-Wright, Emery and Robinson. *Nature*, 1946, **157**, 628.
(94) Rickes, Brink, Koniusky, Wood and Folkers. *Science*, 1948, **107**, 396.
(95) Smith. *Nature*, 1948, **161**, 638.
(96) Shorb. *Science*, 1948, **107**, 397.
(97) Ungley. *Brit. Med. Journ.*, 1948, *ii*, 154 ; *ibid*, 1949, *ii*, 1370.
(98) Smith and Parker. *Biochem. Journ.*, 1948, **43**, Proc. *viii*.
(99) Fantes, Page, Parker and Smith. *Proc. Roy. Soc.*, 1949, B, **136**, 592.
(100) Smith. *Brit. Med. Journ.*, 1949, *ii*, 1367.
(101) Martin and Synge. *Biochem. Journ.*, 1941, **35**, 1358.
(102) Smith. *Proc. Roy. Soc. Med.*, 1950, **43**, 535.
(103) Rickes, Brink, Koniusky, Wood and Folkers. *Science*, 1948, **108**, 134.
(104) Smith. *Nature*, 1948, **162**, 144.
(105) Martin. *Proc. Nutrition. Soc.*, 1944, *i*, 195.
(106) Rickes, Brink, Koniusky, Wood and Folkers. *Science*, 1948, **108**, 634.
(107) Smith. *Brit. Med. Journ.*, 1951, *i*, 151.
(108) Ungley and Campbell. *Brit. Med. Journ.*, 1951, *i*., 152.
(109) Chalmers. *Brit. Med. Journ.*, 1951, *i*, 161.
(110) West. *Science*, 1948, **107**, 398.
(111) Berk, Denny-Brown, Finland and Castle. *New Eng. Journ. of Med.*, 1948, **239**, 328.
(112) Ungley. *Brain*, 1949, **72**, 382.
(113) Jacobson and Bishop. *Journ. Clin. Invest.*, 1949, **28**, 791.
(114) Abbasy, Hill and Harris. *Lancet*, 1936, *ii*, 1413.
(115) Kaiser. *New York Journ. Med.*, 1938, **38**, 868.
(116) Campbell and Cook. *Brit. Med. Journ.*, 1941, *i*, 360.
(117) Glazebrook and Thomson. *Journ. Hyg. Camb.*, 1942, **42**, 1.
(118) Bourne. *Lancet*, 1942, *ii*, 661.
(119) Harris. *Proc. Roy. Soc. Med.*, 1942, **35**, 618.
(120) Harris and Ray. *Lancet*, 1935, *i*., 71, 462.
Abbasy, Harris, Ray and Marrack. *Lancet*, 1935, *ii*, 1399.
(121) Harris and Abbasy. *Lancet*, 1937, *ii*, 1429.
(122) Ungley. *Lancet*, 1938, *i*, 875.
(123) Lund and Crandon. *Journ. Amer. Med. Assocn.*, 1941, **116**, 663.
(124) Tumulty and Howard. *Journ. Amer. Med. Assocn.*, 1942, **119**, 233.
(125) Albright. *Journ. Amer. Med. Assocn.*, 1941, **117**, 527.
(126) Karrer, Salomon and Frietsche. *Helv. Chim. Acta*, 1938, **21**, 520.
(127) Bergel, Copping, Jacob, Todd and Work. *Journ. Chem. Soc.*, 1938, 1382.
(128) Currie. *Brit. Med. Journ.*, 1937, *ii*., 1218.

(129) DRUMMOND. *Lancet*, 1939, *i*, 699.
(130) BICKNELL. *Lancet*, 1940, *i*, 10.
(131) DEMOLE. *Lancet*, 1940, *i*, 431.
(132) WECHSLER. *Journ. Amer. Med. Assocn.*, 1940, **114**, 948.
(133) SHELDON, BUTT and WOLTMAN. *Proc. Mayo Clinic*, 1940, **15**, 577.
(134) DOYLE and MERRIT. *Arch. Neurol. and Psych.*, 1941, **45**, 672.
(135) DENKER and SCHEINMAN. *Journ. Amer. Med. Assocn.*, 1941, **116**, 1893.
(136) FERREBEE, KLINGMAN and FRANTZ. *Journ. Amer. Med. Assocn.*, 1941, **116**, 1895.
(137) FITZGERALD and MCARDLE. *Brain*, 1941, **64**, 19.
(138) BICKNELL and PRESCOTT. "*The Vitamins in Medicine*," 1946, 2nd Edit. Wm. Heinemann, London.
(139) DAM. *Biochem. Journ.*, 1935, **29**, 1273.
(140) SCHØNHEYDER. *Nature*, 1935, **135**, 653.
(141) DAM, SCHØNHEYDER and TAGE-HANSEN. *Biochem. Journ.*, 1936, **31**, 22.
(142) BRINKHOUS, SMITH and WARNER. *Amer. Journ. Med. Sci.*, 1937, **193**, 475.
(143) BINKLEY, MACCORQUODALE, THAYER and DOISY. *Journ. Biol. Chem.*, 1939, **130**, 219.
(144) BINKLEY, MCKEE, THAYER, and DOISY. *Journ. Biol. Chem.*, 1940, **133**, 721.
(145) STEWART. *Surgery*, 1941, **9**, 212.
(146) SMITH and OWEN. *Journ. Biol. Chem.*, 1940, **134**, 783.
(147) FITZGERALD and WEBSTER. *Amer. Journ. Obstet. and Gynec.*, 1940, **40**, 413.
(148) KARK and SOUTER. *Brit. Med. Journ.*, 1941, *ii*, 191.
(149) LYONS. *Nature*, 1945, **155**, 633.
(150) MELLANBY. *Journ. Physiol.*, 1909, **38**, 28 ; **51**, 396.
(151) SELLS, WALKER and OWEN. *Proc. Soc. Exp. Biol. and Med.*, 1941, **47**, 441.
(152) ALMQUIST and KLOSE. *Journ. Biol. Chem.*, 1939, **130**, 787.
(153) MACFIE, BACHARACH and CHANCE. *Brit. Med. Journ.*, 1939, *ii*, 1220.
(154) KARK and SOUTER. *Lancet*, 1940, *ii*, 1150.
(155) DAM, TAGE-HANSEN and PLUM. *Lancet*, 1939, *ii*, 1157.
(156) SANFORD, SCHMIGELSKY and CHAPIN. *Journ. Amer. Med. Assocn.*, 1942, **118**, 697.
(157) NORRIS and BENNETT. *Surg. Gynec. Obstet.*, 1941, **72**, 758.
(158) LEHMANN. *Lancet*, 1944, *i*, 493.
(159) KARK and LOZNER. *Lancet*, 1939, *ii*, 1162.
(160) SHEELY. *Journ. Amer. Med. Assocn.*, 1941, **117**, 1603.
(161) BUTT and SNELL. "*Vitamin K*," 1941, W. B. Saunders Company, Philadelphia and London.
(162) RODERICK. *Amer. Journ. Physiol.*, 1931, 96, 413.
(163) QUICK. *Amer. Journ. Physiol.*, 1937, **118**, 260.
(164) STAHMAN, HUEBNER and LINK. *Journ. Biol. Chem.*, 1941, **138**, 513.
(165) KRUMER and BARKER. *Proc. Staff Meet. Mayo Clin.*, 1944, **19**, 217.
(166) LUCIA and AGGELER. *Proc. Soc. Exp. Biol. and Med.*, 1944, **56**, 36.
(167) FIELD, BAUMANN and LINK. *Cancer Res.*, 1944, **4**, 768.
(168) ALLEN, BARKER and WAUGH. *Journ. Amer. Med. Assocn.*, 1942, **120**, 1009.
(169) ZUCKER. *Journ. Amer. Med. Assocn.*, 1944, **124**, 217.
(170) DAVIS and PORTER. *Brit. Med. Journ.*, 1944, *i*, 718.

(171) Armentano, Bentsták, Beres, Rusznyák and Szent-Györgyi. *Deutsch. med. Woch.*, 1936, **62**, 1325.
(172) Bacharach and Coates. *Analyst*, 1942, **67**, 313.
(173) Scarborough. *Biochem. Journ.*, 1939, **33**, 1400.
(174) Scarborough. *Lancet*, 1940, *ii*, 644.
(175) Scarborough. *Proc. Roy Soc. Med.*, 1942, **35**, 407.
(176) Kugelmass. *Journ. Amer. Med. Assocn.*, 1940, **115**, 519.

CHAPTER VI

THE LIVER

A General Consideration of Hepatitis

Progress is being made in the classification of liver diseases on an ætiological and pathological basis, and studies over the last ten years both in the human patient and in the experimental animal have led to the discarding of many outworn hypotheses (Himsworth (1)).

Acute Parenchymatous Hepatitis. Pathologically the lesions in this condition are of two types: (*a*) zonal hepatitis (*b*) massive hepatitis.

(*a*) The common response of the liver to any mild noxious agent is a centrilobular zonal necrosis, the damage being *pan-hepatic*: such a noxious agent may be chemical, *e.g.* chloroform (Wilcox (2)), micro-biological, *e.g.* the virus of infective hepatitis, or physical, *i.e.* back-pressure in the hepatic veins in heart failure (Boland and Williams (3)). Especially if the disorder is caused by an infection, as well as the necrosis there is a periportal inflammatory cell reaction. If the damage is slight healing will be complete, the centre of the lobules reconstituting from the undamaged peripheral cells: this is the common course. Repeated attacks of zonal hepatitis may, rarely, lead to the development of the diffuse fibrosis type of "cirrhosis". If the attack is severe, due to a very virulent infection, a massive poisoning, or a liver already weakened by dietary deficiency, then the lesion will rapidly progress to a massive hepatitis.

(*b*) In animals a protein deficient diet alone may be sufficient to cause massive hepatic necrosis (Weichselbaum (4)); in man this probably does not occur. The factors responsible are deficiencies of cystine and of tocopherol. The pathological lesion is complete destruction of parenchymal cells over large parts of the liver, with normal areas (in contrast to the picture in zonal hepatitis) left between the damaged areas. In man the condition presents as acute yellow atrophy; many of the cases are due to an extension of a severe zonal necrosis. T.N.T. and cincophen are poisons very likely to cause massive necrosis (Willcox (2), Himsworth and Glynn (5)). In all these cases malnutrition and protein deficiency predispose to an extension of the necrotic process. Findlay (6) has described an epidemic of infective hepatitis occurring in West Africa in which the mortality rate from massive necrosis was 15 times greater in coloured troops than in white troops, the difference being ascribed to discrepancy in nutritional status. Acute massive necrosis may likewise occur in pregnancy, but in most cases of acute yellow atrophy the causative agent is not known. If severe, acute massive necrosis kills; if less severe the patient will develop a subacute hepatitis; complete recovery of liver structure and of the patient's health does not occur.

Subacute Hepatitis. This condition may be compared with the concept of subacute nephritis, in that it may result from previous non-fatal attacks of acute hepatitis (of the massive necrosis type) of known or unknown ætiology, or it may apparently arise *de novo*. In the latter instance there may be a history of severe bacterial infection elsewhere in the body some years previously; the condition may occur following pregnancy or the menopause; or the patient may have been exposed to an epidemic of infective hepatitis without apparently suffering the acute infection (Barker et al. (7)), the virus surviving in the body and wreaking its damage in stealth. Interruption to the vascular supply of the liver in the initial attack of massive necrosis would leave ischæmic areas more liable to damage by any further noxious factors. Patients rarely die in this stage, the condition progressing to the post-necrotic scarring type of cirrhosis. The pathological picture is of a liver showing lesions of every stage, normal lobules, areas of zonal and of massive necrosis, scarring and hypertrophic nodules resulting from previous acute attacks.

Dietary Deficiency and Liver Disease. It is now considered highly probable that alcohol has no direct toxic action on the liver, liver disease in alcoholics being caused by the deficiency in their diets of the lipotropic factors (principally choline and methionine). The principal reasons for this deficiency are a relative poverty (the patient's income being spent on drink) leading to economies being practised by not buying the needed expensive foods of high protein content, and a gastritis caused by the alcohol diminishing appetite and thus intake of food. In rats identical lesions have been produced by keeping the animals on a lipotropic-factor-deficient diet by feeding them either on alcohol or on sucrose (Best et al. (8)). The pathological lesion is a fatty infiltration of the liver cells, which, if continued over many years, will lead to the diffuse fibrosis type of cirrhosis (Rich et al. (9)). Many alcoholic cirrhotics show a terminal picture of mixed fibrosis and post-necrotic scarring; the latter reaction presumably results from the general protein deficiency of the diet.

Much attention has recently been paid to "Kwashiokor" (Waterlow (10)), a complex multiple deficiency syndrome (steatorrhœa, anæmia, dermatoses) occurring in undernourished children in the tropics. A marked feature of the disease is an enlarged fatty liver, which likewise may progress to diffuse hepatic fibrosis. It is thought that the primary lesion is a pancreatic insufficiency possibly due to protein malnutrition, and that the liver disorder and vitamin deficiencies are secondary to this (Davies (11)).

Cirrhosis of the Liver

Classification of the clinical disorders known collectively as cirrhosis of the liver is still a matter for argument. Three main varieties may be distinguished, and mixed types are commonly found.

Biliary Cirrhosis. Obstruction to the bile passages, if continued, leads to an ascending cholangitis and cholangio-hepatitis, with an inflammatory reaction around each portal tract. If the infection is not severe enough to cause death or gross parenchymal damage, then, in the course of years, the lesion develops into a periportal unilobular fibrosis, without any gross disorganisation of lobular architecture or hyperplastic nodules.

Diffuse Fibrosis. As an after-effect of repeated attacks of zonal hepatitis or of fatty infiltration of the liver from any cause fibrosis develops, linking portal and centrilobular tracts. Although the fibrosis is apparently unilobular, it differs from biliary cirrhosis as the fibrous bands intersect the individual lobules and disorganise the architectural structure. Unless complicated by associated sequelæ of subacute hepatitis, hyperplastic nodules are absent. Clinically the condition may take ten years or more to develop, and when discovered (*e.g.* by the appearance of portal hypertension) is usually compatible with several more years of active life; the liver is not grossly enlarged and its surface is only finely granular.

Post-necrotic Scarring. Subacute hepatitis generally progresses to a classical coarse cirrhosis. The liver is irregularly intersected by bands of fibrous tissue, separating hyperplastic nodules of regenerated parenchyma from the occasional normal lobule. Clinically the condition usually develops within ten years of the initial lesions, and once portal hypertension sets in the prognosis is poor. The liver is often grossly enlarged and the surface very irregular.

Cirrhosis of the Liver in Syphilis. In this disease two characteristic types of cirrhosis may be met, unrelated to the main classification, a diffuse pericellular fibrosis in congenital syphilis, and *hepar lobatum* in tertiary syphilis.

Infective Hepatitis

Relationship to Catarrhal Jaundice. Epidemics of jaundice have been described for many years. In 1912 Cockayne (12) writing on sporadic and epidemic catarrhal jaundice, gave a historical review of epidemic catarrhal jaundice, one of the earliest references being to an outbreak in Minorca in 1745. In the British Isles epidemics have been recorded since the Birmingham outbreak in 1852. Each major war has witnessed similar epidemics; they were recorded in the siege of Paris in 1870, in the Boer War, in Gallipoli during the 1914–18 war, and again in the 1939–45 war, chiefly in the Mediterranean theatre of operations.

Cockayne concluded that simple catarrhal jaundice, usually ascribed to gastro-duodenal catarrh, is, except in a comparatively small number of cases, the sporadic or endemic form of epidemic catarrhal jaundice. He thought that the infection was air-borne, that the incubation period was short, about five days, and that there was often a preliminary stage of naso-pharyngeal catarrh. Cockayne further considered that the liver was probably infected through the blood stream, and that inflammation may spread down the bile duct giving rise to catarrhal changes with obstruction. This corresponds very closely with the view now held by many that catarrhal jaundice is a sporadic form of infective hepatitis, and that in all cases the liver is affected by a blood-borne icterogenic agent, probably a virus.

The evidence, however, still exists that isolated cases of catarrhal jaundice are due to gastro-duodenal or bile duct catarrh, and we should not readily accept *ex-cathedra* statements to the contrary. Virchow (13) in 1865 supported the view that in catarrhal jaundice there is a state of duodenal catarrh involving the ampulla of Vater, with plugging of the orifice of the common bile duct with mucus. In 1908 Eppinger (14) described the post-mortem findings in a girl nineteen years of age who committed suicide by throwing herself out of a third floor window during an attack of jaundice associated with gastro-enteritis. The liver was enlarged and icteric and showed typical changes of mechanical jaundice. The common bile duct contained dark coloured and very viscous bile. The mucous membrane of the stomach showed hæmorrhages. The walls of the duodenum were catarrhal, and its contents colourless. The papilla of Vater was prominent. Bile could not be forced through the common bile duct by strong pressure on the distended gall-bladder. Eppinger thought the obstruction was due to swollen lymphoid tissue near the ampulla of Vater and also at the junction of the cystic duct with the common bile duct.

On clinical grounds also certain authorities consider that catarrhal jaundice differs from infective hepatitis, for in catarrhal jaundice prodromal symptoms, apart from depression, are slight, the patient first taking to his bed when the jaundice is manifest. In infective hepatitis, on the other hand, the patient is ill, feverish, and confined to bed for several days before the jaundice appears.

More recently, Dible, McMichael and Sherlock (15), by aspiration biopsy observations on the liver, have found changes in sporadic cases of jaundice identical with those met with in infective hepatitis. Further, Van Rooyen and Gordon (16) by duodenal intubation studies in 11 cases of infective hepatitis found no evidence of duodeno-biliary catarrh. These experiments offer no proof that catarrhal jaundice, due to primary extra-hepatic catarrhal obstruction of the bile ducts, is a myth, as some would have us believe. All they show is that the cases investigated, which were assumed to be representative of catarrhal jaundice, were in reality examples of inflammatory hepatitis. It seems probable therefore that we should not be wise in abandoning Virchow's concept of catarrhal jaundice, and that, as Boyd (17) writes, " the basis of catarrhal jaundice may be (1) catarrhal obstruction of the opening of the bile duct, (2) toxic necrosis of the liver, and (3) cholangitis. Providing these lesions are transient, the jaundice will be catarrhal in type."

Epidemiology. Attention was again drawn to outbreaks of jaundice in England by Pickles (18) in 1930. He gave an account of 250 cases of epidemic jaundice in Wensleydale. The characteristic features were a pre-icteric phase, lasting from four to ten days, during which the patient suffered from nausea, vomiting, and pains in the back and limbs. This was followed by an icteric stage of about fourteen days. Pickles considered that the incubation period varied from twenty-six to thirty-five days, that the period of infectivity was short, and that the method of spread was respiratory, probably by droplet infection. In 1942 Newman (19) described an outbreak in the Lavant valley, in Sussex, but he did not hold that the droplet theory of infection was entirely satisfactory. Fraser (20) in 1931 had brought forward evidence that the disease might be spread by water, and further evidence in favour of this view will be referred to later. Cookson (21) in 1944 reported an epidemic of 246 cases in Gloucestershire, chiefly amongst children attending elementary schools, or living in nurseries. He rejected the idea that the infection was water-borne. During the 1939–45 war, outbreaks of infective hepatitis occurred, especially amongst the troops in Syria, North Africa and Italy. An interesting account of over 1,000 cases of infective hepatitis amongst American troops in the Mediterranean area was given by Barker, Capps and Allen (7) in 1945. The epidemic occurred between February and November, 1944.

Ætiology. It has not been found possible to transmit the disease to animals, although Anderson (22) and Hallgren (23) reported the successful transmission of infective hepatitis to the pig, but other observers have failed to repeat the experiment. It is usually thought that the icterogenic agent is a virus. Hallgren (23) in 1942 published an account of epidemic hepatitis in the county of Västerbotten in Northern Sweden. In an outbreak at the Hällnäs Sanatorium evidence was obtained that the infection was water-borne, a corroded sewer having contaminated the well from which the drinking water was obtained. Thirty-four days after the infected well had been excluded, the epidemic came to an end. No new cases developed amongst 188 fresh patients who arrived after the exclusion of the well, although they were in contact with large numbers of sufferers from infective hepatitis. It was found that 32% of those exposed to infection were susceptible. A pig was given water from the polluted well and subsequently killed. Microscopical examination revealed necrotic and inflammatory liver changes resembling those of infective hepatitis, whereas nine control pigs showed normal livers. Cameron (24) injected intramuscularly six volunteers with 1 to 2 ml. of whole blood or serum obtained from patients suffering from infective hepatitis in Palestine. One man developed jaundice in a month, one within two months, and the other four within six months. As there was infective hepatitis in the district it was not possible to say that all the cases were due to the inoculations. Sheehan (25) in 1944 suggested that the icterogenic agent was conveyed by biting insects, but this view has not been supported by other workers.

Neefe and Stokes (26) recorded an outbreak of infective hepatitis in a summer camp for boys and girls in the Pocono mountains, near Philadelphia. Out of a population of 573 there were 350 cases. It was shown that the water of the girls' well was contaminated by fæces from cesspools. Healthy volunteers were then inoculated with serum, naso-pharyngeal washings, urine, fæces and the infected water. It was shown that the icterogenic agent was present in the serum, fæces and infected water. The serum produced the disease in the human volunteers only when given orally, and not when injected parenterally. The incubation period was similar to that occurring in the epidemics. The agent in the fæces passed through a Seitz filter. No evidence was obtained of the transmission of the infection by biting insects. It was concluded that it was improbable that the infection was transmitted to the majority of persons by air, fomites, food, milk or directly from infected persons. Havens et al. (27) in 1945 also showed that the icterogenic agent is present in fæces, and that the disease can be reproduced in man by feeding such material in gelatin capsules or by spraying it into the nasal and pharyngeal passages. Further, jaundice can be produced by feeding serum from cases of infective hepatitis. The average incubation period was twenty-eight days. The ætiological agent, probably a virus, is in the blood stream before the onset of, and during the jaundice. It is present in the fæces during the acute stage of the disease, and it probably also occurs in the nasal washings. It is filtrable, and markedly heat-stable, resisting a temperature of 56° C. for half an hour. Infection can probably be spread by flies contaminated by infected excreta, as is the case with typhoid fever. Findlay and Willcox (28) also showed that the oral ingestion of fæces or urine, derived from spontaneous cases of infective hepatitis will cause typical icteric and sub-icteric cases of the disease. Seventeen volunteers were given to drink 30 to 50 ml. of urine mixed with an equal quantity of milk, and 5 developed hepatitis. Further, 3 g. of fæces were ground up in 250 ml. of milk and 50 ml. were given to each volunteer to drink on an empty stomach. Positive results were obtained in 11 out of 47 cases.

Alcohol appears to play a part predisposing to infective hepatitis. In the Services the disease had a higher incidence amongst officers than amongst other ranks, possibly due to the greater amount of spirits consumed by the former. Hartfall (29) gives examples of the deleterious effects of alcohol " upon an individual who is incubating the disease, in provoking an overt attack, or in worsening or prolonging an attack otherwise mild, and in causing a relapse or second delayed attack of jaundice ".

Pathology. The disease is probably a systemic infection with a predilection for the liver. Dible, McMichael and Sherlock (15) studied the pathology of acute hepatitis in 56 cases by aspiration biopsy, and found no histological criteria for differentiating the lesions resulting from epidemic hepatitis, arsenotherapy and serum inoculations. The cells of the hepatic lobules show evidence of necrosis and autolysis. In the areas around the central veins there is rarefaction due to the disappearance of liver cells. Small mononuclear cells of the histiocytic class, with some polymorphonuclears and eosinophils, tend to accumulate in the portal zones. These infiltrations may spread around the periphery of the lobules. There is enlargement and hyperplasia of the sinusoidal " endothelial " cells. There does not appear to be any fatty change in the cells. In over a third of the cases proliferation of the bile ducts was seen in the portal tracts. It appears that in the early stages the lesion is chiefly limited to the portal zone, with little destruction of the liver lobule. The liver inflammation probably begins with the prodromal symptoms. Bile thrombi may be seen in the intralobular bile canaliculi. In some cases a permanent cirrhosis develops, in others there is a mild residual fibrosis, which may ultimately completely resolve.

Clinical Findings. The mode of onset, course and severity of the illness are variable. Four clinical modes of onset have been recognised: (1) Insidious, with anorexia and gastro-intestinal symptoms; there is a low grade pyrexia, usually under 100° F., and jaundice appears after three or four days. (2) Febrile, the temperature rising suddenly at the onset to 101° to 103° F. Jaundice occurs two to four days later. (3) Ambulatory, the patient continuing with his work until he is noticed to be jaundiced. (4) Hepatitis without any manifest jaundice. Hartfall (29) in Malta observed that in 53% the onset was insidious, and in 30% it conformed to the febrile type. Barker, Capps and Allen (7) in the Mediterranean theatre found that amongst American troops in over 80% of cases there was an acute febrile onset, the temperature rising to 100° to 103° F., associated with malaise, headache, lassitude, anorexia, nausea and vomiting. The patient complained of chilly sensations, rarely of rigors, with abdominal discomfort and pains and tenderness in the epigastrium and right hypochondrium. Urticaria, morbilliform rashes and arthralgia were occasionally met with. After three or four days the temperature fell to normal, the liver gradually enlarging and becoming tender. The spleen was rarely palpable. Constipation and diarrhœa were equally common. This pre-icteric stage was followed five to ten days later by the icteric stage, the temperature again rising. Nausea and abdominal discomfort were more marked, the jaundice lasting from two to four weeks or in some cases for three months or even longer. In the average case recovery was complete in from six to eight weeks. In this outbreak the stools were rarely clay-coloured, in other epidemics pasty stools were the rule. Cameron (24) in an outbreak in Palestine amongst the troops found the liver enlarged in 97 out of 170 patients, and the spleen enlarged in forty-six cases. Clay-coloured stools were found in half the cases, in 12 cases the stools were normal in colour, in the remainder they were light coloured. In fatal cases, which are rare, the jaundice becomes more intense, hæmorrhages may be seen in the skin, or there may be pulmonary or intestinal bleeding, and, in some cases, ascites develops. The patient becomes irrational and dies in coma.

Nervous complications are uncommon, but meningitis, encephalitis, polyneuritis, myelitis and upper motor lesions of the pyramidal and striatal type have been described by Lescher (30), Byrne and Taylor (31), and Stokes, Owen and Holmes (32). In none of these cases could it be proved that the nervous lesions were in reality due to the icterogenic agent, in all they might have been due to intercurrent causes. The death rate from infective hepatitis is very low, but in the Mediterranean area it was higher in native than in white troops. Relapses are rare, but we have seen one patient who had three relapses and died suddenly from hæmorrhage due to ruptured œsophageal varices.

Infective hepatitis may not be the innocuous disease that was once thought and, as described above, the sequence of pathological changes leading to one or other form of cirrhosis of the liver has been reported by many workers. Wang (33) found that of 447 autopsies of cirrhosis of the liver over a period of sixteen years, 42 could be definitely attributed to previous hepatitis. Similarly Rosenak et al. (34) elucidated a history of jaundice in 14 out of 106 cases of cirrhosis and Howard and Watson (35) confirm the high proportion compared with a control series. Further pathological studies of cirrhosis following hepatitis are reported by Wyllie and Edmunds (36) on 5 fatal cases in children ; they conclude that it is impossible to tell in the icteric stage which cases will go on to cirrhosis : Sherlock (37) stresses the value of liver biopsy as a guide to progesss in a study of 9 cases of cirrhosis following acute hepatitis.

Laboratory Findings. *The Blood.* The white cell count is normal or there is a slight leucopenia. A leucocytosis would indicate that the diagnosis is probably incorrect, and leucocytosis is a feature of Weil's disease. The sedimentation rate of the red cells was found by Miles (38) to be usually normal during the icteric stage of the disease, but often raised in the pre-icteric period and during convalescence. This author suggests that an excess of bile salts in the blood is responsible for the low sedimentation rate during the active phase of infective hepatitis. Barker, Capps and Allen (7) also reported that the sedimentation rate is usually normal in the presence of jaundice. Evans (39) found that the sedimentation rate may remain raised for some weeks after an attack. Hoagland and Shank (40) in a series of 163 cases found that the sedimentation rate was normal or only slightly raised, during the first days of the disease, but frequently raised to values of 25 to 55 mm. per hour during convalescence and gradually falling to normal late in the period of recovery. The serum bilirubin is generally normal during the pre-icteric stage, rising later to levels of 10 mg./100 ml. or higher, according to the intensity of the jaundice. The Van den

Bergh test usually gives a positive direct and indirect reaction falling to normal after about forty days or less.

The Urine. During the pre-icteric stage urobilinogen may, or may not be found in the urine; with the onset of overt jaundice bilirubinuria occurs.

Liver Function Tests. Pollock (41) using the intravenous hippuric acid test found that the synthesis was to a large extent correlated with the severity of the attack and the stage of the disease, but varied only partly and indirectly with the serum bilirubin concentration. The hippuric acid synthesis was noted to be improving while the bilirubin level was still rising, and it appeared that liver damage was probably present in the pre-icteric period. Gordon (42) employing the oral hippuric acid test found evidence of impaired liver function in all of 14 cases examined during the first three weeks of jaundice. Barker, Capps and Allen (7) observed that the bromsulphthalein test was positive in all cases examined during the first five weeks of the illness, and the colloidal gold test was usually positive during the icteric stage. Hallgren (23) found that the galactose tolerance test was positive in 12% of cases. Britton (43), using his special technique for the Takata-Ara test, found a positive reaction beginning within two to three days of the onset of the jaundice, the strength of the reaction following closely the severity of the liver damage and the course of recovery.

Differential Diagnosis. During the pre-icteric stage infective hepatitis may be mistaken for influenza, gastro-enteritis, sand-fly fever, malaria, meningitis, acute appendicitis, enterica group infections, or an alchoholic " hang-over ".

Treatment. *Prophylactic.* Gamma globulin, obtained from large pools of adult human serum, was found by Stokes and Neefe (44) to be a potent agent in the prevention or attenuation of infective hepatitis, if injected during the incubation period. Gellis et al. (45) confirmed this view in two epidemics in the Mediterranean theatre of operation. This beneficial effect is possibly due to neutralising antibodies present in the gamma globulin. Over 1,700 men were inoculated intramuscularly with 10 ml. of globulin, and more than 10,000 men served as controls. The inoculated belonged to units in which the disease was already rife. The incidence of hepatitis in those injected was 0·6%, but of the uninoculated 3% became infected.

Curative. Complete rest in bed from the onset appears to shorten the course of the disease in the majority of cases. It is usually advised that the diet should be high in protein (200 g.) and in carbohydrate (400 g.) and low in fat (40 g.). Darmady (46), on the other hand, considered that there is no difference in the results of treatment whether a high or a low protein diet is given. A light diet with plenty of milk, from which the top layer of cream has been removed, is usually perfectly suitable. During the acute stage the patient should take fluids up to 5 pints a day. If this amount cannot be taken by mouth, 10% dextrose in water should be given intravenously, or if vomiting persists 5% dextrose in saline should be transfused to make up the deficiency. If there are hæmorrhages or if the plasma prothrombin content is low, vitamin K should be injected intramuscularly in doses of 5 mg. daily, and for serious hæmorrhage a blood transfusion should be given. The patient should take no alcohol during the disease or for a year subsequently. Methionine, an essential amino-acid, and a lipotropic factor which promotes the transfer of fat from the liver to the storage depots, has been recommended as an aid to treatment, but Wilson, Pollock and Harris (47) giving 5 g. of methionine daily by mouth to alternate patients in a series of 100 cases of infective hepatitis found that the methionine, as judged by clinical and biochemical criteria, had no significant effect upon the severity or duration of the disease, or the incidence of relapses. Similar results were obtained by Higgins et al. (48). Aureomycin has been tried in the treatment of infective hepatitis. It appears to have no curative effect in the acute phase, but was reported as being somewhat beneficial in the treatment of coma or of chronic liver disease. (Farquhar et al. (49); Shaffer et al. (50)). Finally, the patient should not be allowed to get up until the temperature is normal, the liver has returned to its accustomed size and is no longer tender, there are no symptoms such as lassitude and nausea, and the serum bilirubin has been normal for a week.

Treatment of the cirrhotic stage is the same as treatment of cirrhosis of the liver of other ætiology—rest and a basic diet (containing ample quantities of the vitamin B complex) are probably still the most important factors (Klatski and Yesner (51)). Ralli et al. (52) report that treatment of cirrhosis for three years with intravenous liver extract resulted in a 44% survival rate, against 12% in an untreated control series. Schemm and Layne (53) found a high fluid intake and an acid ash and low sodium diet valuable in the removal of ascites, whilst infusion of salt-poor human albumin is not generally recommended (Faloon et al. (54)). Rosenak et al. (55) used testosterone propionate in doses of 25–100 mg. three times weekly: this caused a marked improvement in their patients' feeling of general well-being.

Homologous Serum Jaundice

It is believed that homologous serum jaundice results from the introduction of an icterogenic substance into man by the injection of human blood, serum, or plasma. The amount of serum injected may be very small, as little as 0·05 ml.

As far back as 1885 Lurman (56) reported an outbreak of jaundice following vaccination against small-pox with "glycerinated humanised" lymph. Out of 1,289 workers so vaccinated, in a ship-building yard at Bremen 191 developed jaundice several weeks later, whereas 500 others, vaccinated with a different batch of lymph, were unaffected.

We now know that homologous serum jaundice may arise in a variety of ways, of which the following are the most important:—By the injection of yellow fever vaccine prepared with human serum; as the result of prophylactic inoculation with measles convalescent serum or mumps convalescent plasma; and following transfusion with whole blood, plasma or serum. It may also result from the use of syringes contaminated with infected blood, and employed either for intravenous, intramuscular or subcutaneous injections, or for removing blood by venepuncture. This latter group includes post-arsenical jaundice occurring in veneral disease clinics, jaundice following the injection of penicillin or Pentothal, and occasional outbreaks of jaundice in clinics for the treatment of diabetes mellitus and arthritis, or in sanatoria. These varieties will now be considered in more detail.

Jaundice following Yellow Fever Vaccination. Findlay and MacCallum (57) in 1937, and subsequently, drew attention to the occurrence of jaundice following immunisation against yellow fever with a vaccine consisting of yellow fever virus suspended in human serum. They observed 89 cases among 3,100 persons immunised over a period of five years, the latent period varying between thirty-six days and seven months, and averaging between two and three months. They showed that the occurrence of the jaundice was not directly due to an infection with the yellow fever virus, and considered that there was presumptive evidence that the post-inoculation jaundice was identical with infective hepatic jaundice. Findlay, MacCallum and Murgatroyd (58) later showed that the icterogenic agent bore no relationship to the strain of yellow fever virus used, but that experiments suggested the presence of an extraneous virus in the human serum used in the preparation of the vaccine. In 1939 Fox, Manso, Penna and Para (59) published an account of an outbreak of inoculation jaundice in Brazil, after over a million people had been inoculated there against yellow fever. Out of a group of 304 persons inoculated with one batch of vaccine, 27% developed jaundice four to five months later, one case proving fatal. The occurrence between January 1st and July 1st in 1942 of 28,585 cases of jaundice, 62 of which proved fatal, out of between two and two and a half million American troops inoculated against yellow fever, was commented on in Editorials in the American medical press (60). Widespread attention was directed to this variety of jaundice, which was again shown to be due to the presence of an icterogenic agent in the serum used as a vehicle in the preparation of the vaccine. The latent period in this series varied between twelve and eighteen weeks. In 1944 Findlay, Martin and Mitchell (61) reported on a series of 689 cases of jaundice following yellow fever vaccine injections given during 1942, the average latent period being 101·5 days. There was one fatal case. Human serum is no longer used in the preparation of the vaccine and this type of jaundice has now ceased.

Jaundice following Measles Convalescent Serum. In the Annual Report of the Chief Medical Officer of Health for 1937 (62) there was a brief account of the occurrence of 37 cases of jaundice, 7 of which proved fatal, 16 to 100 days after the injection of measles convalescent serum from two small batches into between 82 and 109 recipients. Propert (63) in 1938 drew attention to the cases of 7 children inoculated with convalescent measles serum of the same batch, who all developed jaundice 78 to 83 days later, 3 cases proving fatal. The pooled serum used was the same as that referred to in the Ministry of Health report. A fuller account was reconstructed from contemporaneous records and published in a Memorandum from the Ministry of Health in 1943 (64), as the matter was now considered to be one of major importance. It was thought that the jaundice was due to the injection of human blood products, and that probably further cases would occur, particularly after transfusion, and such indeed has proved to be the case. Cockburn et al. (65) have reported some cases of homologous serum hepatitis following measles prophylaxis, using dried human plasma. Ten children were inoculated using a batch of plasma which was subsequently found to be icterogenic. Seven of the children developed a severe form of jaundice, and three of the seven died. One of the fatal cases had symptoms of encephalitis without apparent jaundice.

Jaundice following Mumps Convalescent Plasma. Beeson, Chesney and McFarlan (66) in 1944 reported the occurrence of 101 cases of jaundice following the inoculation of 266 men with mumps convalescent plasma. The onset was in the majority of cases between the fifty-ninth and ninety-fourth day after inoculation. The jaundice was considered to be due to a hepatoxic agent in two batches of plasma.

Jaundice following Transfusion. Cases of jaundice following at an interval of about three months after blood transfusions were recognised in England in 1942. Morgan and Williamson (66) reported that 9 patients who were treated with large transfusions of plasma or serum, 7 suffering from intermittent claudication, 1 from diabetes mellitus with gangrene of the toes, and 1 from calcinosis circumscripta, developed jaundice seven to ten weeks later. It was not possible to trace the icterogenic agent to definite batches of serum or plasma. The authors stated that the jaundice might be due to a virus or to some toxic chemical substance, such as altered plasma protein, but there was no evidence to favour one or other of these hypotheses. Beeson (68) in America, in 1943, reported 7 cases of jaundice occurring one to four months after the transfusion of whole blood or plasma, and concluded that isolated cases may not infrequently be met with. Steiner (69) also recorded 5 cases of jaundice following transfusions with whole blood or human plasma, given to soldiers when they were wounded two to three months previously. There was no proof in any case that an icterogenic agent was transferred by the transfusion, the evidence being purely presumptive.

In a series of 760 recipients of transfusion of "large-pool" plasma, Lehane et al. (70) found 54 cases (11·9%) in whom jaundice was a sequela: in their opinion 0·35% of donors carry the icterogenic virus.

We now pass on to the other type of serum jaundice, in which it is believed that the causative agent is transmitted by contaminated syringes.

Post-arsenical Jaundice. Bigger (71), in 1943, drew attention to the increased incidence of post-arsenical jaundice in venereal disease clinics. In one of these the case incidence rose from 4·2% in 1941 to 16·5% in 1942. Beattie and Marshall (72) found an incidence of over 50% of post-arsenical jaundice at a clinic in 1942 and 1943, the jaundice usually developing between the ninety-first and one hundred and sixty-sixth day from the first injection. Bigger (71) showed that the icterogenic agent was probably transmitted by syringes contaminated by a trace of blood from an infective patient, and hence the term "syringe jaundice" or "syringe-transmitted hepatitis" came into use. When an intravenous injection is given a minute amount of blood enters the syringe after the needle is put into the vein, and Bigger, using in his experiments citrated blood contaminated with staphylococci, showed that the methods in use at the clinics for sterilising the syringes, such as soaking in 1/1,000 biniodide of mercury, and washing in four changes of water, were not adequate to remove minute quantities of infected material. He recommended that the syringes should be boiled between each patient. It was subsequently proposed by the Medical Research Council Syringe Sterilisation Committee that all-glass syringes should be sterilised by dry heat at 160° C. for an hour. Salaman, King, Williams and Nicol (73) suggested that the increase in post-arsenical jaundice during these years might be due to a variety of causes, such as a shortage of syringes and an increase in the number of patients, with a consequent diminution of the time the syringes could be soaked in disinfectants, and also to an increased incidence of infective hepatitis, if we accept the theory that the blood from patients incubating infective hepatitis is the source of the icterogenic agent. There is a further possibility, the low protein content of the war-time diet or increased alcoholic consumption may have diminished the resistance of the liver to the icterogenic agent. Sheehan (25) observed that some orderlies at a venereal disease clinic, who helped in the injections and had their hands contaminated with blood from the patients, developed jaundice, presumably through scratches in the skin. Beattie and Marshall (72) tried to lower the incidence of post-arsenical jaundice at a clinic by giving the patients a casein digest, a casein digest with cystine, or methionine. These measures had no effect on the over-all incidence of liver damage and jaundice, but tended to shift its incidence to later in the course of treatment, and to render the jaundice less severe.

Jaundice following the Injection of Pentothal and Penicillin. Darmady and Hardwick (74) observed 6 cases of jaundice following the intravenous injection of Pentothal between thirty-one and one hundred and fifty-one days previously, and 4 cases sixty-four to one hundred and thirteen days after the intramuscular injection of penicillin for the treatment of gonorrhœa or syphilis. They suggested that here again the jaundice resulted from the use of " dirty " syringes. They further considered that some cases of transfusion hepatitis may be due to the same cause and not to the blood injected, Pentothal or penicillin having been given at the time of the transfusion. Howells and Kerr (75) treated 47 patients suffering from jaundice, who had previously received injections of penicillin, the average latent period being 97 days. Of these cases, 41 had been given penicillin for the treatment of gonorrhœa or syphilis. They concluded " that penicillin is not the direct cause of the hepatitis, which may be due to some icterogenic agent—*e.g.* a virus—transmitted by faulty injection technique ".

Jaundice following the Withdrawal of Blood. Graham (76) was puzzled by the occurrence of 28 cases of jaundice developing during a period of two and a half years in patients suffering from diabetes mellitus, treated at hospital, none being noted in private patients during the same period. He wrote, " I have come to the conclusion that the jaundice must be due to an infective agent passed from patient to patient at hospital." He suspected that the infection was conveyed by the syringes. This might have occured when blood was removed for sugar estimations, or when insulin was injected. Droller (77) described an outbreak of jaundice in a diabetes clinic in which 62 patients were affected during a period of two years, 4 of the cases proving fatal. Blood was collected for sugar estimations in syringes which were not boiled, and it was thought that small amounts of infective material might have contaminated the needles. Damodaran and Hartfall (78) observed cases of jaundice in a clinic at which patients suffering from arthritis were treated with gold injections. They do not state whether blood was removed for sedimentation readings. In 1935 there were no cases of jaundice, but later, when there was a sparse outbreak of infective hepatitis, up to 9·4% of the patients at the clinic developed jaundice. They did not recognise infected syringes as a possible cause of the jaundice. Sheehan (25) in the same year reported cases of jaundice occurring in a sanatorium. It was noted that a patient who developed jaundice had had a vein puncture for the estimation of the sedimentation rate of the red cells about three months earlier, and on the same day as another patient in the ward who was destined to develop jaundice a month or two later, the incubation period being therefore about twelve weeks. In all these cases it is is probable that the syringe was contaminated by a small quantity of blood containing the icterogenic agent, and that, as was shown by Mendelssohn and Witts (79), on removing the needle from the vein, if the tourniquet is released before the needle is withdrawn, a small quantity of blood is sucked back from the needle and the syringe into the vein. If the syringe, therefore, is not sterile, the patient is exposed to infection.

The Nature of the Icterogenic Agent. It has been suggested that infective hepatitis and homologous serum jaundice are both due to the same agent, a virus, but there is no proof of this view. There is, indeed, evidence that the two conditions are dissimilar and result from different causes.

The icterogenic agent has been found to behave in many respects like a virus ; it passes through Seitz filter-pads, and resists freezing and drying for long periods, but it has never been transmitted to the lower animals. Findlay and Martin (80) in 1943 instilled nasal washings from patients suffering from jaundice following yellow fever inoculation intranasally into volunteers. In 3 out of 4 instances jaundice resulted at intervals of twenty-eight, thirty and fifty-six days. They suggested that infective hepatitis and homologous serum jaundice are due to the same virus, the difference in the incubation period being due to the infection occurring intranasally in infective hepatitis, and by subcutaneous injection in homologous serum jaundice Findlay, Martin and

Mitchell (61) in 1944 failed to produce jaundice in volunteers by the intranasal instillation of whole blood or the subcutaneous injection of whole blood from patients suffering from post-inoculation jaundice. MacCallum and Bauer (81) showed that serum from a presumed case of homologous serum jaundice was icterogenic when inoculated subcutaneously or intramuscularly into a volunteer, on the seventh day after the onset of jaundice, but not so fifty-nine and one hundred and thirty-four days later. A further point in favour of the view that infective hepatitis and serum jaundice are manifestations of the same disease is afforded by the work of Dible, McMichael and Sherlock (15). They examined microscopically specimens obtained by liver puncture, and could detect no difference in the appearance of the liver in infective hepatitis, post-arsenical jaundice, and serum jaundice. On the other hand there is evidence that infective hepatitis and serum jaundice are not due to the same virus. Homologous serum jaundice does not afford immunity against infective hepatitis. Sufferers from serum jaundice have not been proved to infect contacts, although there is some evidence that this may very occasionally happen. The incubation period of the two diseases is very different, about thirty days for infective hepatitis, and about one hundred days for serum jaundice. Some authorities have also pointed out differences in the clinical features, especially the occurrence of erythema multiforme, stiff joints, splenomegaly, and the usually apyrexial course in serum jaundice. MacCallum (82) has summed up the position as follows : "There are many debatable points in favour of and against the identity of infective hepatitis and homologous serum jaundice, but there is no conclusive evidence one way or the other. It is essential to find a satisfactory susceptible experimental animal before much further knowledge can be obtained."

Liver Puncture Biopsy

Historical. One of the earliest recorded examples of diagnostic liver puncture is that performed by Stanley (83) in 1833 for drainage of a hepatic abscess. In 1895 Lucatello (84) introduced the practice of exploratory puncture of the liver using a needle 1 mm. in diameter. The little fragments withdrawn were then lacerated and examined fresh, but it was not possible to establish a histo-pathological diagnosis of the disease process. Von Hansemann (85) in 1904 used a special trocar to obtain small fragments of liver tissue, and by this method made a diagnosis of syphilis of the liver. In 1927 Shupfer (86) employed a special bevelled needle with an internal diameter of 1·4 mm. attached to a 10 ml. syringe. By this means he obtained specimens of liver up to 2 cm. in length, which were usually sufficient for a histological diagnosis. Iversen and Roholm (87) in 1939 introduced their method of liver puncture, with a cannula of 2 mm. bore, through which they aspirated specimens of liver tissue, suitable for paraffin sections and histological examination. This has lead to a widespread use of aspiration liver biopsy as a reliable aid to diagnosis.

The Indications. Aspiration, or, as it is sometimes called, needle liver biopsy, is of value in enabling the nature of pathological changes in the liver to be determined during life, without the necessity of a laparotomy. By this procedure many conditions affecting the liver may be diagnosed, amongst which may be mentioned infective hepatitis, obstructive jaundice, cirrhosis, neoplasms, fatty changes, amyloidosis, sarcoidosis, leukæmia, Gaucher's disease, reticuloses, miliary tuberculosis, Kala-azar, schistosomiasis, hæmochromatosis, infectious mononucleosis, and brucellosis.

The Contra-indications. Because of the risk of spreading infection it is wise not to perform liver puncture in suspected cases of liver abscess or hydatid disease, or if there is infection in the lungs or pleura. It is contra-indicated if there is severe anæmia or a tendency to bleeding which does not respond to treatment. It is also best avoided when the liver dulness cannot be delineated by percussion owing to emphysema, or in ascites, unless the fluid has been previously removed. It should never be attempted if the patient is uncooperative, and unwilling or unable to hold his breath. Some authorities, such as Cogswell et al. (88), consider it unwise to perform liver biopsy in passive congestion due to heart failure, owing to the possibly increased risk of bleeding.

The Method. The prothrombin, bleeding and clotting times and the blood group of the patient should be determined, and two pints of compatible blood should be at hand with facilities for transfusion in case of hæmorrhage following the puncture. Twenty mg. of Synkavit are injected intramuscularly daily for three days, or longer if necessary, before the biopsy is performed. The puncture should not be made until or unless the prothrombin, bleeding and clotting times are normal. If there is ascites the fluid should be aspirated so that the liver comes in close apposition to the chest wall. It is usually recommended that morphine sulphate gr. 1/6 to 1/4 should be injected subcutaneously half an hour before the operation, but in cases of advanced cirrhosis such a dose of morphine may prove dangerous or even fatal, and should not be given. In such instances sodium phenobarbitone gr. 1 in 1 ml. of water may be injected intramuscularly half an hour before the puncture. The patient lies in bed on his back, with his right hand behind his head, the side of the chest parallel with the edge of the bed, and the left buttock raised on a pillow, so as to tilt the body slightly to the right. The upper limit of the hepatic dulness is percussed out, with the breath held in full expiration, and the puncture site selected one intercostal space below the upper border of the liver dulness, just behind the anterior axillary line. This is usually the seventh intercostal space. The skin over the proposed site of puncture is painted with iodine, and the skin, subcutaneous tissues, intercostal muscles, pleura, diaphragm and peritoneum, down to the capsule of the liver, are freely infiltrated with at least 10 ml. of 2% procaine hydrochloride solution. The patient should now be instructed how to breathe in, breathe out deeply, and then stop breathing. It is explained that he will be told to do this when the puncture is being made, and that he must hold his breath in full expiration until the word is given that he may breathe again.

For the puncture a trocar with a handle and cannula are used. The cannula is 15 cm. long, with a bore of 1·8 mm., and its end is bevelled and sharp. It is fitted with a metal guard, and can be attached by an adaptor to a 20 ml. all-glass syringe. The skin at the site of the puncture is nicked with a tenotomy knife, and the sterilised trocar and cannula are pushed slowly through the intercostal space until the transmitted respiratory movements indicate that the diaphragm has been reached. The guard is now adjusted to allow the cannula to be pushed 3 cm. into the liver, the trocar is withdrawn and the syringe is fitted to the cannula. The patient is now told to breathe in, breathe out fully, and stop breathing. It is essential for him to realise that he must hold his breath until told he may breathe again. The cannula is now inserted sharply, and with a slight twisting movement, into the liver until the guard is in contact with the skin. The syringe plunger is withdrawn, and the cannula and syringe removed, maintaining suction as this is done. The patient is now told he may breathe again. The cannula is only in the liver for about five seconds. The biopsy specimen is found either in the cannula or in the syringe and is placed in a specimen bottle containing 10% formol in saline. The wound is sealed with collodion, and the patient instructed to lie flat for twenty-four hours. The pulse rate should be taken every fifteen minutes for two hours and every hour for twenty-two hours, and if it rises the physician must be sent for. If there are signs of internal hæmorrhage a blood transfusion is given. There may be pain on the right side of the chest or at the top of the right shoulder requiring an analgesic such as aspirin or Veganin.

Variations in Technique. A cannula of 2 mm. bore with three sharp teeth was used by Iversen and Roholm (87) but this may increase the risk of tearing the liver capsule with subsequent hæmorrhage. Sherlock (89) uses a trocar and cannula with a bore of 1 mm. and inserts the cannula into the liver for ½ inch before removing the trocar, and then pushes the cannula into the liver a further 4 to 5 cm. Silverman (90) in 1938 introduced a split needle for obtaining liver specimens. It consists of an outer needle or cannula of 16 gauge, and an inner needle of 18 gauge which is split longitudinally down to the hub. The outer needle or cannula, with obturator in place, is inserted into the liver. The obturator is then removed and the split needle inserted in its place and pushed into the liver, cutting a cylinder of tissue between its prongs. The cannula is now advanced over the split needle into the liver for a distance of about ½ inch. The entire instrument is then rotated slightly and the inner needle withdrawn with the specimen. A Vim-Silverman needle was employed by Cogswell et al. (88) the fragment of liver tissue removed being 1–2 mm. in diameter and 1–2 cm. long. Terry (91) used a modified Gillman needle, in which the stylet is attached to the plunger of the syringe. The needle has a diameter of 1·8 mm. with a bevelled point internally bored to give a knife-like edge. Other sites of puncture are sometimes preferred. Thus Iversen and Roholm (87) punctured the ninth intercostal space in the posterior axiliary line, Gillman and Gillman (92) the costo-xiphoid angle between the xiphoid and the right costal margin, and Davis et al. (93) used the subcostal route. The needle, either a

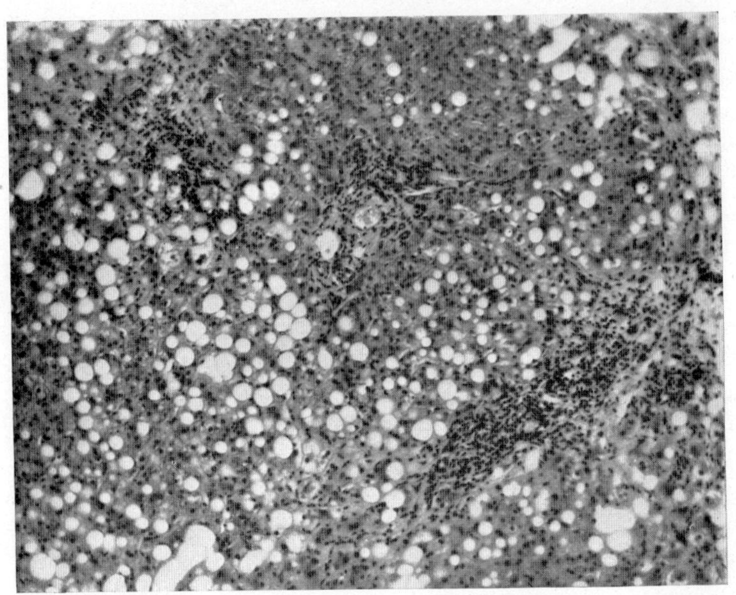

FIG. 7. Liver biopsy showing fatty changes.

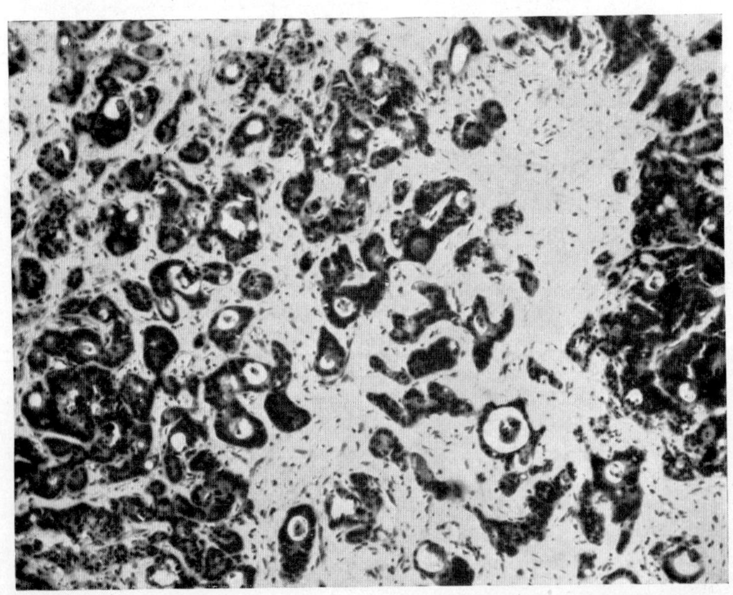

FIG. 8. Liver biopsy showing secondary carcinoma.

To face p. 139.]

Silverman or a Roth-Turkel needle, with small saw teeth, was inserted a few centimetres to the right of the xiphoid process and below the costal margin, and directed upwards and to the right toward the centre of the liver.

Some Difficulties and Complications. Failure to obtain a satisfactory specimen of liver may be due to the presence of ascites increasing the mobility of the liver. The chief difficulty in detaching and removing a suitable piece of liver is met with in cirrhosis. The risk of fatal hæmorrhage has diminished with improvements in technique and with the use of vitamin K. Terry (91) refers to 2,469 biopsies performed between 1939 and 1948 in which there were 7 deaths. Cogswell et al. (88) performed 403 biopsies on 345 patients without any serious reaction. Other complications include pneumothorax, hæmothorax, empyema and air embolism. Davis et al. (93) performed biopsies by the subcostal route on 68 patients without serious complications, but state that the risks include extensive bleeding into the peritoneal cavity and abdominal wall, perforation of the large or small intestine or gall bladder, introduction of infection or spread of localised infection into the general peritoneal cavity, and injury to the kidney, adrenal or pancreas.

Conclusions. Liver biopsy is usually, but not invariably, not dangerous or painful when performed by a skilled physician and when due precautions are taken, but it should not be undertaken sporadically by the uninitiated. We have found it of value in distinguishing between obstructive jaundice of short duration and jaundice due to hepatitis. In the former the biopsy reveals accumulation of the bile in the liver canaliculi near the centre of the lobules, in the latter there is loss of lobular structure, ballooning of the polygonal cells and focal areas of small mononuclear cell infiltration. The early fatty changes in cirrhosis are well shown (see Fig. 7) and enable a diagnosis to be made when the changes are still reversible with adequate dietetic treatment. We have also found the method of value in the diagnosis of secondary carcinoma of the liver (see Fig. 8), thus avoiding an unnecessary laparotomy. At times also a correct diagnosis may be made in obscure cases of hepatomegaly.

Liver Function Tests

Investigation of the Pigmentary Function of the Liver. Hæmoglobin, released from erythrocytes destroyed in the reticuloendothelial system, is converted to bilirubin and biliverdin which are excreted in the bile. The probable route is (i) the porphyrin ring is opened leading to the formation of a "verdohæmoglobin"—probably a biliverdin - globin-iron complex, Lemberg et al. (94); (ii) the iron is split off to travel thereafter with the β-globulin fraction of the plasma proteins, and some of the (green) biliverdin is reduced to (orange) bilirubin, which remains in association with globin.

Authorities disagree regarding the nature of the protein-binding of the plasma bilirubin, and regarding changes taking place in this linkage when the bilirubin-protein complex passes through the liver (Watson (95)). The subject is critically discussed by With (96). The consensus of present-day opinion is that the pre-hepatic (type A, indirect, type I) bilirubin is closely bound to protein: it is converted to post-hepatic (type B, direct-reading, type II) bilirubin probably in the Küppfer cells and is excreted by the parenchymal cells (Schaffner et al. (97)). This bilirubin is only loosely associated with protein, and is probably in the form of a sodium salt.

In the intestines bilirubin is reduced by bacterial action to urobilinogen (a mixture of two colourless chromogens, mesobilirubinogen and stercobilinogen). Some of the urobilinogen is excreted in the fæces, and is oxidised by the air to urobilin: the remainder is absorbed into the portal circulation and returned to the liver, where a part is excreted unchanged, a part re-oxidised and excreted as bilirubin, and a part returns to the general circulation and is excreted by the kidney.

Types of Jaundice and the van den Bergh Reaction

In view of the easily available literature (*e.g.* McNee (98)), only the briefest summary of this important work will be given here. Jaundice, at the time of Virchow, was considered to fall under two headings, hepatogenous and anhepatogenous. Thus, in the hepatogenous variety the condition resulted from obstruction of the biliary tract, whilst in the second, anhepatogenous variety, the bile pigment was thought to originate in tissues other than the liver. Later, owing to certain experimental work which need not be detailed here, the possibility of anhepatogenous jaundice was excluded. Thus Eppinger (99) stated that all jaundice was obstructive, and in those cases where obvious obstruction could not be seen the seat of the trouble was said to be in the fine bile capillaries. Later, however, the work of Aschoff (100), and his co-workers, pointed rather to the original separation of jaundice into hepatogenous, or obstructive, and hæmolytic, or anhepatogenous. His work has completely changed the views on the formation of bile pigments from hæmoglobin. Thus it used to be thought that this change was effected by the polygonal cells of the liver, but in the newer conception it is held that these simply pass the pigment on from another group of cells to the lumen of the bile capillary.

Jaundice may be classified either, according to the site of the primary disturbance, into obstructive post-hepatic, hepatic, or pre-hepatic (McNee (98)); or, alternatively, depending on the path taken by the excess bilirubin, into retention jaundice if the bile has not passed through the liver cells, and regurgitation jaundice if this has taken place. A combined classification is shown in the table after Lichtman (101).

SITE	CAUSE	TYPE OF JAUNDICE
Pre-hepatic .	Excessive destruction of R.B.C.s	Retention
Hepatic:		
Intralobular .	(i) familial hyperbilirubinæmia, Meulengracht (102), due to sub-normal hepato-cellular function	Retention
	(ii) parenchymal cell necrosis or œdema (toxic or infective hepatitis)	Regurgitation
	(iii) cholangiolitis	Regurgitation
Extralobular .	(iv) cholangitis	Regurgitation
	(v) distortion of cell-canalicular continuity (as in " cirrhosis ")	Regurgitation
Post-hepatic .	Obstruction to biliary outflow (stone, carcinoma, etc.)	Regurgitation

In retention jaundice the excess bilirubin is principally type A, in regurgitation jaundice type B. A chemical reaction to distinguish between these would have diagnostic value.

This has been devised by Hijmans van den Bergh (103), who employs Ehrlich's azo reaction. This consists in adding to the solution of bilirubin a diazonium salt in acid solution, causing the appearance of a purple compound, azo-bilirubin. The diazonium compound is provided by mixing a solution of sulphanilic acid in HCl with sodium nitrite. Van den Bergh noted that icteric sera, when treated in this manner, either gave an immediate colour, or else a very delayed reaction. He was able to assert that the first type of reaction was given by bilirubin which had passed through the liver cells, and that the delayed reaction resulted with pigment formed without the agency of the polygonal cells, *i.e.* absorbed direct from the Küpffer cells. The present-day view is that colour developing within a minute of adding the diazo reagent to the serum (prompt direct reaction) is probably a measure of bilirubin type B: colour developing when the mixure is allowed to stand, or on adding alcohol (Ducci and Watson (104)) or on adding caffeine and urea (Gray and Widbourne (105)) is a measure of total bilirubin (A + B).

Interpretation of the Results. Normal serum contains both bilirubin A and B, approximately 30% being type B. In clinical work the only significant observations are of total serum bilirubin (as measured by any suitable method), and of the presence of a prompt direct reaction, a visible colour appearing within a minute of adding the diazo reagents to the serum. "Biphasic" and "delayed direct" reactions have no significance. Many workers such as Klatski and Drill (106) consider that a positive direct reaction, or alteration of the prompt total serum bilirubin ratio is of no diagnostic significance; whilst, contrariwise, Schaffner et al. (97) find that the average percentage of bilirubin B is significantly higher in obstructive jaundice and toxic hepatitis than in infective hepatitis. In our experience a raised total serum bilirubin with a negative prompt direct reaction indicates retention jaundice: if the prompt direct reaction is positive (more than 45% being type B), then there is regurgitation jaundice. The total serum bilirubin level serves to follow the progress of the disease, as clinical jaundice may not be noticeable for several days after the serum level is raised, and the pigment will remain in the skin for a little while after the serum level has returned to normal. Jaundice generally appears when the serum bilirubin is in the range 1·5–2 mg. %. In retention jaundice the range is 0·5–1 mg. % higher, for bilirubin type A.

Icterus Index. As this measures only the colour of the serum, and not chemically its bilirubin content, other materials (*e.g.* carotenoids, hæmatin) are also detected and the test is of little value except as a simple method for the small laboratory to follow the degree of jaundice. It may have value in the control of biliverdin jaundice (Larson et al. (107)) in cases of long standing obstruction or of receding jaundice, for biliverdin does not give a Van den Bergh reaction.

Biliary Pigments in the Urine. The kidney does not excrete bilirubin type A (hence the term "acholuric jaundice") whilst bile pigments can be detected in the urine by simple tests when the total serum bilirubin level in cases of regurgitation jaundice is more than approximately 2 mg. %. This "threshold" is not a true one and in hepatitis urinary bile pigments can be found at serum bilirubin levels of about 1 mg. %.

Normally a small quantity of urobilinogen is detectable in freshly passed urine by the use of Ehrlich's aldehyde reagent. In retention jaundice (due to overproduction of bilirubin) the urine and fæcal urobilinogen are greatly increased; in the obstructive type of regurgitation jaundice urobilinogen is absent from both urine and fæces. In early liver damage, *e.g.* in infective hepatitis, one of the first hepatic functions to be altered is the power to oxidise urobilinogen to bilirubin, hence an increased urinary urobilinogen is a sensitive sign of minimal impairment. As the liver damage proceeds an obstructive element supervenes and the urinary urobilinogen disappears, to return on recovery. Watson (108) discusses urobilinogen excretion in greater detail and gives quantitative details of the findings in various diseases.

The Bilirubin Excretion Test. The measurement of the excretion of bilirubin, injected intravenously, as a means of estimating hepatic function was originated by Eilbott (109). The technique described below is that of Soffer and Paulson (110). The test is, however, rarely used today.

A total amount of bilirubin equal to 1 mg. per kg. of body-weight, but not exceeding 70 mg., is dissolved in 15 ml. M/10 sodium carbonate, which previously has been boiled and then cooled to 80° C. A control sample of blood is collected in a dry syringe to prevent hæmolysis, after which, with the needle *in situ,* the bilirubin solution is injected. Further specimens of blood are taken five minutes later and after four hours. Two ml. of plasma from the control and from the four-hour specimens are treated with 2 ml. of acetone and centrifuged, while 1 ml. of the plasma from the five-minute specimen is treated with 4 ml. of acetone. The supernatant fluids are filtered and promptly matched against suitable standards. These are prepared from stock 1 in 2,000 solution of potassium dichromate, which yields a colour identical with that of 1 mg. of circulating bilirubin per 100 ml. plasma. Suitable standards contain the equivalent of 0·9, 0·8, 0·7, 0·6, 0·5, 0·4, 0·3 and 0·2 mg. of circulating bilirubin per 100 ml. of plasma, and are made by diluting 9, 8, 7, 6, 5, 4, 3 and 2 ml. of the 1 in 2,000 dichromate to 10 ml. with water. When acidified with one drop of dilute hydrochloric acid, these standards are stable for some time and may be kept in sealed tubes.

Calculation. 200 × (mg. % bilirubin found in four-hour filtrate — mg. bilirubin found in control filtrate) divided by (5 × mg. % bilirubin found in five-min. filtrate — 2 × mg. % bilirubin found in control filtrate) gives the percentage of bilirubin retained.

Findings. Normally not more than 5 to 6% of the injected bilirubin should be retained at the end of four hours. An advantage of the test is that the liver is given a natural pigment, bilirubin, to excrete, although this substance is expensive and difficult to procure. It should be borne in mind that the test is inapplicable to patients with jaundice and is most useful in cases in which the bilirubin does not exceed 1 mg. per 100 ml. plasma. Several workers have reported favourably on the reliability and delicacy of the bilirubin test. Thus Soffer (111) found that the normal retention of bilirubin was exceeded in recovering cases of diffuse hepatitis in which the jaundice had subsided, as well as in cases of cirrhosis and malignancy. Sweet, Gray and Allen (112) concluded that the test was more delicate than the galactose tolerance, bromsulphthalein and hippuric acid tests in the detection of hepatic damage in cases of minimal or no symptomatic evidence of cirrhosis of the liver.

Investigation of the Antitoxic Powers of the Liver

The Oral Hippuric Acid Excretion Test. This test, which was devised by Quick (113), depends on the ability of the liver to conjugate benzoic acid with glycine. It has now been largely replaced by the intravenous test.

The Intravenous Hippuric Acid Test. In 1938 Quick et al. (114) showed that hippuric acid is synthesised in man following the intravenous injection of sodium benzoate. 1·77 g. of sodium benzoate is dissolved in 20 ml. of distilled water and injected slowly intravenously, taking five minutes over the injection. The bladder is emptied before the test and the urine is collected one hour after the injection. The hippuric acid is estimated in the urine. Normally 0·7 g. to 0·95 g. is excreted as hippuric acid in the first hour.

Findings. Mateer et al. (115 and 116) using this test, compared it with the oral method and found that the intravenous test is more delicate, yielding positive results (diminished hippuric acid excretion) in 85% more cases of liver damage than does the oral test. The test is sensitive, but has the disadvantages that the degree of "positivity" is not proportional to the extent of liver damage, and that false low outputs of hippuric acid are found if there is renal damage, dehydration or obstructive anuria. The test is applicable to jaundiced and non-jaundiced patients; it is not very reliable if used in the differential diagnosis of hepatic from post-hepatic jaundice, as minor degrees of obstruction generally give a positive result.

Investigation of the Capacity of the Liver to Excrete Foreign Substances

The Bromsulphthalein Test. Rosenthal and White in 1924 (117 and 118) proposed a liver function test based on the ability of the liver to remove bromsulphthalein (phenoltetrabromphthalein disodium sulphonate) from the blood. The dye in the plasma is bound loosely to albumin, and the rate of removal from the plasma by the liver is a constant proportion of the plasma level, and depends on the blood flow to the liver and the functional capacity of the parenchymal cells. Ingelfinger et al. (119) discuss variation in this "percentage disappearance rate", normally 10–16%/min. In very severe liver damage there is some extra-hepatic bromsulphthalein uptake (Mendeloff et al. (120)).

For clinical purposes a simple satisfactory method of estimating bromsulphthalein clearance is as follows. The test is performed with the patient fasting and at rest. Inject intravenously bromsulphthalein solution, 5 mg./kg. body-weight. Some authorities use a 2 mg./kg. dose; this does not give a sufficient load to the parenchymal cells, and we have not observed any of the reported toxic effects of the higher dose. At five minutes and at forty-five minutes after the injection withdraw 10 ml. samples of blood for estimation of the dye content of the sera.

Analysis of the five-minute sample serves as a check on the correctness of the quantity injected, normally it contains between 15% and 85% (compared with the 100% standard). At forty-five minutes the dye content of the serum is normally between 0 and 5%: a value above 10% indicates definite liver damage, and the height of the forty-five-minute level is proportional to the degree of damage.

This test is sensitive, and is most satisfactory for the detection and investigation of diffuse hepatocellular damage in the absence of jaundice: it should be noted that in children bromsulphthalein excretion does not follow that of bilirubin. The test cannot be used to differentiate hepatic disease and post-hepatic obstruction (which equally causes retention of dye): mildly positive results are often also found in heart failure and febrile states. At the time of writing the dye was obtainable only from the U.S.A. and the cost of material per injection was about 15*s*.

Investigation of the Metabolic Functions of the Liver

Carbohydrate. Of the three sugars that could be used in tests of tolerance, glucose and lævulose are not satisfactory for liver function tests because of their extra-hepatic utilisation. MacLagan (121 and 122) has used galactose with consistent results.

Galactose Tolerance Test. This sugar is absorbed freely from the gut, and readily stored as glycogen by the normal liver. More satisfactory results are obtained if the patient is fasting. Take a resting blood sample; the patient then empties the bladder completely and drinks a solution of 40 g. galactose in lemon water: blood samples are taken every thirty minutes for two hours, and the total urine excretion collected over five hours. Normally the blood galactose level reaches a peak, at sixty minutes, of 10–40 mg./100 ml.: the sum of the 4 blood galactose values—termed the "galactose index"—is normally about 70 mg.; an index over 160 indicates hepatocellular damage. Normally the urinary excretion in five hours is less than 3 g.: an excretion of over 4 g. must be regarded with suspicion: an excretion of over 6 g. indicates severe hepatocellular damage.

This test is moderately sensitive, and has the advantage of giving normal results in most cases of uncomplicated mechanical obstructive jaundice (Bensley (123)). The test gives invalid results if there is malabsorption of the carbohydrate from the gut, as in the sprue syndrome or myxœdema.

Protein. The plasma proteins are made in the liver. In chronic hepatitis damage to the liver cells results in changes in the plasma proteins detectable by the normal methods of quantitative analysis; the albumin level being decreased and the globulins increased. In acute parenchymal hepatitis (*e.g.* infective hepatitis) the changes in the proteins are not detectable by methods of routine analysis; there is a qualitative alteration in the albumin, and an increase of the γ-globulin fraction.

In order to detect these qualitative alterations of the plasma proteins, tests are used in which the patient's serum is added to a suitable colloidal system: conditions are arranged so that normal (but generally not hepatitic) albumin stabilises the system and inhibits flocculation, whereas, generally speaking, γ-globulin in excess (especially hepatitic globulin) destroys the stability and flocculation or precipitation results (MacLagan (124)). A very large number of such tests have been developed, depending on the nature of the precipitant and the conditions of the test: amongst those in use are tests employing zinc sulphate (Kunkel (125)), cadmium sulphate (Wunderly and Wuhrmann (126)) and "colloidal red" (Ducci (127)).

The tests that we employ are as follows:—

Thymol Turbidity (MacLagan (128)). The reagent used is a buffered solution of thymol: the resultant turbidity is read in comparison with artificial standards. (Normal 0–4 units.) Precipitation occurs with excess β and γ globulins, and with a lipoid factor, and is inhibited by normal albumin.

Colloidal Gold. (MacLagan (128)). The reagent used is a colloidal gold solution as employed for the Lange test on cerebrospinal fluid. When the test is done using serum, instead of a colour change precipitation occurs and degrees of precipitation 0–5 are distinguished. (Normal 0–1.) Precipitation occurs with excess γ-globulin, and is inhibited by normal α and β globulins, and by albumins only slightly.

Cephalin-Cholesterol (Hanger (129), Steinberg (130)). The reagent now used in our laboratories is an artificial emulsion of desoxycholic acid + cholesterol, replacing the original emulsion of brain extract + cholesterol. Complete precipitation is termed 4 +: (normal 0–1 +). Precipitation occurs with excess γ-globulin and hepatitic α and β-globulins, and is inhibited by albumin.

These tests in general give parallel results, and are much used in the differential diagnosis of hepatic from post-hepatic jaundice. In hepatic disease the tests give positive results, in an uncomplicated obstruction the tests tend to be normal.

When used in the investigation of liver function the cephalin-cholesterol test is the most sensitive, and best employed in the detection of liver damage in the absence of jaundice. It is unsuitable for differential diagnosis, as it frequently yields a positive result in apparently uncomplicated obstructive jaundice. If the thymol or gold test is positive in obstructive jaundice then there is superimposed liver damage. The flocculation tests are frequently negative in carcinomatosis or "compensated cirrhosis of the liver".

The thymol turbidity test is often positive in diseases associated with hyperlipæmia in the absence of any protein changes, and has been sometimes found to give positive results in glandular fever. The colloidal gold test tends especially to yield "false positives" in rheumatoid arthritis, and the cephalin-cholesterol in rheumatic heart disease and malaria; though all these tests are sensitive to such miscellaneous diseases (with possibly some secondary liver damage) associated with changes in the globulins.

Lipoid. Alterations in the serum levels of free and ester cholesterol occur in various types of liver disease (Albrinke et al. (131)), however these changes are not generally employed for diagnostic purposes.

Obstructive jaundice : free cholesterol greatly increased : ester cholesterol increased.

Hepatocellular damage : free cholesterol variable : ester cholesterol greatly diminished.

In jaundice due to chemical agents (*e.g.* NAB), and during recovery from acute parenchymal damage, an hypercholesterolæmia is frequently found.

Investigations on Enzymes

The Plasma Alkaline Phosphatase. Roberts (132) was the first to note an increase in the plasma alkaline phosphatase in some cases of obstructive jaundice. The reason for this alteration is not known for certain. The main hypotheses are that during obstruction the enzyme, normally excreted in the bile, is forced back into the general circulation; that the parenchymal cells fail to excrete the enzyme; or that the parenchymal cells are "stimulated" by the back-pressure of the pent-up biliary secretions to produce excess of the enzyme.

The methods of assay generally in use in this country (modifications from King and Armstrong (133)) involve incubation of the serum with a buffered phenyl-phosphate solution; then estimating the phenol liberated under standard conditions—the normal being 3–13 King-Armstrong units in adults. In the U.S.A. the method of Bodansky (134) is commonly employed involving the measurements of phosphorus liberated from glycerophosphate, the normal being 1–4 units in adults.

This estimation is valuable in the differential diagnosis of obstructive from hepatocellular jaundice, especially when used in combination with the simple flocculation tests. In an obstructive jaundice the level is generally above 35 units (King-Armstrong), whilst in hepatocellular jaundice it is usually between 10 and 25 units. High values are also found in cirrhosis of the liver, more especially in biliary cirrhosis, and sometimes in widespread carcinomatosis. It must be remembered in interpreting alkaline phosphatase levels that the enzyme is also produced by osteoblasts and high values are obtained in such bone diseases as rickets, hyperparathyroidism, primary and secondary malignant disease and Paget's disease.

The Prothrombin Time. Prothrombin is synthesised in the parenchymal cells of the liver. The production depends on the amount of vitamin K reaching the cells, and on the functional state of the cells. Accordingly in liver disease the production of prothrombin may be diminished for two reasons: (i) damage to parenchymal cells, (ii) absence of bile salts from the intestine leading to diminished absorption of vitamin K.

Estimation of the prothrombin time by itself is not satisfactory as a liver function test. To differentiate between low prothrombin times resulting from liver damage and from deficient absorption of vitamin K recourse may be had to the intramuscular injection of a suitable preparation of vitamin K (*e.g.* 2 mg. of 2 methyl 1 : 4 naphthaquinone: Lord and Andrus (135)): this returns the prothrombin time to normal when deficiency is caused by malabsorption, but not when caused by hepatocellular damage.

The Serum Cholinesterase. This enzyme, which destroys acetylcholine, is a protein synthesised by the liver; and attention has been paid in recent years to its estimation as an index of liver function (McArdle (136)). The serum cholinesterase level is decreased in hepatocellular jaundice, and is normal in uncomplicated obstructive jaundice. The estimation is technically difficult, and the units of measurement depend on the method employed. Vorhaus et al. (137) describe studies using a simplified technique.

Conclusions. The choice of liver function tests to be performed on a patient depends on the purpose for which the tests are to be done. As an aid to the differential diagnosis of jaundice the urine and fæces should be tested for bile and urobilinogen, the Van den Bergh reaction and total serum bilirubin estimated, and the combination of analyses for serum alkaline phosphatase and a flocculation test (*e.g.* colloidal gold) considered. For the estimation of liver insufficiency the bromsulphthalein clearance, the estimation of total and differential serum proteins, and a flocculation test (*e.g.* cephalin-cholesterol) are suitable.

There is no single comprehensive test for liver function and the tests described each deal with limited functions of the liver. Extension of abnormality detected in one aspect of liver metabolism to the conclusion that there is global damage to the liver is not always justifiable. It must be emphasised that only when considered in conjunction with the more important clinical evidence can reliable conclusions be drawn from the results of liver function tests.

REFERENCES

(1) HIMSWORTH. "*Lectures on the Liver and its Diseases*," 2nd Edit., 1950. Blackwell Scientific Publications, Oxford.

(2) WILLCOX. *Lancet*, 1931, *ii*, 1, 57, 111.

(3) BOLAND and WILLIAMS. *Arch. Int. Med.*, 1938, **62**, 723.

(4) WEICHSELBAUM. *Quart. Journ. Exp. Physiol.*, 1935, **25**, 363.

(5) HIMSWORTH and GLYNN. *Lancet*, 1944, *i*, 457.

(6) FINDLAY. *Bull. Ministry of Health*, 1948, Jan.–Feb.

(7) BARKER, CAPPS and ALLEN. *Journ. Amer. Med. Assocn.*, 1945, **128**, 997.

(8) BEST, HARTROFT, LUCAS and RIDOUT. *Brit. Med. Journ.*, 1949, *ii*, 1001.

(9) RICH, BERTHRONG and GERMUTH. *Trans. Assocn. Amer. Physicians*, 1948, **61**, 263.

(10) WATERLOW. *Med. Research Council, Special Reports*, 1948, **263**.

(11) DAVIES. *Lancet*, 1948, *i*, 317.

(12) COCKAYNE. *Quart. Journ. Med.*, 1912, **6**, 1.

(13) VIRCHOW. *Virchow's Arch.*, 1865, **32**, 117.

(14) EPPINGER. *Wien. klin. Woch.*, 1908, **21**, 480.

(15) DIBLE, MCMICHAEL and SHERLOCK. *Lancet*, 1943, *ii*, 402.

(16) VAN ROOYEN and GORDON. *Journ. Roy. Army Med. Corps*, 1943, **79**, 213.

(17) BOYD. "*A Text-book of Pathology*." 4th Edit., Reprinted, 1945. Henry Kimpton, London.

(18) Pickles. *Brit. Med. Journ.*, 1930, *i*, 944.
(19) Newman. *Brit. Med. Journ.*, 1942, *i*, 61.
(20) Fraser. *Canad. Publ. Health*, 1931, **22**, 396.
(21) Cookson. *Brit. Med. Journ.*, 1944, *i*, 681.
(22) Andersen. *Acta. med. Scand.*, 1937, **93**, 209.
(23) Hallgren. *Acta. med. Scand.*, 1942, Supp. 140.
(24) Cameron. *Quart Journ. Med.*, 1943, **36**, 139.
(25) Sheehan. *Lancet*, 1944, *ii*, 8.
(26) Neefe and Stokes. *Journ. Amer. Med. Assocn.*, 1945, **128**, 1063.
(27) Havens, Paul, Van Rooyen, Ward, Drill and Allison. *Lancet*, 1945, *i*, 202.
(28) Findlay and Willcox. *Lancet*, 1945, *ii*, 594.
(29) Hartfall. *Brit. Med. Journ.*, 1944, *ii*, 21.
(30) Lescher. *Brit. Med. Journ.*, 1944, *i*, 554.
(31) Byrne and Taylor. *Brit. Med. Journ.*, 1945, *i*, 477.
(32) Stokes, Owen and Holmes. *Brit. Med. Journ.*, 1945, *ii*, 642.
(33) Wang. *Nord. Med.*, 1946, **32**, 2634.
(34) Rosenak, Moser and Howell. *Journ. Indiana State Med. Assocn.*, 1949, **42**, 897.
(35) Howard and Watson. *Arch. Int. Med.*, 1947, **80**, 1.
(36) Wyllie and Edmunds. *Lancet*, 1949, *ii*, 553.
(37) Sherlock. *Lancet*, 1948, *i*, 817.
(38) Miles. *Brit. Med. Journ.*, 1945, *ii*, 767.
(39) Evans. *Brit. Med. Journ.*, 1942, *ii*, 446.
(40) Hoagland and Shank. *Journ. Amer. Med. Assocn.*, 1946, **130**, 615.
(41) Pollock. *Brit. Med. Journ.*, 1945, *ii*, 878.
(42) Gordon. *Brit. Med. Journ.*, 1943, *ii*, 807.
(43) Britton. *Middlx Hosp. Journ.*, 1945, **45**, 29.
(44) Stokes and Neefe. *Journ. Amer. Med. Assocn.*, 1945, **127**, 144.
(45) Gellis, Stokes, Brother, Hall, Gilmore, Beyer and Morrissey. *Journ. Amer. Med. Assocn.*, 1945, **128**, 1062.
(46) Darmady. *Brit. Med. Journ.*, 1945, *i*, 795.
(47) Wilson, Pollock and Harris. *Brit. Med. Journ.*, 1945, *i*, 399.
(48) Higgins, O'Brien, Peters, Stewart and Witts. *Brit. Med. Journ.*, 1945, *i*, 401.
(49) Farquhar, Stokes, Whitlock, Bluemle and Gambescia. *Amer. Journ. Med. Sci.*, 1950, **220**, 166.
(50) Shaffer, Bluemle, Sborov and Neefe. *Amer. Journ. Med. Sci.*, 1950, **220**, 173.
(51) Klatski and Yesner. *Journ. Clin. Invest.*, 1949, **28**, 723.
(52) Ralli, Leslie, Stueck, Shorr, Robson, Clarke and Laken. *Medicine*, 1949, **28**, 301.
(53) Schemm and Layne. *Gastroenterology*, 1947, **9**, 705.
(54) Faloon, Eckhardt, Murphy, Cooper and Davidson. *Journ. Clin. Invest.*, 1949, **28**, 583.
(55) Rosenak, Moser and Kilgore. *Gastroenterology*, 1947, **9**, 695.
(56) Lurman. *Berl. klin. Woch.*, 1885, **22**, 20.
(57) Findlay and MacCallum. *Trans. Roy. Soc. Trop. Med. Hyg.*, 1937, **31**, 297. *Proc. Roy. Soc. Med.*, 1938, **31**, 799.
(58) Findlay, MacCallum and Murgatroyd. *Trans. Roy. Soc. Trop. Med. Hyg.*, 1939, **32**, 575.
(59) Fox, Manso, Penna and Para. *Amer. Journ. Hyg.*, 1942, **36**, 68.

(60) *Journ. Amer. Med. Assocn.*, 1942, **119**, 1110 ; *ibid*, 1942, **120**, 51.
(61) Findlay, Martin and Mitchell. *Lancet*, 1944, *ii*, 301, 340, 365.
(62) *Ann. Rep. Chief. Med. Officer, Min. of Health*, 1938, p. 39.
(63) Propert. *Brit. Med. Journ.*, 1938, *ii*, 677.
(64) Memorandum Med. Officers Min. of Health. *Lancet*, 1943, *i*, 83.
(65) Cockburn, Harrington, Zeitlin, Morris and Camps. *Brit. Med. Journ.*, 1951, *ii*, 6.
(66) Beeson, Chesney and McFarlan. *Lancet*, 1944, *i*, 814.
(67) Morgan and Williamson. *Brit. Med. Journ.*, 1943, *i*, 750.
(68) Beeson. *Journ. Amer. Med. Assocn.*, 1943, **121**, 1332.
(69) Steiner. *Brit. Med. Journ.*, 1944, *i*, 110.
(70) Lehane, Kwantes, Upward and Thompson. *Brit. Med. Journ.*, 1949, *ii*, 572.
(71) Bigger. *Lancet*, 1943, *i*, 457.
(72) Beattie and Marshall. *Brit. Med. Journ.*, 1944, *ii*, 651.
(73) Salaman, King, Williams and Nicol. *Lancet*, 1944, *ii*, 7.
(74) Darmady and Hardwick. *Lancet*, 1945, *ii*, 106.
(75) Howells and Kerr. *Lancet*, 1946, *i*, 51.
(76) Graham. *Lancet*, 1938, *ii*, 1.
(77) Droller. *Brit. Med. Journ.*, 1945, *i*, 623.
(78) Damodaran and Hartfall. *Brit. Med. Journ.*, 1944, *ii*, 587.
(79) Mendelssohn and Witts. *Brit. Med. Journ.*, 1945, *i*, 625.
(80) Findlay and Martin. *Lancet*, 1943, *i*, 678.
(81) MacCallum and Bauer. *Lancet*, 1944, *i*, 622.
(82) MacCullum. *Proc. Roy. Soc. Med.*, 1944, **37**, 449.
(83) Stanley. *Lancet*, 1833, *i*, 189.
(84) Lucatello. Lavori del 6⁰ Congress. Ital. di med. int., Roma, 1895.
(85) Von Hansemann. "*Lehrbuch den klinischen Untersuchungemethoden und ihrer Andwendung auf die specielle ärztliche Diagnostik.*" d'Eulenburg, Kolle et Weintrad, Vienne, 1904.
(86) Shupfer. *La Semaine Médicale*, 1927, 27me Ann., 229.
(87) Iversen and Roholm. *Acta. med. Scand.*, 1939, **162**, 1.
(88) Cogswell, Schief, Safdi, Richfield, Kumpe and Gall. *Journ. Amer. Med. Assocn.*, 1949, **140**, 385.
(89) Sherlock. *Lancet*, 1945, *ii*, 397.
(90) Silverman. *Amer. Journ. Surg.*, 1938, **40**, 671.
(91) Terry. *Brit. Med. Journ.*, 1949, *i*, 657.
(92) Gillman and Gillman. *South African Journ. Med. Sci.*, 1945, **10**, 53.
(93) Davis, Scott and Lund. *Amer. Journ. Med. Sci.*, 1946, **212**, 449.
(94) Lemberg, Lockwood and Legge. *Biochem. Journ.*, 1941, **35**, 363.
(95) Watson. *Blood*, 1946, **1**, 99.
(96) With. *Acta. med. Scand.*, 1949, supp. 234.
(97) Schaffner, Popper and Steigman. *Amer. Journ. Med. Sci.*, 1950, **219**, 307.
(98) McNee. *Quart. Journ. Med.*, 1923, **16**, 390.
(99) Eppinger. *Ergeb. der. inner. med. v. Kinderheilk*, 1908, **1**, 1107.
(100) Aschoff. *Münch. med. Woch.*, 1922, **69**, 1352.
(101) Lichtman. "*Diseases of the Liver, Gallbladder and Bileducts,*" 2nd Edit., 1949. Henry Kimpton, London.
(102) Meulengracht. *Klin. Wschr.*, 1939, **18**, 118.
(103) Van Den Bergh. "*Der Gallenfarbstoff in Blute,*" 1918. Leiden.
(104) Ducci and Watson. *Journ. Lab. Clin. Med.*, 1945, **30**, 293.

(105) Gray and Widbourne. *Biochem. Journ.*, 1946, **40**, 81.
(106) Klatski and Drill. *Journ. Clin. Invest.*, 1950, **29**, 660.
(107) Larson, Evans and Watson. *Journ. Lab. Clin. Med.*, 1947, **32**, 481.
(108) Watson. *Arch. Int. Med.*, 1937, **59**, 196, 206.
(109) Eilbott. *Zeitschr. f. klin. Med.*, 1927, **106**, 529.
(110) Soffer and Paulson. *Amer. Journ. Med. Sci.*, 1936, **192**, 535.
(111) Soffer. *Medicine*, 1935, **14**, 185.
(112) Sweet, Gray and Allen. *Journ. Amer. Med. Assocn.*, 1941, **117**, 1613.
(113) Quick. *Amer. Journ. Med. Sci.*, 1933, **185**, 630.
(114) Quick, Ottenstein and Weltchek. *Proc. Soc. Exp. Biol. and Med.*, 1938, **38**, 77.
(115) Mateer, Baltz, Marion and Hollands. *Amer. Journ. Digest. Dis.*, 1942, **9**, 13.
(116) Mateer, Baltz, Marion and MacMillan. *Journ. Amer. Med. Assocn.*, 1943, **121**, 723.
(117) Rosenthal and White. *Journ. Pharm. Exp. Therap.*, 1924, **24**, 265.
(118) Rosenthal and White. *Journ. Amer. Med. Assocn.*, 1925, **84**, 1112.
(119) Ingelfinger, Bradley, Mendeloff and Kramer. *Gastroenterology*, 1948, **11**, 646.
(120) Mendeloff, Kramer, Ingelfinger and Bradley. *Gastroenterology*, 1949, **13**, 222.
(121) Maclagan. *Quart. Journ. Med.*, 1940, **33**, 151.
(122) Maclagan. *Brit. Med. Journ.*, 1944, *ii*, 363.
(123) Bensley. *Canad. Med. Assocn. Journ.*, 1935, **33**, 360.
(124) Maclagan. *Brit. Med. Journ.*, 1948, *ii*, 892.
(125) Kunkel. *Proc. Soc. Exp. Biol. and Med.*, 1947, **66**, 217.
(126) Wunderly and Wuhrmann. *Schweiz. Med. Wschr.*, 1945, **75**, 1128.
(127) Ducci. *Journ. Lab. Clin. Med.*, 1947, **32**, 1273.
(128) Maclagan. *Brit. Journ. Exp. Path.*, 1944, **25**, 15, 234.
(129) Hanger. *Journ. Clin. Invest.*, 1939, **18**, 261.
(130) Steinberg. *Journ. Lab. Clin. Med.*, 1949, **34**, 1049.
(131) Albrinke, Man and Peters. *Journ. Clin. Invest.*, 1950, **29**, 781.
(132) Roberts. *Brit. Med. Journ.*, 1933, *i*, 734.
(133) King and Armstrong. *Canad. Med. Assocn. Journ.*, 1934, **31**, 376.
(134) Bodansky. *Journ. Biol. Chem.*, 1933, **101**, 93.
(135) Lord and Andrus. *Arch. Int. Med.*, 1941, **68**, 199.
(136) McArdle. *Quart. Journ. Med.*, 1940, **33**, 107.
(137) Vorhaus, Scudamore and Kark. *Gastroenterology*, 1950, **15**, 304.

CHAPTER VII

THE STOMACH

X-ray Examination

Examination of the stomach and of the duodenum by means of the X-rays after the ingestion of an opaque meal is a useful adjunct in the differential diagnosis of ulcers of these organs.

Investigations should be made both under the screen and with films. The opaque meal used in the screen examination usually consists of 3 oz. of barium sulphate in half a pint of milk. By this means the shape of the stomach and its filling properties can be investigated.

The motor power and rate of stomach emptying are better studied with a more solid meal, such as porridge or bread and milk containing barium sulphate. There should be no residue of such a meal in the stomach after six hours.

Persistent deformity in the outline of the stomach or duodenum affords some radiological indication of ulcer. Thus in gastric ulcer the barium may be seen filling a niche in the wall of the stomach, or there may be a definite organic hour-glass appearance. In the duodenum a persistent alteration in the shape of the duodenal cap may be seen. The X-ray examination will also reveal pyloric obstruction.

Variations in tone or in the position of the stomach are not diagnostic of ulceration. Subsequent examination after the administration of belladonna is of value in distinguishing between constriction of the stomach due to spasm and that due to cicatrisation.

Study of the relief pattern of the gastric and duodenal mucous membrane has been stimulated by the work of Berg (1). Cordiner and Calthrop (2) have published details of this method as applied to the radiography of the duodenal cap, and they emphasise its importance.

Gastroscopy

The introduction of the flexible gastroscope in 1932 by Schindler and Wolf, and of the Hermon Taylor (3) model with controllable flexibility in 1941 has further advanced the study of gastric diseases.

A biopsy attachment to the Wolf-Schindler instrument has been developed in America. The patient should be examined fasting, using 2% Anethaine as a local anæsthetic. A preliminary subcutaneous injection of morphin. sulph. gr. ¼ and atropin. sulph. gr. 1/120 is given three-quarters of an hour before instrumentation, and a gr. 1½ Anethaine pastille is sucked thirty minutes later. If the pharynx is still sensitive, 3 ml. of 2% Anethaine are used in addition as a gargle. Overdosage may result in toxic symptoms. Rodgers (4) gives the following indications for gastroscopy: When the skiagram has shown some abnormality but no definite diagnosis has been made, or when, a diagnosis having been made, some additional information is required. It is helpful in cases of dyspepsia in which the skiagram has revealed no abnormality. In certain cases of anæmia its use is of interest, although of little practical value. There are also contra-indications, which include local conditions such as trismus, œsophageal stenosis, enlarged mediastinal glands, an aneurysm or severe curvature of the spine. A large carcinoma near the cardiac orifice may render the examination impossible, and it should not be performed within a few days of a severe hæmatemesis. The abolition of the "blind area" in the stomach has been largely effected by the use of the Hermon Taylor gastroscope. In some cases of doubtful X-ray diagnosis of carcinoma a definite diagnosis, either positive or negative, may be made by gastroscopy. On the other hand, a lesion which has been seen through the gastroscope and diagnosed as an ulcer, may be proved by operation to be a carcinoma some weeks later. Like most methods of investigation, gastroscopy is not infallible. Gastric ulcers may frequently be visualised and be seen to heal under medical treatment. In some cases an ulcer may be seen which is not demonstrable radiologically and the converse is also true. Lintott (5) found that gastroscopic healing of gastric ulcers did not occur until one to several weeks after the disappearance of all X-ray deformity. A gastro-jejunal stoma is not always easy to see.

It is in the diagnosis of gastritis that gastroscopy appears most useful as has been emphasised by Bank and Renshaw (6) and by Freeman (7). During the active stages of inflammation the mucous membrane shows hyperæmia, œdema, exudation, hæmorrhages and superficial ulceration. The results of inflammation are granularity of the mucous membrane, narrowing and distortion of the folds, and atrophy. Gill et al. (8) examining 217 service cases of dyspepsia gastroscopically found gastritis as an isolated lesion in 32%, and gastritis was present as an associated lesion in 80% of cases of gastric ulcer, and in 60% of cases of pyloric and duodenal ulcer. Berry (9) studied gastroscopically 100 alcohol addicts, and found that only 35% had unequivocal alcoholic gastritis.

In pernicious and simple achlorhydric anæmias the mucous membrane is thin, pale and, as described by Hartfall (10), the most characteristic feature in pernicious anæmia " is the presence of branching submucosal vessels which impart a bluish network to the thin, pale, wash-leather background ". The pallor is probably due to anæmia and is much less marked after adequate treatment, but the mucous membrane remains thin and does not appear to regenerate. The changes in the simple achlorhydric anæmias are very similar, but the atrophy is less severe. There does not appear to be any evidence of a preceding gastritis.

Principles of Treatment of Gastric and Duodenal Ulcers

Varous modifications in the treatment of ulcers of the stomach and duodenum have been introduced during recent years. From the practical point of view the subject can be considered under the following headings :—

The treatment of hæmatemesis due to gastric or duodenal ulceration.

The medical treatment of ulcers not at the time complicated by hæmorrhage.

The indications for surgical treatment of gastric and duodenal ulcers, not complicated by hæmorrhage.

Hæmatemesis. It is probable that between 10% and 30% of all peptic ulcers bleed, but the hæmorrhage is not necessarily severe, and the average death rate from hæmorrhage has been variously estimated as follows : Cullinan and Price (11) give a mortality of 10% in a series of 105 cases of the hospital class, 4 of which were treated surgically, all dying. Hurst and Ryle (12) in 677 cases of the private practice class had a mortality of 1·5%. Three of their cases were treated surgically and all died. Meulengracht (13) records a mortality of 1·3% in 368 cases of the hospital class treated by early feeding. The more recent mortality figures are not so good. Thus Avery Jones (14) in 1947 recorded a mortality rate of 8% in a series of 687 cases admitted to hospital between 1940 and 1947. Baker (15) in a series of 576 cases admitted to Selly Oak Hospital between 1940 and 1945 found 13·4% proved fatal, and Lewin and Truelove (16) in 1949 showed a mortality figure of 19% in a series of 305 cases admitted as emergencies. Needham and McConachie (17) have analysed the records of 476 cases of hæmatemesis admitted as emergencies to the Aberdeen Royal Infirmary from January 1941 to December 1948. The mortality rate was 13·9%.

Discussions at the Royal Society of Medicine, London, in 1924, and again in 1934 (18) emphasised that the immediate treatment of acute hæmatemesis due to gastric or duodenal ulcer is almost always medical. It has usually been considered that the likelihood of death rises with the recurrence of hæmorrhage, a primary hæmorrhage not being so dangerous as a subsequent one. This view is not borne out by statistics from Seattle (U.S.A.). Thus Blackford and Allen (19) in 1942 recorded 120 deaths in men, and 31 deaths in women from bleeding peptic ulcer. Seventy-seven per cent of all fatalities occurred during the first hæmorrhage, and only 8 deaths occurred in patients under forty-five years old. Needham and McConachie's (17) figures do not support this view. They found the risk of dying was eight to ten times greater in the recurrent group. In patients under forty years of age fatalities are almost unknown, but the mortality rate rises steeply after middle age. The surgical view-point will be referred to later.

Medical Treatment of Severe Hæmatemesis. It must be clearly understood that the type of patient for whom this treatment is required is so desperately ill that he is not able to take feeds by mouth. (*a*) The patient is put to bed, kept warm and very still. (*b*) Morphine sulphate gr. $\frac{1}{4}$ and atropine sulphate gr. $\frac{1}{100}$ are injected subcutaneously. This may be repeated up to a total of morphine gr. 1 in twenty-four hours. Willcox (20) has drawn attention to the danger of morphine in cases of hæmatemesis due to cirrhosis of the liver, when the detoxicating power of the liver may be so diminished that even gr. $\frac{1}{4}$ may cause death; our experience supports this view. (*c*) Nothing is given by mouth for one to two days. Ice should not be sucked, but attention must be given to the toilet of the mouth, it being rinsed out from time to time with water. (*d*) An hourly pulse chart should be kept. (*e*) The blood pressure and hæmoglobin percentage should be determined every twelve to twenty-four hours. (*f*) The blood urea should be estimated, and, if raised, determinations should be made daily until it falls to normal. (*g*) The bowels should not be opened for four to seven days, an enema then being given. (*h*) Rectal salines of 6 to 8 oz. with dextrose 2% should be given every four hours, or a rectal drip may be used with a Murphy vulcanite rectal nozzle, which allows free escape of flatus backwards along the tube to the reservoir, as described by Marriott and Kekwick (21). Six to 8 pints of water, normal or isotonic saline (0·85% sodium chloride) or isotonic dextrose (5% dextrose) may be run in slowly every twenty-four hours, resting the bowel every other hour by interrupting the flow. (*i*) Blood transfusion is indicated, according to Witts (22), if the hæmoglobin is below 40%, the systolic blood pressure below 90 mm. Hg., the pulse rate over 140, or the blood urea over 100 mg. per 100 ml. Needham and McConachie (17), however, found that in many patients who died the pulse rate did not rise as high as 120. The transfusion may be either a small one of 250 ml. repeated as required, or the drip method advocated by Marriott and Kekwick (23) may be used. The amount of blood given by either method should raise the hæmoglobin to about 80%. One pint of blood administered to an adult will increase the hæmoglobin by about 10%. By the drip method this 10% increase should be achieved every four hours. (*j*) The value of hæmostatics is open to question. Five or 10 ml. of "Stypven" containing 0·5 mg. or 1 mg. of Russell's viper venom may be given by mouth, or 5 ml. calcium gluconate (10%) intramuscularly once daily.

After periods of one to two days, and when the bleeding has been arrested, as judged by absence of hæmatemesis and the general condition of the patient, 4 oz. of half-strength normal saline (0·42% sodium chloride) should be given by mouth every four hours for twelve hours. Milk feeds may now be begun, first with milk 1 oz., water 1 oz. and emulsio mag. oxid. m. 30, every two hours, and then milk 2 oz. every two hours and gradually increasing the milk feeds to 5 oz. every two hours. Tincture of belladonna (m. 10–15) should be given before three feeds, and olive oil (½ fl. oz.)

alternately before three other feeds. A teaspoonful of an alkaline powder (*see* p. 163) or of Aludrox should be given after five feeds, and a double dose at night. Ferri et ammon. citrat. gr. 30 should be given three times a day between the feeds. The subsequent medical treatment is as for the treatment of ulcer not complicated by hæmorrhage, and is detailed later.

Routine Medical Treatment of Hæmatemesis. In the majority of cases of hæmatemesis the patient can tolerate early feeding and does better with it. The stomach is not rested by starvation. The starvation treatment is now being generally abandoned except in the very severe cases, as mentioned above. With a turn of the wheel we are back where we were in 1904 when Lenhartz (24) introduced his diet for immediate feeding in hæmatemesis, which was described in earlier editions of this book. Meulengracht (13) has published figures showing a lower mortality rate than has been obtained by other methods of treatment, and he advocates a liberal dietary from the first day of bleeding. The routine he recommends is as follows: 6 *a.m.* Tea, white bread and butter. 9 *a.m.* Oatmeal with milk, white bread and butter. 1 *p.m.* A selection from: meat balls, timbale, broiled chops, fish balls, vegetable gratin, fish gratin, mashed potatoes, vegetable purée, vegetable soups, cream of vegetables, stewed apricots, apple sauce, gruel, rice and tapioca puddings. 3 *p.m.* Cocoa. 6 *p.m.* White bread and butter, sliced meats, cheese and tea. The patients are allowed as much as they like. In addition, one teaspoonful of the following powder is given: Sod. bicarb. gr. 30, mag. carb. lev. gr. 30, ext. hyoscyam. sicc. gr. 4, and ferri lact. gr. 5, t.i.d.

We have tried this method with satisfactory results in a few cases, but in others it has proved impracticable as the patient could not take the diet. We doubt whether the true Meulengracht diet is now ever employed in this country, the fact being that we can seldom stomach it. There are, indeed, numerous modifications thereof which masquerade under the name of Meulengracht and cause much confusion. Witts (22) recommends a diet which is more fluid than that of Meulengracht and contains no meat, but which conforms to the principles of feeding by mouth on the first day of the hæmorrhage. This has proved of great value in the treatment of many cases of hæmatemesis. Thus Pickering (25) writing in 1942 says that during the last six years he has treated all his patients (over 40 in number) suffering from gastric and duodenal hæmorrhage by the diet recommended by Witts, with only one death, and he supports Witts' view that " the results of

Dietetic Treatment of Gastro-duodenal Hæmorrhage arranged for Two-hourly Feeding

Feeds by Day	Food	Day 1	Day 2	Day 3 and subsequent
1	Whole milk (fresh or dried) . oz.	5	5	5
	Patent barley or strained porridge .	Portion	Portion	Portion
2	1 egg beaten up in milk . oz.	5	5	5
	Buttered rusks or cream crackers .	–	1	2
3	Whole milk (fresh or dried) . oz.	5	5	5
	Marmite to taste	–	–	–
	Barley sugar . . . . oz.	1	1	1
	Thin crustless white bread and butter slices	–	1	2
4	Strained orange or tomato juice oz.	1	1	1
	Vegetable purée	Portion	Portion	Portion
	Pudding	,,	,,	,,
	Cream . . . . . . oz.	1	1	1
	Boiled or steamed fish . . .	–	–	Portion
5	1 egg beaten up in milk . oz.	5	5	5
	Barley sugar . . . . oz.	1	1	1
	Buttered rusks or cream crackers .	–	1	2
6	Whole milk (fresh or dried) . oz.	5	5	5
	Fruit purée	Portion	Portion	Portion
	Pudding	,,	,,	,,
	Cream . . . . . . oz.	–	1	1
	Thin crustless white bread and butter slices	–	1	2
7	1 egg beaten up in milk . oz.	5	5	5
	Black treacle or barley sugar . oz.	1	1	1
	Buttered rusks or cream crackers .	–	1	2
8	Whole milk (fresh or dried) . oz.	5	5	5
	Fruit purée	Portion	Portion	Portion
	Pudding	,,	,,	,,
Feeds at night (when awake)	1. Whole milk (fresh or dried) oz.	5	5	5
	2. 1 egg beaten up in milk . oz.	5	5	5
Between feeds	Strained orange or tomato juice oz.	1	1	1
	Approximate caloric value . .	2,545	3,118	3,624

immediate feeding, supplemented when necessary by transfusion, are much superior to starvation or operation ". The advocates of early feeding to the exclusion of the mouth starvation method must, however, remember that in Witts' original series of cases he found that not all the patients could take even his fluid diet from the start. The diet is as shown on p. 160.

The milk is not citrated, but may be flavoured with Horlick's malted milk or Ovaltine. Vitamin C is given as fruit juice or as ascorbic acid tablet 50 mg. t.i.d. Sips of water or of dextrose solution or half strength normal saline are allowed between feeds, up to 5 oz. an hour. The total fluid intake in the twenty-four hours should be about 5 pints. Neutralising substances or alkalis are only given if there is abdominal pain, which is unusual. No purgatives are given, and if the bowels are not opened an enema is given on the seventh day. Transfusion is given according to the criteria laid down above. Woldman (26) treated 21 cases of hæmatemesis, admitted to St. Luke's Hospital, Cleveland, Ohio, by the continuous intragastric aluminium hydroxide drip method and they all recovered. In addition, during the first twenty-four hours the patients were given by mouth 2 oz. of milk and cream every two hours, and after that the diet included cooked cereals, gelatine, custard, cream soup, and rice and tapioca puddings. Morphine was not used, but barbiturates and other sedatives were administered as required. Woldman considers the drip is a further advance on the principle of early feeding. This compares favourably with the 38 cases of hæmatemesis, admitted to the hospital during the previous five years, who were not treated by the drip, for 11 of these cases died.

The Surgical Treatment of Hæmatemesis. Gordon-Taylor (27) urges that the surgeon should not be excluded from consultation until the last desperate stage of ulcer hæmorrhage, and supports the view expressed by Finsterer (28) that the first forty-eight hours is the optimum period for operation. The practical difficulty is to decide in any individual case whether death will occur if medical treatment is adopted, and whether life could be saved by an early operation. Further, it is often impossible to decide at this stage whether the patient has an acute or chronic ulcer or chronic gastritis. The chief indications for operation are (*a*) The erosion of a large vessel. (*b*) Concomitant hæmorrhage and perforation of the stomach. (*c*) Hæmorrhage which cannot be controlled by blood transfusion. (*d*) A primary hæmorrhage may require surgical treatment in elderly people whose vessels are thickened and blood pressure raised. Needham and McConachie

(17) consider that surgical treatment is indicated in the majority of patients over 50 who suffer a further hæmorrhage after admission to hospital. An operation is rarely, if ever, advisable in primary hæmorrhage under other circumstances, and acute ulceration of the stomach probably never requires surgical treatment.

The position with recurrent hæmorrhages is somewhat different. Previous X-ray investigation will probably have been carried out. With a large penetrating ulcer, a fibrotic ulcer, with pyloric or duodenal stenosis or with mid-gastric narrowing, an operation may be required to prevent further bleeding. It should not be performed until the hæmoglobin has been raised to 60% by blood transfusion. In no case should an operation be advised unless very skilled surgery is available with adequate facilities for blood transfusion, for the mortality rate for operation for active hæmorrhage from chronic ulcer is at the best about 10%. In all cases in which the patient is under forty-five years of age an operation is best avoided.

The Medical Treatment of Ulcers not Complicated by Hæmorrhage. The modified Sippy treatment is now usually employed.

The Sippy Treatment (modified) or The Alkali Treatment. Sippy (29), of Chicago, introduced this treatment in 1915. Its object is to protect the ulcer from hydrochloric acid. This is accomplished by giving large doses of alkalis after, and of belladonna before the feeds, and by using as the basis of the diet milk and cream.

Modifications of the Sippy treatment have been found to yield good results and are more easily carried out than the original method. The feeds are given at two or two and a half hourly intervals, an alkaline powder or neutralising substance is taken one hour after, and olive oil or belladonna before the feeds. There is some difference of opinion as to the best alkalis or neutralising substances for the purpose. Sippy (29) recommended sodium bicarbonate, heavy magnesia and bismuth carbonate. All carbonates have the disadvantage of liberating CO_2 and causing gaseous distension, which proves distressing in some cases. Sodium bicarbonate and magnesium oxide provoke a secondary secretion of gastric juice. Bismuth carbonate has no neutralising power and theoretically is of little value, as it is improbable that it forms a protective coat to the ulcer. It is, however, out of fashion now owing to its expense, to the slaty colour it gives to the fæces which interferes with the detection of blood, and because it is said neither to relieve pain nor to neutralise acidity. Clinically, however, bismuth undoubtedly exerts a sedative effect. Magnesium oxide and magnesium hydroxide are both powerful neutralising agents. Sodium and potassium citrate, tribasic calcium phosphate and tribasic magnesium phosphate neutralise hydrochloric acid without producing an alkaline solution (30, 31). Crohn (32) in 1929 introduced colloidal aluminium hydroxide as an antacid. Six daily doses of 60 to 120 m. of a preparation such as Aludrox (5·8% aluminium hydroxide) in water may be given between feeds. Fauley et al. (33) have shown that aluminium hydroxide gel in relatively large doses interferes with the absorption of phosphates in man and dog, and that it may produce a phosphorus deficiency in the presence of a relative deficiency of pancreatic juice, of diarrhœa or of a low phosphorus diet. This is, however, not likely to occur with a patient on an ordinary ulcer diet. They also showed that aluminium phosphate gel will prevent the formation of a peptic ulcer in Mann-Williamson dogs (in which a gastro-jejunostomy is performed and the pancreatic juice and bile are diverted into the last 20 to 25 cm. of the ileum). In such dogs a jejunal ulcer develops with death in about eleven weeks. Aluminium phosphate gel does not interfere with phosphate absorption. Aluminium hydroxide gel did not prevent ulcer formation in these dogs. The use of aluminium phosphate gel in a few cases of patients suffering from peptic ulcer indicated that it was as effective as any other neutralising agent, and it is probably preferable to aluminium hydroxide gel in cases asssociated with pancreatic deficiency or diarrhœa. Mutch (34) has obtained good results with a synthetic hydrated magnesium trisilicate in doses of gr. 5 to 21 (anhydrous weight) between each feed. It possesses antacid and general adsorbent properties. Cohn et al. (35) record the case of a granuloma of the stomach following the ingestion of a medication containing hydrated aluminium silicate which the patient had been taking for a long time for a duodenal ulcer.

There is some risk of producing alkalosis if large doses of magnesia or sodium bicarbonate are given, but this risk is diminished if magnesium trisilicate or colloidal aluminium hydroxide are employed.

Milk is the best neutralising food substance, and the addition of sodium citrate, gr. 3 to the ounce, not only prevents curds forming, but also increases the neutralising effect. Fatty substances tend to diminish gastric secretion, carbohydrates have little neutralising power.

During the stage of healing of the ulcer the patient must be kept in bed and feeds given at not more than two to two and a half hourly intervals during the day; by night a feed should only be given if the patient wakes. The time for an ulcer to heal, as judged by X-ray appearances and negative tests for occult blood in the fæces, varies according to its size from four to eight weeks. It is improbable that a deeply excavated and adherent ulcer could heal so quickly. Although some authorities maintain that it is irrational to increase the diet until the ulcer is healed, in our experience this can be done with advantage by carefully graduated changes.

The treatment we adopt is as follows :—

Healing Stage (Diet 1). *Weeks* 1 *and* 2. Feeds of 5 oz. are given at 7 a.m., 9 a.m., 11 a.m., 1 p.m., 3 p.m., 5 p.m., 7 p.m., 9 p.m., 11 p.m., and once during the night, if awake. The feeds consist of milk (warm and containing 3 gr. soldium citrate to the ounce), Horlick's malted milk or Benger's food. At least five of the feeds should be of milk which may be coloured with tea. Sugar may be added to the feeds as desired. If the patient is hungry the feeds may be increased to 6 oz., or even 8 oz., and ½ oz. of glucose taken 3 times a day. Strained orange or tomato juice, 1 oz., should be given daily thoughout the treatment to supply vitamin C.

Week 3. Add one raw egg to two of the milk feeds, if available. A little thin bread and butter is given with one feed and a rusk or plain biscuit may be taken with the other feeds. In addition, the patient may be given once a day a little of one of the following: sweet jelly, milk jelly, custard or junket. The feeds are still given two-hourly.

Week 4. The feeds are given every two and a half hours, from 7 a.m. to 10 p.m. They consist of 5 oz. of citrated milk every other feed with one egg in two of the feeds, if available, the thin bread and butter, rusk or plain buscuit and sugar, as in week 3. The alternate feeds are composed of a similar quantity of potato soup, arrowroot, cornflour, or milk pudding (sago or tapioca), and once a day a little sweet jelly, milk jelly, custard, junket, apple or prune purée or honey.

Week 5. The feeds are given every two and a half hours. The milk may now be reduced to three times a day, at 7 a.m., 5 p.m. and 10 p.m. Additions to the diet are a small helping of porridge made from very fine oatmeal, pounded fish 2 oz., lightly boiled egg, crisp toast or rusk (well chewed) with butter, sponge or Madeira cake.

Week 6. Feeds still every two and a half hours. Add 2 to 4 oz. minced meat daily.

Take immediately before three feeds, $\frac{1}{2}$ oz. of olive oil, and immediately before three other feeds, tinct. bellad. m. 5–10, aq. chlorcf. ad fl. oz. $\frac{1}{2}$, or atrophine sulphate gr. $\frac{1}{200}$ in m. 60 of water. Take one teaspoonful of the magnesium trisilicate or of Aludrox one hour after five feeds during the day and two teaspoonfuls the last thing at night, in a little water, during the first two weeks of the treatment.

During the third and fourth weeks take a teaspoonful of the powder or of Aludrox three times a day after feeds and two teaspoonfuls at night. In the fifth to eighth weeks take a teaspoonful of the powder or of Aludrox twice a day after feeds and two teaspoonfuls at night. It is very important to neutralise, as far as possible, the gastric secretion during the night. The patient should always have a milk feed by his bed to drink if he wakes. The mouth should be cleaned after each feed with bicarbonate of soda solution, gr. 60 to 5 oz. of water. This is important, as parotid suppuration may occur if it is neglected. No smoking is allowed.

Convalescent Stage (Diet 2). During this period of about a month the patient is allowed up for gradually increasing periods, and additions are made to the dietary.

7.30 *a.m., Breakfast.* One egg (lightly boiled, if available), or 2 oz. of steamed fish, thin bread and butter or crisp toast buttered when cold (to be well chewed), honey or apple jelly, sugar and milky tea.

10 *a.m.* Milk 5 oz. (containing 15 gr. of sodium citrate) or Horlick's malted milk or Benger's food.

12.30 *p.m., Lunch.* Milk soup (potato or artichoke), fresh white fish (boiled or steamed), or rabbit, chicken or tender mutton, mashed potato. Custard or milk pudding or stewed apples (with no pips, skin or core), or prune purée, and the juice of an orange, if available.

3 *p.m.* Thin bread and butter, or biscuits and butter, or one small slice of sponge or Madeira cake, and milky tea.

5.30 *p.m.* Milk 5 oz. (containing 15 gr. sodium citrate) or Horlick's malted milk.

8 *p.m.*, *Dinner.* As for lunch.

10.30 *p.m.* Milk 5 oz. (containing 15 gr. sodium citrate) or Benger's food.

The neutralising powder or Aludrox should be taken, one teaspoonful after breakfast and two teaspoonfuls last thing at night, and the olive oil or belladonna before breakfast, lunch and dinner. The meals should be small and eaten slowly. No smoking is allowed.

After Treatment (Diet 3). 8 *a.m.*, *Breakfast.* A selection from porridge, made from very fine oatmeal; egg, boiled, poached or scrambled; white fish, grilled or steamed; cold ham; tongue; toast, crisply made and well chewed; breakfast biscuits; honey; apple jelly; butter; sugar; and milky tea or coffee.

11 *a.m.* A tumbler of milk, Ovaltine, Horlick's malted milk, or Benger's food and a biscuit.

1 *p.m.*, *Lunch.* A selection from soup, made from milk and vegetables, such as potato or artichoke. Fresh white fish, boiled, grilled or steamed with white sauce, or fish soufflé. Meat, such as minced fresh beef, mutton, rabbit, liver or veal, grilled lamb cutlet, boiled or roast chicken. If the meat is not minced, it must be well masticated. Cheese soufflé. Vegetables, such as mashed potato, steamed or boiled green vegetables, marrow, peas (if tender). Sweets, such as custard, boiled or baked, junket, milk pudding very well cooked, cornflour, stewed apples (with no pips, core or skin), chocolate soufflé, plain steamed or baked pudding. Crisp toast, butter, and the juice of one or more oranges.

4 *p.m.* A cup of milky tea, thin bread and butter, jelly jam or honey, sponge or plain cake.

7 *p.m.*, *Dinner.* As for lunch.

10 *p.m.* A feed as at 11 a.m.

The breakfast, lunch and dinner should be small meals, well chewed and eaten slowly. The patient should rest for half an hour after meals. No condiments should be eaten, and nothing taken which cannot be reduced to a soft pulp in the mouth. If it is impossible to obtain the liquid feeds between all the meals, a biscuit or some chocolate should be eaten. A teaspoonful of the neutralising powder or of Aludrox should be taken every night on retiring to bed. No smoking is allowed.

The following articles of food are forbidden: Smoked salmon, kippers, whitebait, tough meat, pork, high game, sausages, brawn, curry, made-up dishes, fried foods, cheese (except cream cheese), meat extracts and meat soups, pickles, spices, ginger, salads, uncooked vegetables, celery, carrots, cucumber, onions or any fibrous vegetables, new or wholemeal bread, buns, Ryvita, Vita-wheat, digestive and oatmeal biscuits, hot buttered toast, unripe or raw fruit, rhubarb, plums, nuts, raisins, sultanas, figs, jam with pips, marmalade with peel, strong tea or coffee, aerated drinks and alcohol.

The Danger of Alkalosis. Large doses of alkalis, especially of sodium bicarbonate, magnesium oxide and carbonate, may produce toxic symptoms (Hardt and Rivers (36)). Alkalosis is liable to occur in cases of gastric stasis especially associated with duodenal ulcer or renal insufficiency. It would appear that this observation is difficult to reconcile with the rationale of the alkali treatment of nephritis, for renal insufficiency usually tends to produce acidosis. The symptoms are headache, vertigo, loss of appetite, distaste for milk, malaise, nausea, vomiting, drowsiness or coma. A determination of the alkali reserve of the blood is of value in confirming the diagnosis. All alkalis should be stopped, dextrose given by mouth or in rectal salines, ammon. chlor. 0·5 g. (stearettes) should be administered by mouth every six hours, or by rectum in doses of 4 g. every six hours, and an intravenous injection made of collosol calcium (1 ml.), repeated next day if necessary.

Continuous Intragastric Drip Treatment. Winkelstein (37) in 1932 determined the gastric acidity during the night in cases of duodenal ulcer, gastric ulcer and normal controls. A Rehfuss tube was inserted in the stomach at 7 p.m. and specimens of gastric juice removed every two hours during the night. He found a high continuous acid secretion in cases of duodenal ulcer, a moderate acid secretion in gastric ulcer, but in the controls the curve was very low, and in 4 out of every 6 cases no free hydrochloric acid was secreted during the night. He introduced a continuous Murphy drip through a Rehfuss tube for the treatment of peptic ulcer, using alkalinised milk. Woldman and Rowland (38) in 1936 published their results in cases of peptic ulcer treated with a continuous intragastric drip of 200 ml. of 7% colloidal aluminium hydroxide mixed with 600 ml. of water. These authors (39) reported further that gastric and duodenal ulcers which were quite apparent radiologically disappeared after about seven to fourteen days' treatment; further, only 3 or 4 small bland feeds a day were required such as milk, cream, junket, custard, jelly, cereals, etc. Rutherford and Emery (40) in 1939 and 1940 used Creamalin (5·5% aluminium hydroxide), 1 part, to 3 parts of water, as a drip, running at 15 drops a minute. They treated 28 severe cases of peptic ulcer, which had previously failed to respond to medical or surgical treatment, or to both. They gave the drip usually for a week and subsequently the aluminium hydroxide was administered by mouth for several months. In a follow-up fifteen months later, of 14 of their original 28 very severe cases, they reported that 8 were well, 2 doubtfully improved and 4 were unsatisfactory. We use a mixture of milk 1 pint, dextrose 2 oz. and sod. citrate gr. 10. A Ryle's tube is passed through the nose into the stomach and joined by a glass connection to rubber tubing attached to the drip. The fluid flows at the rate of 40 drops a minute, day and night, *i.e.* 6 pints in twenty-four hours. If the tube blocks it is flushed through with a syringeful of milk. A specimen is removed every four hours for the first twenty-four hours, and titrated for free HCl; if it is present ½ fl. oz. of Aludrox is added to each pint of milk. If the patient is hungry the amount of dextrose is increased. The Ryle's tube is changed every other day, cleaned and boiled, and the rubber tubing and glass connections are washed and boiled. We have found that some cases of gastric or duodenal ulcer which have not healed after six to eight weeks' treatment in bed on the conventional Sippy lines have healed after treatment by the drip method in periods of three to seven weeks.

Whatever form of treatment is adopted, it is important that, as soon as the patient is in a fit state, a search should be made for any possible focus of infection, which should be eradicated when found. The teeth should be X-rayed, the nose and sinuses examined, and pyorrhœa should be treated. A search for signs of appendicitis or infection of the gall-bladder or uro-genital tract should also be made.

The Medical Treatment of Chronic Ulcers. This is in all essentials similar to that detailed above for acute ulceration of the stomach or duodenum; in fact, apart from the history of the duration of the case, it is difficult to distinguish between the two conditions.

It will be noticed that throughout this section gastric and duodenal ulcers have been considered together, as if their treatment were the same. Duodenal ulcers are of much more frequent occurrence, and are more easy to diagnose.

The Surgical Treatment of Ulcers not Complicated by Hæmorrhage. While, on the one hand, it is clear that in certain circumstances medical measures are of no avail in the treatment of gastric and duodenal ulcers, yet patients are frequently seen who have had operations for these conditions and who have received no permanent benefit. Indeed, their last state is not infrequently worse than their first. It is, therefore, profitable to endeavour to decide what are the indications for surgical treatment. In this way patients should derive the maximum benefit possible, and not be subjected to operations which either give no relief or are followed by only a temporary amelioration of the symptoms.

The following are the chief indications for operations :—

Surgical treatment is imperative in cases of perforation or of perigastric abscess, although some cases of perforation have been successfully treated by continuous gastric suction.

Ogilvie (41) makes the following further recommendations :—

Gastric Ulcer. Operation is required for the following reasons : (*a*) Organic stenosis causing delay in emptying. (*b*) If cancerous transformation of the ulcer is suspected. (*c*) If medical treatment fails, as will occur if a chronic ulcer becomes fixed to neighbouring structures. The acid secretion in gastric ulcer is not usually raised, and gastrectomy is generally the most satisfactory operation.

Duodenal Ulcer. Operation is required for organic stenosis. A posterior gastro-enterostomy or a gastro-duodenostomy should be performed. As the gastric acidity is usually low, owing to the presence of chronic gastritis, recurrent anastomotic or jejunal ulceration is unlikely to ensue. Recurrent ulceration of this type is probably due to the operation of gastro-enterostomy being performed in the presence of high gastric acidity. Further, the average time for the appearance of the recurrent ulcer is several years. Gastro-jejunostomy alone is, therefore, absolutely contra-indicated when the gastric acidity is high and the rate of stomach emptying is rapid, with the following exception. In a patient over the age of fifty, if symptoms of duodenal ulcer persist, usually because the patient will not adhere strictly to his medical treatment, a short-circuiting operation may be performed, even if there is no stenosis. The gastric acidity tends to fall progressively after the age of fifty, and so the chance of a recurrent ulcer is slight.

Vagotomy

Division of the vagus nerves to eliminate gastric secretion due to nervous stimuli would appear to be a sound procedure in cases of peptic ulcer, as such ulceration is believed to result from the corroding effect of unneutralised gastric hydrochloric acid. Vagotomy will not influence the gastric secretion which results from hormonal influences and which accompanies the taking of food. The presence of the meal in the stomach, however, probably protects the gastric mucosa from the effects of the hydrochloric acid. The nervous secretion occurs as the result of psychic stimulation at the thought or sight of a meal and also accounts for the considerable secretion of gastric juice which is poured out during the night. By diminishing or abolishing such nocturnal secretion vagotomy should exert a powerful influence both in the healing of peptic ulcers, and in preventing their recurrence.

As far back as 1814 Brodie (42) showed that the intravenous injection of arsenic in dogs causes the stomach to be filled with mucus and watery fluid. If the vagi were cut before the arsenic was injected the stomach remained empty. In 1894 Pavlov (43) found that division of the vagi in dogs prevented the gastric secretion of hydrochloric acid. In 1923 Carlson (44) pointed out that although vagotomy abolished the neurogenic secretion, there still remained the humoral secretion due to the formation of gastrin in the pyloric mucosa, which is carried by the blood-stream to the stomach. In 1930 Dragstedt and Ellis (45) isolated the stomach in dogs, keeping the blood and nerve supplies intact, and maintaining intestinal continuity by an oesophago-jejunostomy. The gastric secretions were collected through a gold-plated cannula. Chlorides had to be supplied to keep the animals alive. In such animals gastric ulcers developed. When the vagi were divided the amount of gastric secretion was reduced from 1,000 to 2,500 ml.

per twenty-four hours to 300 to 600 ml. per twenty-four hours, and gastric ulcers did not develop. The gastric acidity was also lowered. It was this experiment which led Dragstedt to divide the vagi in man for the treatment of peptic ulcer. Since then vagotomy has been more extensively used as a therapeutic measure, especially as so much emphasis is now laid on the effect of nervous stress, emotion, and frustration in the production of peptic ulcers. Vagotomy results in the abolition both of gastric hypersecretion and hypermotility, and gastric acidity and secretion tend to return to normal.

In 1946 Dragstedt (46) reported very promising results from vagotomy in the treatment of peptic ulcer and observed no recurrence of ulcers, although he cautiously stated " a longer period of observation and a more extensive series of patients are obviously necessary to provide final answers". Thorek (47) reviewed in 1947 the anatomical nerve supply of the stomach, and emphasised the relative merits of the transabdominal and transthoracic methods of approach. He concluded that the operation appeared to be indicated in duodenal and stomal ulcers which do not respond to medical treatment. He advised that gastric ulcers should be resected owing to their tendency to malignant degeneration. The transabdominal operation has the advantage that the lesion can be inspected and a gastro-enterostomy performed to compensate for obstructive or atonic complications. It has been shown by many observers that if all the vagal fibres are not divided the gastric acidity tends to return to its previous values. Thompson and James (48) believe the vagi can be more completely divided by the transthoracic approach. They report satisfactory results in 4 patients with severe and recurrent peptic ulceration. Orr and Johnson (49) have tried vagotomy as an alternative to gastro-jejunostomy, which they state is a failure as a routine procedure, for it does not cure more than half the patients and has an operative mortality rate of about 2%. Gastrectomy, they say, is more successful if sufficiently radical, but has a mortality rate of about 5%, and a recurrent ulceration rate of 2 to 9%. These surgeons performed vagotomy or vagal resection on 50 patients without a death. The operation they prefer is post-hiatal vagal resection from below. A gastro-enterostomy may subsequently be necessary if the stomach does not recover sufficient tone to drive the meal through the narrowed pylorus. They consider that vagal resection is particularly indicated in young subjects who suffer from relapses of duodenal ulcer, whereas gastrectomy is the operation of choice for gastric ulcer. Vagal resection may also be used with advantage in cases of stomal ulcer, either with or without other operative procedures.

The insulin test is of value in determining whether the vagal fibres have been adequately divided. With an intact vagal supply the intravenous injection of 16 units of insulin causes a sharp rise in the free and total acidity of the gastric juice. This is due to hypoglycæmia, affecting the vagal nerve centre, and is not a primary insulin effect. After vagal resection no such rise occurs.

Walters et al. (50) in 1948 reported the results of vagus nerve resection in 118 cases of gastro-duodenal and jejunal ulceration. The authors operated on patients suffering from duodenal ulcer, when treatment had failed. Such cases they would formerly have considered suitable for partial gastrectomy. Vagotomy was combined with gastro-enterostomy, when indicated. Relief of pain and healing of the ulcer is much more likely to occur with duodenal than with gastric ulcer. Rob (51) has recounted a case of recurrence of symptoms of duodenal ulcer six months after complete freedom of symptoms following bilateral vagotomy. The insulin test indicated that the vagal resection was adequate, and there was no evidence of nerve regeneration when the symptoms recurred. Rob found that in a series of 37 operations for peptic ulcer the results were very good in 5 cases with secondary ulceration following gastrectomy or gastro-enterostomy. In the other 32 cases, with duodenal ulcer, there were numerous early complications, such as temporary severe dysphagia, persistent diarrhœa, and eructations of foul gas. Beattie (52) reviewed in 1950 the results of gastrectomy and vagotomy in duodenal ulcers. The after results of gastrectomy for duodenal ulcers are often disappointing. He says that the stomach is too small to hold a sufficiency of food or to digest it properly, and recurrent gastro-intestinal upsets occur in about a sixth of the cases, which are sufficiently severe to upset the patient's economic life. In a series of 3,000 successful vagotomies performed during an eight-year period up to 1950 it was found that recurrent ulceration is extremely rare when the insulin test has shown complete nerve section. Secondary pylorospasm, due to overaction of the sympathetic nerves, however, frequently caused recurrent ulcer symptoms. Beattie had to operate again on 54 of his 103 cases of simple vagotomy to relieve retention symptoms. In order to prevent these Beattie advises performing pylorectomy together with vagotomy, and considers that gastrectomy should be reserved for those less common cases in which the ulcer has penetrated deeply into the surrounding viscera.

Conclusions. Vagotomy offers a physiological method of reducing the gastric acidity which leads to the formation of peptic ulcers, and is now being more extensively used, especially when combined with some other operation. The disturbances of motor function and the tendency to the secondary development of pyloric spasm may lead to a recurrence of ulcer symptoms causing considerable distress and requiring a subsequent gastro-enterostomy. It is not yet possible to say whether vagotomy will become the operation of choice in the majority of cases of duodenal ulcer, but it does seem probable that vagotomy should be combined with some other procedure to eliminate the probable delay in stomach emptying. Although the physician should understand what types of operation are available for the treatment of peptic ulcer, the ultimate choice is the responsibility of the surgeon.

REFERENCES

(1) Berg. "*Rontgenuntersuchungen am innenrelief des verdauungskanals,*" 1930. Thieme, Leipzig.
(2) Cordiner and Calthrop. *Brit. Journ. of Surg.*, 1936, **23**, 700.
(3) Taylor. *Lancet*, 1941, *ii*, 276.
(4) Rodgers. *Proc. Roy. Soc. Med.*, 1938, **32**, 519.
(5) Lintott. *Proc. Roy. Soc. Med.*, 1938, **32**, 533.
(6) Bank and Renshaw. *Journ. Amer. Med. Assocn.*, 1939, **112**, 214.
(7) Freeman. *Journ. Amer. Med. Assocn.*, 1939, **112**, 217.
(8) Gill, Berridge and Jones. *Lancet*, 1942, *i*, 727.
(9) Berry. *Journ. Amer. Med. Assocn.*, 1941, **117**, 2233.
(10) Hartfall. *Proc. Roy. Soc. Med.*, 1938, **32**, 527.
(11) Cullinan and Price. *Bart's Hosp. Rep.*, 1932, **65**, 185.
(12) Hurst and Ryle. *Lancet*, 1937, *i*, 1.
(13) Meulengracht. *Acta med. Scand.*, 1934, Supplement 59, 375; *Lancet*, 1935, *ii*, 1220; *Wien. klin. Woch.*, 1936, **49**, 1481; *Münch. med. Woch.*, 1937, **84**, 1565.
(14) Jones. *Brit. Med. Journ.*, 1947, *ii*, 441, 477.
(15) Baker. *Guy's Hosp. Rep.*, 1947, **96**, 1.
(16) Lewin and Truelove. *Brit. Med. Journ.*, 1949, *i*, 383.
(17) Needham and McConachie. *Brit. Med. Journ.*, 1950, *ii*, 133.
(18) *Proc. Roy. Soc. Med.*, 1924, **17**, 1; 1934, **27**, 1437.
(19) Blackford and Allen. *Journ. Amer. Med. Assocn.*, 1942, **120**, 811.
(20) Willcox. *Lancet*, 1924, *i*, 544.

(21) Marriott and Kekwick. *Practitioner*, 1937, **139**, 250.
(22) Witts. *Brit. Med. Journ.*, 1937, *i*, 847.
(23) Marriott and Kekwick. *Lancet*, 1935, *i*, 977.
(24) Lenhartz. *Deutsch. med. Woch.*, 1904, **30**, 412.
(25) Pickering. *Lancet*, 1942, *i*, 631.
(26) Woldman. *Amer. Journ. Med. Sci.*, 1937, **194**, 333.
(27) Gordon-Taylor. *Brit. Journ. of Surg.*, 1937, **25**, 403.
(28) Finsterer. *Journ. de Chir.*, 1933, **42**, 673 ; *Lancet*, 1936, *ii*, 303.
(29) Sippy. *Journ. Amer. Med. Assocn.*, 1915, **64**, 1, 625.
(30) Freezer, Gibson and Matthews. *Guy's Hosp. Rep.*, 1928, **78**, 191.
(31) Hurst. *Brit. Med. Journ.*, 1928, *ii*, 779.
(32) Crohn. *Journ. Lab. and Clin. Med.*, 1929; **14**, 610.
(33) Fauley, Freeman, Ivy, Atkinson and Wigodsky. *Arch. Int. Med.*, 1941, **67**, 563.
(34) Mutch. *Brit. Med. Journ.*, 1936, *i*, 143 ; *ibid*, 1936, *i*, 254.
(35) Cohn, White and Weyrauch. *Journ. Amer. Med. Assocn.*, 1941, **117**, 2225.
(36) Hardt and Rivers. *Arch. Int. Med.*, 1923, **31**, 171.
(37) Winkelstein. *Amer. Journ. of Surg.*, 1932, **15**, 523.
(38) Woldman and Rowland. *Amer. Journ. Digest. Dis.*, 1936, **2**, 733.
(39) Woldman and Rowland. *Review of Gastroenterology*, 1936, **3**, 27.
(40) Rutherford and Emery. *New Eng. Journ. of Med.*, 1939, **220**, 407.
(41) Ogilvie. *Lancet*, 1935, *i*, 419 ; *ibid.*, 1938, *ii*, 295.
(42) Brodie. *Phil. Trans. Roy. Soc. London*, 1814, **104**, 102.
(43) Pavlov. *Trudi Obsh. russk. vrach.*, 1894–95, **61**, 298.
(44) Carlson. *Physiol. Rev.*, 1923, **3**, 1.
(45) Dragstedt and Ellis. *Amer. Journ. Physiol.*, 1930, **93**, 407.
(46) Dragstedt. *Minnesota Med.*, 1946, **29**, 597.
(47) Thorek. *Journ. Amer. Med. Assoc.*, 1947, **135**, 1141.
(48) Thompson and James. *Lancet*, 1947, *ii*, 44.
(49) Orr and Johnson. *Lancet*, 1947, *ii*, 84.
(50) Walters, Neibling, Bradley, Small and Wilson. *Journ. Amer. Med. Assoc.*, 1948, **136**, 742.
(51) Rob. *Lancet*, 1948, *ii*, 730.
(52) Beattie. *Lancet*, 1950, *i*, 525.

CHAPTER VIII

THE CARDIOVASCULAR SYSTEM

Cardiac Irregularities

Potain (1), in 1867, obtained tracings from the jugular vein in man. He used as a receiver of its pulsations a glass funnel which was connected by a rubber tube with a Marey sphygmograph, and recorded at the same time tracings from the apex beat, carotid and radial arteries. In 1892 Sir James Mackenzie (2), using a small metal cup as a receiver, devised the instrument originally called a phlebograph, by means of which simultaneous tracings of the pulsations of the jugular vein and radial artery were obtained. The records were taken upon smoked paper, but by the use of inked pens the polygraph was evolved.

Our knowledge of the essential nature of the different forms of cardiac irregularity is mainly due to Sir James Mackenzie's pioneer work with this instrument, by means of which he obtained records representing the activities both of the auricle and of the ventricle. Further light has been thrown upon this subject and upon myocardial disorders by the use of the electrocardiograph.

The chief varieties of cardiac irregularity are as follows: (1) Sinus arrhythmia; (2) premature systoles; (3) heart-block; (4) auricular flutter; (5) auricular fibrillation; (6) paroxysmal tachycardia; and (7) pulsus alternans.

The Electrocardiograph

The electrical currents produced by the contraction of the human heart were first recorded by Waller (3) in 1887 by means of the capillary electrometer. With this instrument the movements of a fine column of mercury are photographed on a moving plate.

The string galvanometer was later introduced by Einthoven (4) in 1903, and modifications of it are now known as the electrocardiograph.

Immersion electrodes have been largely replaced by small electrodes of German silver plate, about 3 square inches in size. Cambridge electrode jelly is smeared over the electrode and rubbed

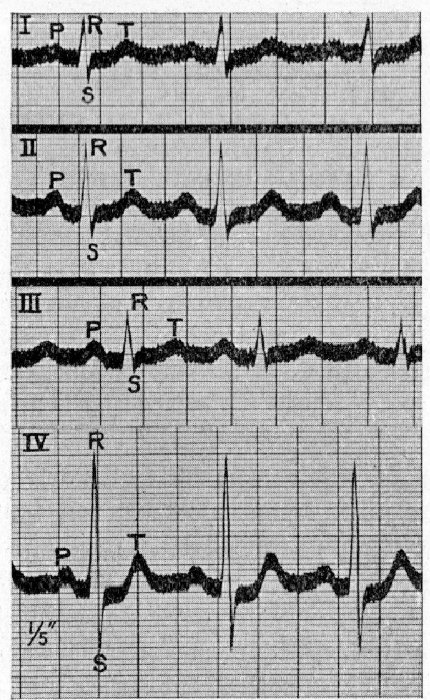

FIG. 9. Normal Electrocardiogram (Lead IV R, left arm electrode anteriorly, right arm electrode on right arm).

gently into an area of skin, corresponding with the size of the electrode.

The leads usually adopted are as follows :—

Lead I (transverse). Right and left hands.

Lead II (axial). Right hand and left foot.

Lead III (left lateral). Left hand and left foot.

Lead IV (chest leads). See p. 189.

Unipolar leads. See p. 190.

Curves representing the changes in potential caused by the heart's beat are photographed. A single beat from the normal heart shows the following waves (see Fig. 9) :—

P is due to auricular systole, and constitutes the auricular complex. **QRST** occur during ventricular systole, and constitute the ventricular complex. **Q** and **S** are often absent. **T–P** represents diastole.

Certain time relations are important:—

The **P–R** interval is normally 0·14 second. Prolongation of this indicates delay in conduction in the A–V node or the upper part of the bundle of His.

The **QRS** interval is normally just under 0·10 second. Prolongation of this occurs in the various grades of heart-block and in ectopic ventricular beats.

The **R–T** interval is normally 0·32 second. Prolongation of this occurs especially in complete A–V block.

The **QRST** curves are produced by currents originating in the two ventricles, and represent the algebraic sum of the waves produced by the two ventricles contracting separately.

The characteristic appearance of the deflections in the first three leads should now be studied (see Fig. 9). The **R** wave is normally greatest in Lead II, and $\mathbf{R}_1$ and $\mathbf{R}_3$ are together approximately equal to $\mathbf{R}_2$. (The figures below the waves indicate the leads in which the waves occur.) The **P** and **T** waves are also usually larger in Lead II than in Leads I or III.

The Significance of certain Alterations in the Form of the Deflections. *The P Wave.* This may be inverted, indicating that the impulse originates at a new focus in the auricle (at times in the A–V node as in paroxysmal tachycardia and in nodal extrasystoles). The **P** wave may be absent, or replaced by a small series of oscillations of a fine or coarse variety, as is seen in auricular fibrillation. It may be abnormally large and notched, indicating auricular hypertrophy, as may occur in mitral stenosis. $\mathbf{P}_3$ may be greater than $\mathbf{P}_2$, as may be seen in auricular flutter.

The R Wave. A maximum **R** wave in Lead I indicates left axis deviation, which, when present to a high degree, is most often due to left ventricular preponderance. It may also be associated with an unduly transverse lie of the heart, associated with a high diaphragm. In right axis deviation, which also includes right ventricular preponderance, the **R** wave is greatest in Lead III.

Normally the left ventricle is 1·8 times heavier than the right.

The S Wave. A maximum **S** wave in Lead I indicates right axis deviation, whereas a maximum **S** wave in Lead III is a sign of left axis deviation.

The T Wave. It is held that the $\mathbf{T}_2$ wave is of great importance as indicating the condition of the ventricular muscle. A negative

$\mathbf{T_2}$ wave is always pathological and a negative $\mathbf{T_1}$ wave usually indicates a pathological condition. With full doses of digitalis the **S–T** segment is usually depressed and the **T** wave inverted in all leads. A negative $\mathbf{T_3}$ wave is not necessarily pathological.

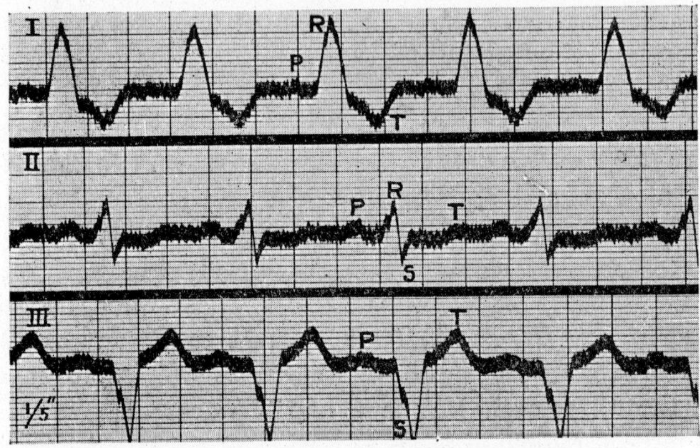

Fig. 10. Bundle-Branch Block (Type I).

Prolongation of the QRS Complex. In the condition known as bundle-branch block, the right or left branch of the bundle of His is impaired and fails to conduct. The **QRS** complex is prolonged or spread out, and lasts longer than the normal maximum of 0·10 second. The **R** wave may be notched. The **T** wave is in the opposite direction to the main initial deflection (**R** or **S**), and is usually of a greater amplitude than normal. The ventricular complex is therefore diphasic.

Two types of curves are met with in patients suffering from bundle-branch block, depending on which branch of the bundle is obstructed. The old classification was based on animal experiments, and according to the type of curve obtained right or left bundle-branch block was diagnosed. Later work on human subjects has thrown doubt on the applicability to man of these conclusions drawn from animal experiments, and there is therefore uncertainty as to which type of curve corresponds with right or left bundle-branch block. The curves are referred to now simply as Type I and Type II.

Type I Bundle-Branch Block (old terminology, right). The main

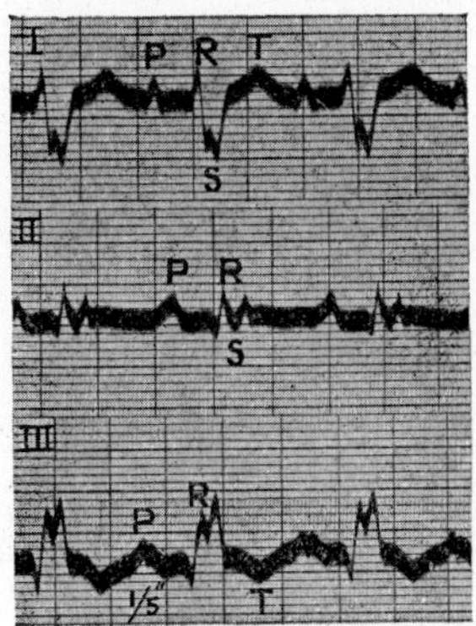

FIG. 11. Bundle-Branch Block (Type II).

initial deflection (**R**) is positive in Lead I and negative (**S**) in Lead III (see Fig. 10). This is the common variety.

Type II Bundle-Branch Block (old terminology, left). The main initial deflection (**S**) is negative in Lead I and positive (**R**) in Lead III (see Fig. 11). **Type IIa.** This was described by Wilson and his co-workers (5) in 1934, and in 1937 was called by Evans and Turnbull (6) "the newer electrocardiogram denoting right bundle-branch block". It is more common than the hitherto standard Type II curve. The distinctive features are: Lead I. **R** and **S** almost equal in size. **R** narrow. **S** broad and notched. **T** upright. Lead II. **S** broad and deep. **T** usually upright. Lead III. **Q** or **S** usually deep. **T** inverted (see Fig. 12).

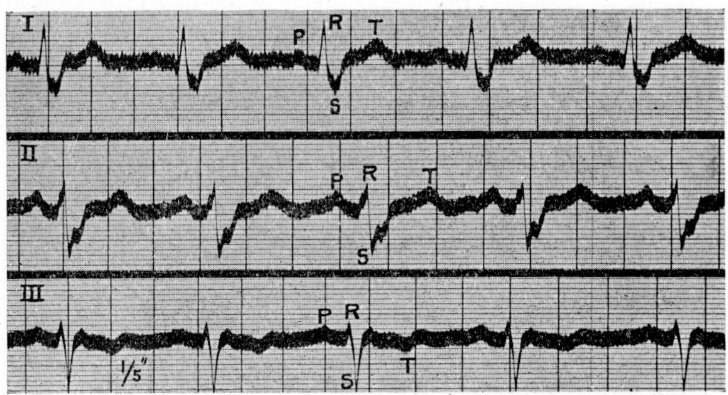

FIG. 12. Bundle-Branch Block (Type IIa).

The **QRS** complex is also prolonged in *intraventricular block*, in which the terminations of the bundles in the ventricular subendothelial tissue are destroyed. The **R** wave is also often notched, and the **T** wave is in the same direction as the initial main deflection.

In *congenital dextrocardia* all the waves in Lead I are inverted, whereas Lead II may represent the normal Lead III, and vice versa.

Absence of the PRT Complex. This occurs in sino-auricular block, in which the stimulus arising in the S–A node at times fails to cause a contraction of the auricle. The whole heart, therefore, misses a beat, but the succeeding contraction occurs at approximately the normal interval. This is not necessarily a serious condition (see Fig. 13).

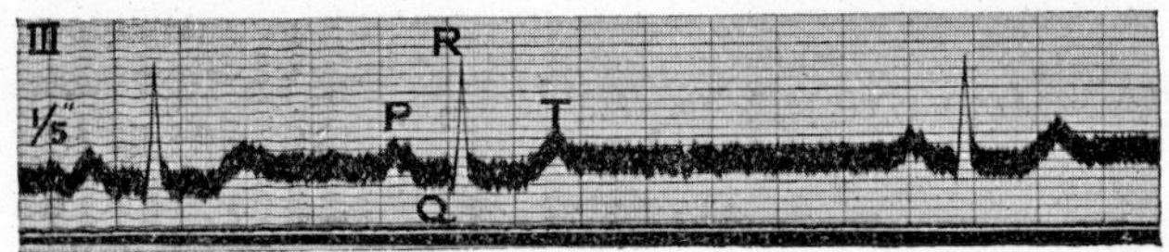

FIG. 13. Sino-Auricular Block.

In addition to the light which the electrocardiograph throws upon the condition of the myocardium and conducting tissue, the various types of cardiac irregularity can be accurately determined.

Sinus Arrhythmia. Variations in the length of the **T–P** intervals are seen, but the auricular and ventricular complexes are normal.

Premature Systoles. *Auricular.* The premature impulse may arise at the S–A node, near it, or some distance away. In the two former instances the **P** wave caused by the premature contraction is in the normal direction, in the latter it is inverted, indicating that the impulse spreads through the auricle along abnormal

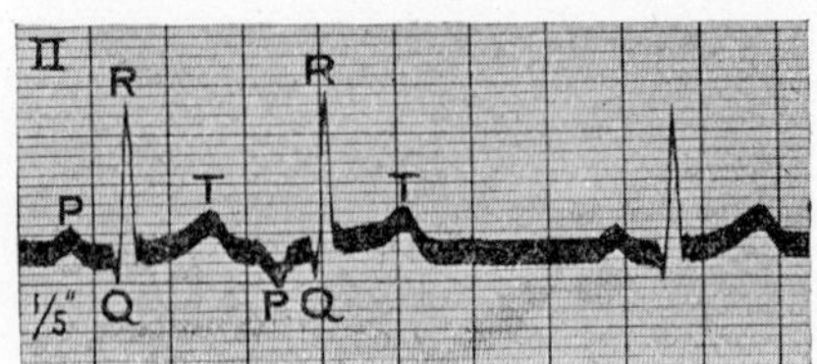

FIG. 14. Premature Auricular Systole.

paths (see Fig. 14). The ventricular complex following the premature auricular stimulus is usually of normal type. The premature **P** wave may occur so early in diastole that it fuses with the previous **T** wave.

Usually the diastole following the premature beat is not fully compensatory.

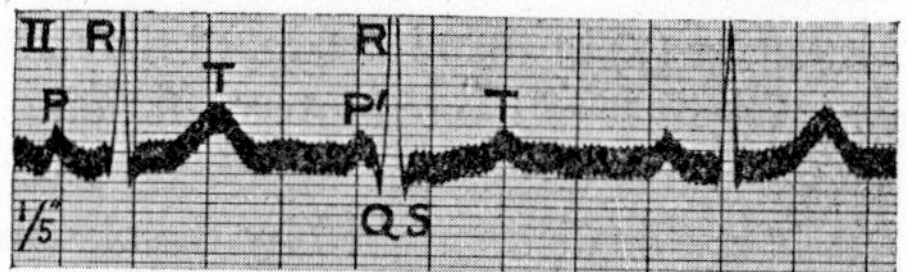

FIG. 15. Premature Nodal Systole.

Nodal. The premature impulse arises in the junctional tissue uniting the auricle and ventricle, *i.e.* in the A–V node or the A–V bundle before division. The ventricular contraction may occur just before, or abnormally shortly after, the auricular, but is seen to be supraventricular in origin because the **QRS** complex is of normal appearance (see Fig. 15).

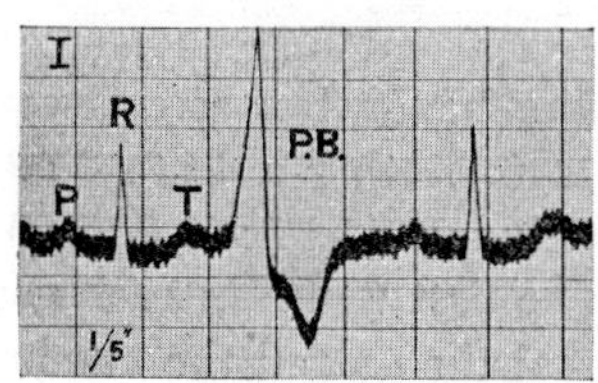

FIG. 16. Premature Ventricular Systole.

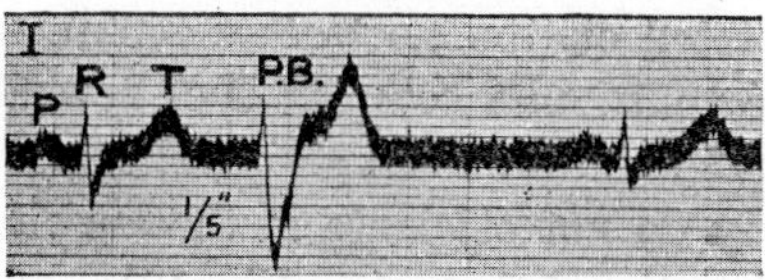

FIG. 17. Premature Ventricular Systole.

Ventricular. A premature stimulus arises in the ventricle below the division of the main A–V bundle. The premature ventricular complex resulting has the same duration as a normal ventricular complex, but its form is altered, the initial deflections of the premature beat being larger than normal. The auricular waves occur at regular intervals, and may be fused with the premature venticular deflections, or appear just after them. The premature ventricular beat is followed by a prolonged diastole and the succeeding pause is thus fully compensatory.

Two types occur (see Figs. 16 and 17) formerly called left and right ventricular premature systoles. As with the site of bundle-branch block, the localisation of ventricular systoles is now a matter of doubt, but of little clinical significance. According to the old terminology, based on experiments on dogs, the main ventricular deflection is upright in Lead I and inverted in Lead III with left ventricular premature systoles and with right bundle-branch block. With right ventricular premature systoles and with left bundle-branch block the deflections occur in the reverse direction. Barker, McLeod and Alexander (7) in 1930 introduced the new terminology which is the exact opposite of the old interpretation.

Heart-block. Various degrees of impairment of conductivity of the heart muscle can be distinguished by the electrocardiograph.

Slight. Prolongation of the **P–R** interval to more than 0·2 second.

Occasional Dropped Beats. The **P–R** interval gradually becomes longer until, finally, the ventricular complex fails to follow its preceding auricular complex. The **P** waves are quite regular, but the ventricular complexes occur at different intervals, and the **P** and **T** waves may at times fuse.

Regular Dropped Beats. Every fourth, third or second ventricular contraction may be omitted, constituting a 4 : 3, 3 : 2, or 2 : 1 heart-block. Other varieties include 8 : 7, 7 : 6, 6 : 5, 5 : 4, 3 : 1, 4 : 1 and 5 : 1 heart-block. The first figure in each couple indicates the number of auricular, and the second the number of ventricular beats.

Complete Heart-block. The ventricle contracts at its own independent rate of about 30 beats a minute. The **P** waves occur regularly, and may be seen isolated on the electrocardiogram or fused with **R** or **T** waves. The ventricular complex is of normal duration and configuration, and so the impulses giving rise to it are supraventricular, but as they do not originate in the auricle, they must be derived from the junctional tissue (see Fig. 18).

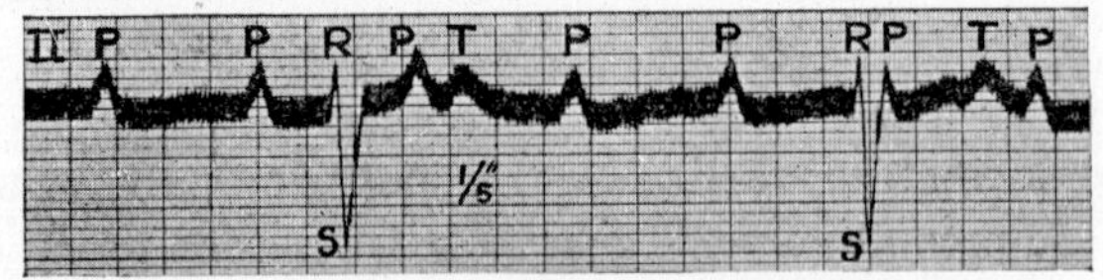

Fig. 18. Complete Heart-block.

Bundle-branch Block and *Intraventricular Block* have already been described (p. 178) (see Figs 10, 11 and 12).

Sino-auricular Block (*Tortoise Heart*). Some of the impulses arising in the S–A node fail to reach the main mass of auricular muscle, and occasional intermittences of the whole heart may occur (see Fig. 13). If the rate is slow, as is usually the case, on exercise it may increase to about double.

When the heart is beating at such a slow rate the ventricle may interpolate a beat on its own (*ventricular escape*), the **P**–**R** interval being shortened, or the **P** and **R** waves may partially fuse.

Nodal Rhythm. The impulse may arise at the A–V node instead of at the S–A node, the auricles and ventricles contract simultaneously, and no **P** waves are seen or they occur shortly after the **R**–**S** complex and are usually inverted (see Fig. 19).

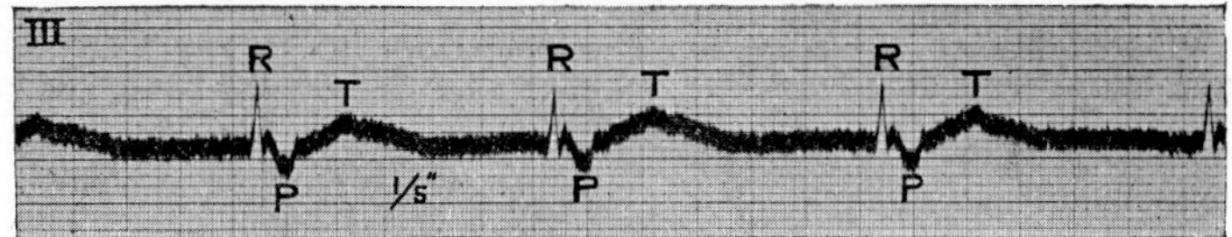

Fig. 19. Nodal Rhythm.

Auricular Flutter. An electrocardiogram shows the auricular contractions occurring at a regular rate, with ventricular complexes superimposed upon the curve at regular or irregular intervals. Heart-block of varying grades is almost invariably present.

The **P** waves occur at regular intervals and have a dome-shaped appearance (see Fig. 20). In some tracings the **T** wave is also apparent.

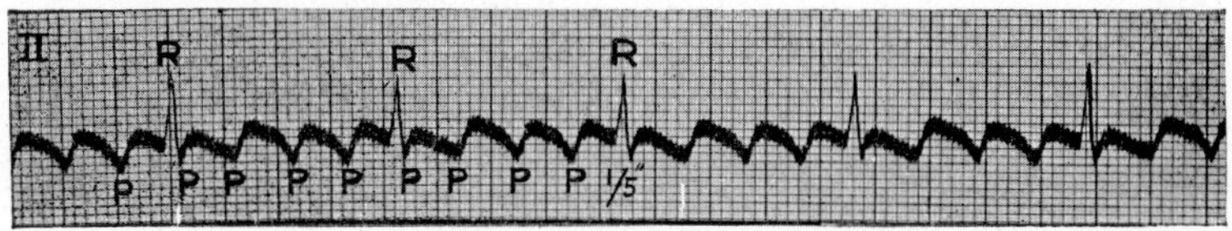

Fig. 20. Auricular Flutter.

Pressure on the vagus in the neck may slow the rate of ventricular contraction, but the **P** waves continue to come through at regular and rapid intervals.

The auricular contraction is no longer believed to pursue an abnormal circular path in the auricle. When the normal rhythm is established, as the result of the administration of digitalis or of quinidine, the gentle undulations of the **P** waves of flutter are replaced by the sharper peaked waves of normal rhythm.

Auricular Fibrillation. Here the **P** waves are absent, **QRS** deflections occur at irregular intervals, and are of varying height. The ventricular complex is of normal form. Oscillations of irregular size may be seen in diastole, caused by the fibrillating auricle; these may be fine or coarse. They are usually best seen in Leads II and III. They also occur during systole, and may alter the shape of the **T** wave, although the **QRS** deflections are not affected. In rapidly beating hearts the oscillations are usually not well seen in diastole, but their effect upon the **T** wave is generally noticeable (see Fig. 21).

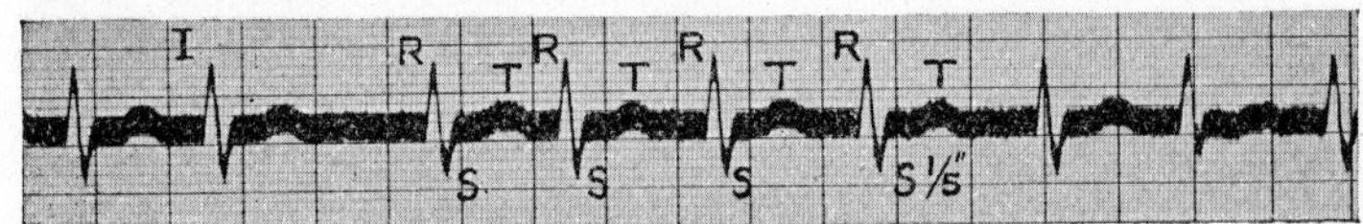

Fig. 21. Auricular Fibrillation.

The **QRS** deflections may occasionally be seen at regular intervals, although the auricle is fibrillating and no **P** waves are present, but oscillations due to fibrillation may be seen in diastole. This occurs when the ventricle has adopted its independent rhythm owing to complete heart-block.

Ectopic beats may arise during fibrillation; they are ventricular in origin. They may occur regularly after each **QRS** deflection, due to a supraventricular stimulus, constituting the coupled beats. This is usually due to excessive digitalis administration, and is a sign for immediate discontinuance of the drug.

Ventricular Fibrillation. Although compatible with life in man, if only of short duration (Gallavardin and Berard (8)), it is the probable cause of sudden death from heart failure, such as occurs under anæsthetics, etc.

Paroxysmal Tachycardia. *Simple Paroxysmal Tachycardia (Auricular).* A succession of ectopic auricular contractions occurs, arising at a new focus in the auricle. This is shown in the electrocardiogram by a rapid regular rhythm of about 150, in which the ventricular complexes are normal. The impulse has, therefore, a supraventricular origin. The **P** wave is often inverted in Leads II and III, and usually modified in Lead I. The auricular impulse is therefore ectopic in origin, and if not inverted in Leads II and III it is usually smaller than normal (see Fig. 22).

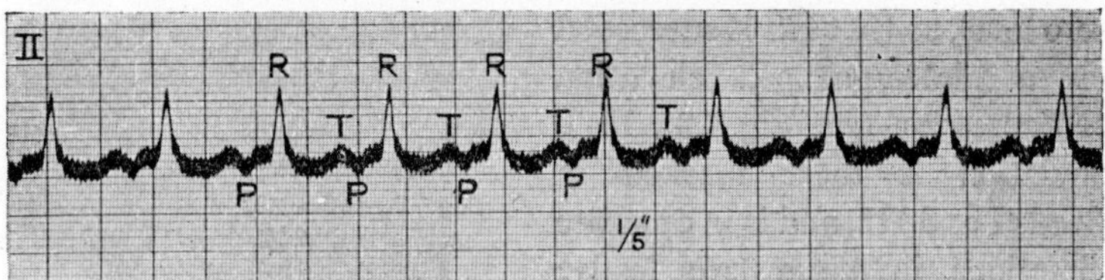

Fig. 22. Simple Paroxysmal Tachycardia, showing inversion of the " P " wave.

When the paroxysm ceases there is a pause, which is immediately followed by the restoration of the normal rhythm.

Auricular Flutter (see p. 183).

Auricular Fibrillation (see p. 184).

Nodal, arising in the A–V node. Here the auricle may contract first and the **P–R** interval be shortened, and **P** inverted, or the auricle and ventricle may contract simultaneously and the **P** and **R** be fused.

Ventricular. A rare condition characterised by a succession of ectopic ventricular systoles.

Pulsus Alternans. This condition, which is revealed by a tracing from the arterial pulse, is not always shown by the electrocardiograph. Thus, the **R** waves may be of equal height although the pulse shows marked alternation. At times the **R** waves may show alternation, but the large **R** waves may correspond with the small pulse waves, and vice versa. Occasionally the electrocardiogram shows alternation of the **R** waves, although the pulse tracing is regular.

Coronary Thrombosis. Besides disturbances in rhythm, coronary thrombosis often causes characteristic changes in the form of the ventricular complexes. These changes were first observed by Smith (9) after experimental coronary occlusion in dogs, and later by Herrick (10) and Pardee (11) in man. Rothschild and his co-workers (12) and Parkinson and Bedford (13) have demonstrated that serial records, at intervals after coronary thrombosis, show that the electrocardiographic changes usually occur in a definite sequence, corresponding with the pathological events in progress in the myocardium.

R–T Deviation. Within a few hours up to a week of the onset, the **T** waves take off from the **RS** waves above or below the zero level, so that **RS** is succeeded by a plateau-shaped elevation or depression (see Fig. 23). **R–T** deviation is most marked in Leads I and III, and is in opposite directions in these two leads; thus **R–T** elevation in Lead I is associated with **R–T** depression in Lead III and vice versa.

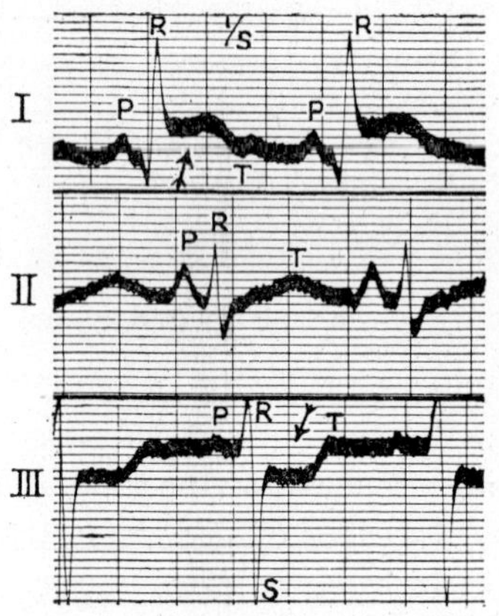

Fig. 23. Electrocardiogram taken four days after coronary thrombosis, showing plateau type of curve; the R–T period is elevated in Lead I and depressed in Lead III, as indicated by arrows. (Parkinson and Bedford.)

T Wave Changes. Within about a week, the **R–T** segment returns to the iso-electric level and **T** waves develop, pointing away from the direction in which **R–T** was displaced in each lead. Thus **R–T** elevation is succeeded by an inverted **T**, and **R–T** depression by an upright **T**. Inversion of **T** occurs either in Lead I or Lead III, but not in both, and often to a lesser degree in Lead II. According to the direction of **R–T** displacement, and consequently to the direction of the **T** waves in Leads I and III, two types of curve are common.

1. *T*1 *Type.* **T** is deeply inverted in Lead I, often slightly inverted or flattened in Lead II, and upright in Lead III (see Fig. 24).

2. *T*3 *Type.* **T** is deeply inverted in Lead III, often slightly inverted or flattened in Lead II, and upright in Lead I (see Fig. 25).

Changes in the direction of normal usually follow in the course of the first six months after the attack. The inversion of **T** diminishes first in Lead II, then in Lead I or Lead III; eventually **T** may become upright in all leads, but in some cases inversion of **T** persists almost unaltered. Evidence is accumulating that the **T1** type of curve corresponds with infarction of the anterior wall or apex of the left ventricle (occlusion of the left anterior descending coronary) and the **T3** type of curve with infarction of the posterior wall of the left ventricle (occlusion of the right coronary (Barnes and Whitten (14)).

Changes in QRS. Notching and widening of **QRS** are quite

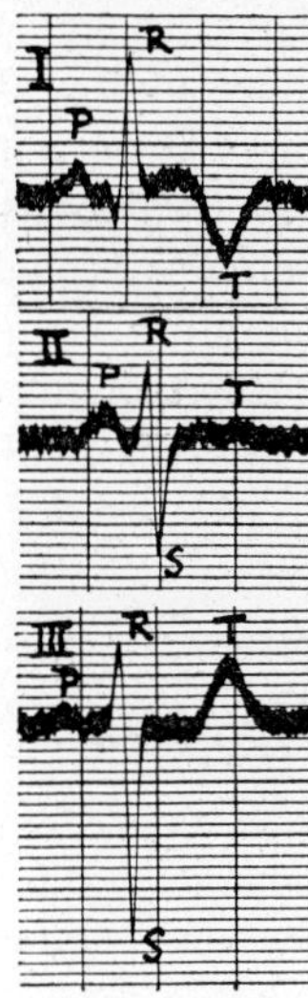

FIG. 24. Electrocardiogram taken three weeks after coronary thrombosis, showing the T1 type of curve. (D. E. Bedford.)

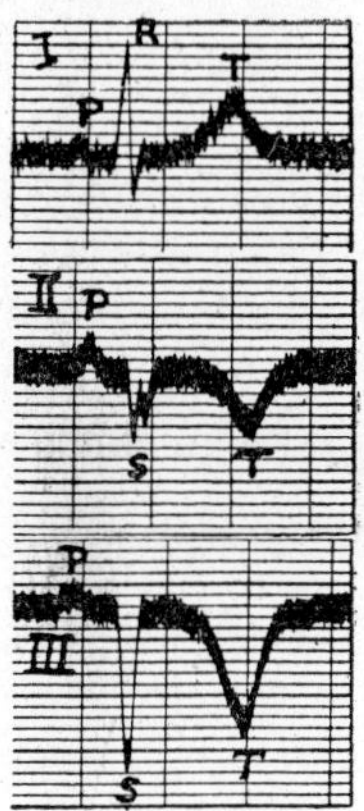

FIG. 25. Electrocardiogram taken one month after coronary thrombosis, showing the T3 type of curve. (D. E. Bedford.)

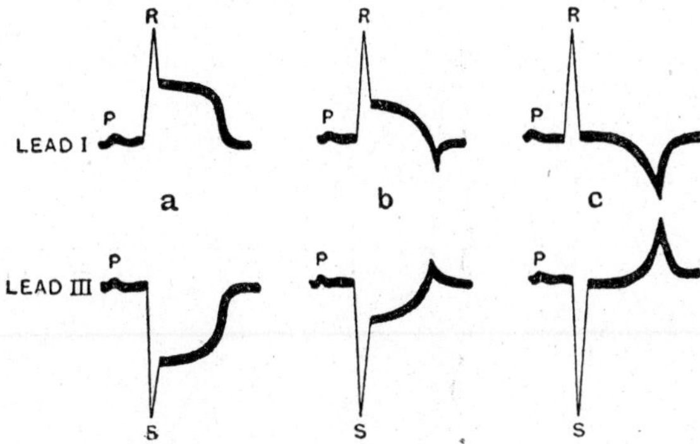

FIG. 26. Diagram illustrating the changes in the ventricular complexes in Leads I and III after coronary thrombosis. (a) R–T deviation; (b) T waves becoming evident; (c) R–T deviation disappeared. The T waves point in the opposite direction to the R–T deviation in each lead. (Parkinson and Bedford.)

frequent in curves after coronary thrombosis, though not in any way special to this condition. Low voltage of the **QRS** waves in all leads is also a common finding. A large **Q** wave in Lead III has been noticed in many cases of coronary thrombosis, and it is regarded as a suggestive sign of coronary disease, though it occurs in the chronic stages and occasionally in other forms of heart disease, or in displacement of the heart. It is thought to indicate damage to the posterior part of the interventricular septum (Pardee (15), Fernichel and Kugell (16)). The reader's attention is also directed to the diagram (see Fig. 26) which illustrates the electrocardiographic changes described above.

Chest Leads in Coronary Disease

Wolferth and Wood (17), in Pennsylvania in 1932, introduced chest leads in the electrocardiographic study of coronary occlusion, as "there are 'silent areas' in the heart where infarction may occur without producing a deviation of the **S–T** interval from the iso-electric line in any of the three conventional leads". The lead which is now commonly employed is IV R or CR IV. The lead switch is turned to Lead I, the left arm terminal is connected with the praecordial electrode and is placed on the extreme outer border of the apex beat as determined by palpation or auscultation. The right arm electrode is placed on the right arm. By this method both **P** and **T** waves are normally upright. If the electrocardiograph cable has four leads the pectoral (**PC**) lead is attached to the praecordial electrode, and the right arm lead attached to the right arm.

The præcordial electrode should be circular, 2 to 3 cm. in diameter, and made of German silver.

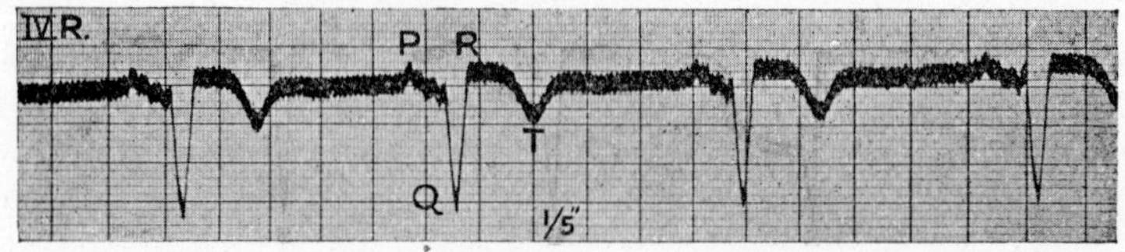

Fig. 27. Lead IV R in T_1 type of coronary thrombosis.

Results in Coronary Thrombosis. In the T_1 type of electrocardiogram (see Fig. 27) which corresponds with an acute anterior infarction, Lead IV shows an abnormal curve in the majority of cases. Thus, using the right arm chest-lead of Roth (Lead IV R), the typical findings are an elevation of the **R–T** segment, with an inverted **T** wave. The **R** wave is small or absent (see Fig. 27).

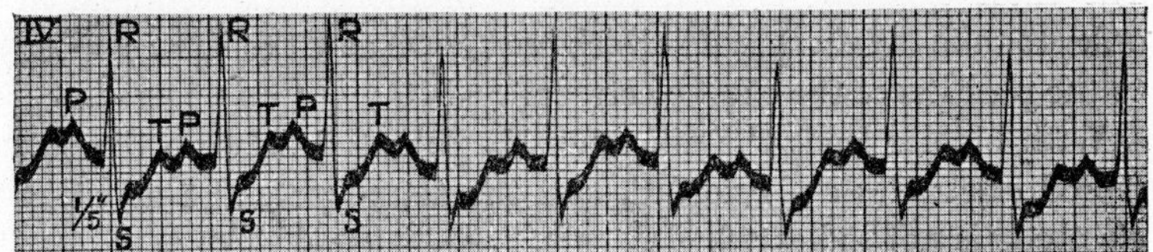

FIG. 28. Lead IV R in T_3 type of coronary thrombosis.

The **T** wave may be huge, over 10 mm. In the T_3 type of electrocardiogram (see Fig. 28) which is met with in acute posterior infarction the changes in the fourth lead are not so constant, and not so characteristic as in the three conventional leads. The **R–T** segment is depressed, and the **T** wave is upright (see Fig. 28).

When acute anterior and posterior infarctions occur simultaneously, Wolferth and Wood (17) have shown that the **R–T** segment is raised in all the limb leads, especially in Lead II. In Lead IV R the **R–T** segment is also elevated. Wood and Wolferth (18) suggest that the huge **T** waves (over 10 mm. in amplitude) in Lead IV, whether positive or negative, indicate localised apical infarction.

Multiple Chest Leads

In 1938 (19) the American Heart Association endeavoured to standardise the use of multiple chest leads, the chest electrode being placed on six different sites over the præcordium and on the left side of the chest. These leads were not then adopted in Britain, but the exact positions now recommended both by the American Heart Association and by the British Cardiac Society for chest leads are described later (see p. 191). With bipolar leads the distal electrode, which is paired with the chest electrode, may be placed on the left leg, the lead then being known as CF 1 to 6, according to the position of the chest lead; or the distal electrode may be placed on the right arm, CR 1 to 6,

Unipolar Leads

In 1934 Wilson and his colleagues (20) introduced the unipolar leads. These are known as V leads. In this method the distal electrodes on the right arm, left arm and left leg are connected, each through a resistance of 5,000 ohms, with a central terminal. The chest electrode is then paired with the central terminal in order to take the chest leads, which are known as V1 to V8 according to the position of the chest electrode.

With bipolar leads the differences in potential between the two paired electrodes are recorded, and the actual potential at either electrode is not indicated.

With unipolar electrodes we have an exploring electrode, placed either on the chest for the chest leads, or on one limb for the limb leads, and an indifferent electrode, resulting from connecting the three limb electrodes to a central terminal. The potential of the indifferent electrode may, for clinical purposes, be taken as zero, although it can never actually become zero otherwise no current would flow. Wilson has shown that the voltage at the so-called indifferent electrode never rises above 0·3 mV. With bipolar electrodes there are therefore two variables of potential, whereas with the unipolar electrodes there is only one variable, that of the exploring electrode.

It was later noted that, with the three distal electrodes connected with a central terminal, in the majority of cases it made no difference in the electrocardiogram if the resistances were omitted from the circuit, and in 1942 Goldberger (21) constructed a unipolar indifferent electrode which could be made in a few minutes at a cost of less than 10 cents. Goldberger further found that he could augment the galvanometric deflection by 50% in the limb leads if the indifferent electrode was left off the limb from which the tracing was made. These augmented limb leads are now generally employed, and were known as aVR, aVL, and aVF; "a" stands for augmented, "V" for voltage, indicating the unipolar lead, and "R", "L" and "F" for right arm, left arm, and left leg respectively. As augmented limb leads are now always employed the "a" is usually omitted.

In order to take the unipolar leads, whether chest or limb leads, the switch on the electrocardiograph is placed in Lead I position. Electrocardiographs are now supplied with a switch which does away with the necessity of disconnecting one of the limb leads, from the right arm, left arm or left leg, when taking the respective limb leads. This disconnection is effected in the switch, so that it is only necessary to turn the switch to the appropriate position, as labelled, in order to obtain all the leads required. The positions on the unipolar lead switch we use, are labelled S, V, aVr, aVl, and aVf. With the unipolar lead switch turned to S, the three standard limb leads can be taken by placing the patient switch on the electrocardiograph to position I, II and III, as for taking the ordinary bipolar limb leads. By turning the patient switch back to the Lead I position, and the unipolar lead switch to position V, the 6 or more unipolar chest leads are taken by moving the chest electrode to the appropriate position. By turning the unipolar switch to positions aVr, aVl, and aVf, the unipolar limb leads are taken.

The standard positions for the chest leads have been laid down by the Committee of the British Cardiac Society (22) in 1949, and they are as follows :—

V1, right margin of sternum, in the fourth intercostal space.
V2, left margin of sternum, at the same level.
V4, mid-clavicular line, in the fifth left intercostal space.
V3, a point midway between 2 and 4.
V5, left anterior axillary line, at the same level as V4.
V6, left mid-axillary line, at the same level as V4.
V7, left posterior axillary line, at the same level.
V8, below the angle of the left scapula, at the same level.
VE, may be used, the electrode being placed over the tip of the xiphoid cartilage.

The corresponding V positions to the right are shown by the letter R, *e.g.* V3R.

If there is hypertrophy of the heart with a forcible impulse visible in the sixth space, V4 must not be placed over the apex beat, but in the position described above, otherwise no information concerning rotation of the heart can be obtained.

As the voltages of V leads are often high, half standardisation may be used (1 mV = 5 mm.). If this reduction is used it should be employed uniformly in all chest leads, and indicated N/2.

The electrode jelly must be carefully applied when recording the chest leads, as positions 2, 3 and 4, are often very close together.

The jelly in each lead must be kept separate, otherwise if there is contact of the jelly the tracings will be distorted.

There is a correlation between the standard limb leads and the unipolar limb leads, for Lead VL $= \frac{I - III}{2}$, Lead VR $= -\frac{I + II}{2}$ and Lead VF $= \frac{II + III.}{2}$

If the position of the heart in the thorax is considered, it will be appreciated that the chest lead in position 1 and 2 is over the right side of the heart, 3 is over the septal region, 4 is over the septum or the left ventricle, and 5 and 6 are over the left side of the heart. With an extensive anterior infarction of the heart, changes may be seen in all the chest leads 1 to 6 ; with an anterolateral infarct changes may occur in leads 4 to 6, and with an anteroseptal infarct in leads 1 to 3 . The British Cardiac Society Committee state that " the full electrical exploration of the heart involves the taking of at least twelve leads, and sometimes more. The twelve basic leads are the three standard limb leads, the three unipolar limb leads, and six unipolar præcordial V leads". For ordinary routine testing the following are recommended, V1 and V2, or V4 and V5, or V5 and V6, according to the size of the heart, together with VL and VF. The right ventricular leads V1 and V2 show best some myocardial infarcts, right bundle-branch block, right ventricular hypertrophy, massive pulmonary embolism and auricular arrhythmias. The left ventricular leads V4 to 6 are used to demonstrate some myocardial infarcts, left ventricular hypertrophy and left bundle-branch block. Myocardial ischæmia is shown by V1 to 6, VL and VF. For practically all purposes the leads taken may be reduced to the three standard leads, with VF, V4 and V6.

Basic Normal V (Unipolar) Lead Patterns

Goldberger (23) described five basic ventricular unipolar lead patterns, depending upon the surface of the heart the lead faces. Further, if the pattern shown in a limb lead is similar to that obtained from a chest lead, it is presumed that the limb faces the surface of the heart from which the corresponding chest tracing is obtained.

Electrocardiographically the ventricular muscle can be divided into three groups, the interventricular septum, and the right and left ventricles. A transverse section through the chest at the level of the 4th costal cartilage shows that the right ventricle faces the anterior chest wall, only a small portion of the right ventricle being found to the right of the sternum. The greater part of the left ventricle lies over the diaphragm, but in health these relationships vary according to the position of the heart. The posterior wall of the heart is composed of the left auricle, the left ventricle faces to the left side of the chest, the right auricle to the right side of the chest, and the interventricular septum runs obliquely from behind, forward to the left, its right ventricular surface facing anteriorly and to the right, its left ventricular surface facing posteriorly and to the left.

The unipolar leads, whether chest or limb, record alterations in potential produced by electrical changes in the ventricular muscle groups.

With the heart in the usual position the chest leads V1, 2 and 3, face the right ventricle, and the right side of the septum, V4, 5 and 6 face the left ventricle and left side of the septum. The limb lead VR faces the cavity of the right ventricle. The limb leads VL and VF are much influenced by changes in the position of the heart.

When a unipolar lead faces the epicardial surface of the left ventricle, the ventricular complex consists of a small **q** wave, followed by a large **R**, and **T** is usually upright. R T q qRT When the lead faces the left ventricle near the septum the **q** wave is absent, but the **R** wave is large. The initial small **q** wave is due to the electrical impulse spreading through the septum from the left to the right, and so travelling away from the lead. As soon as the stimulus spreads outwards through the left ventricle the **R** wave results. The impulse is simultaneously spreading through the right ventricle, which would give a downward deflection, but this potential is too small to affect the **R** wave appreciably. This pattern can be expected with V5 and V6, occasionally with V2, 3, 4 and with VL and VF.

When a unipolar lead faces the epicardial surface of the right ventricle, the ventricular complex consists of a small **r** and a large **S**, or a large **R** and a large **S**. **T** may be up or down. r T S rST

or R T S RST

Thus as the chest lead is moved from the V1 and V2 positions to the V5 and V6 positions, the **S** wave disappears and the **R** wave increases in amplitude up to the V4 position and then diminishes again. The point at which **R** = **S** is called the *transitional point* and indicates the line of the interventricular septum. In some cases the transitional point is situated farther to the right than is shown in V1, or farther to the left than is shown in V6. There is usually a small **q** wave in V6. The **T** wave is often inverted in V1, and it may be inverted in V2 if the heart is vertical. In children with normal hearts the **T** wave may be inverted in V3.

When a unipolar lead faces the cavity of the right ventricle, as in VR the pattern of the tracing is **rS**, with a downward **T**. The **r** wave is due to spread of the impulse through the septum towards the right arm lead, the **S** wave results from the stimulus spreading through the right and left ventricles, away from the lead. r S T rST

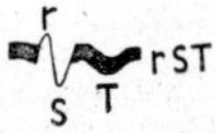

When a unipolar lead faces the cavity of the left ventricle, as in VL or VR or in a lead taken from the upper back of the chest, the pattern is **QS**, with a downward **T**. The **Q** wave is due to the stimulus spreading through the septum away from the lead, the **S** is due to the stimulus spreading through the ventricles still away from the lead. QS T QST

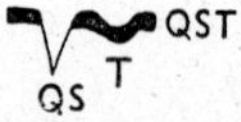

When a unipolar lead faces the back of the heart, with the electrode placed in the interscapular region, it faces the cavity of the left ventricle, through the cavity of the left auricle, and a portion of the epicardial surface of the left ventricle. The pattern is **QR** followed by a downward **T**. The **Q** is due to the lead facing the cavity of the left ventricle, the **R** is caused by the stimulus passing out to the posterior wall of the left ventricle. It will be seen that when the main **QRS** deflection is upward **T** also tends to be upward, and vice versa. A small round or **U** wave may occasionally be seen between the **T** and **P** waves. R Q T QRT

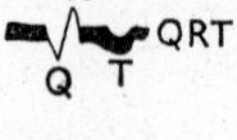

Axis Deviation

The unipolar leads enable a distinction to be made between deviation of the axis of the heart and preponderance of the ventricles. Normally the cardiac axis runs obliquely downwards, forwards and to the left. The three standard leads, six V leads and three unipolar limb leads with the heart in the normal semi-vertical position are shown in Fig. 29. The **R** wave in VF is tall, and the deflections of VF resemble those of the leads from the left of the præcordium, such as V6. When rotation occurs about a horizontal antero-posterior axis, it may be in a clockwise direction towards the vertical, or in an anti-clockwise direction towards the horizontal. The heart may also rotate along its longitudinal axis. If it rotates in a clockwise direction, as looked at from below, the right ventricle becomes more anterior and the left ventricle more posterior. Rotation of the heart around its transverse axis will bring the apex of the heart either nearer to, or farther away from the anterior chest wall, according to the direction of rotation.

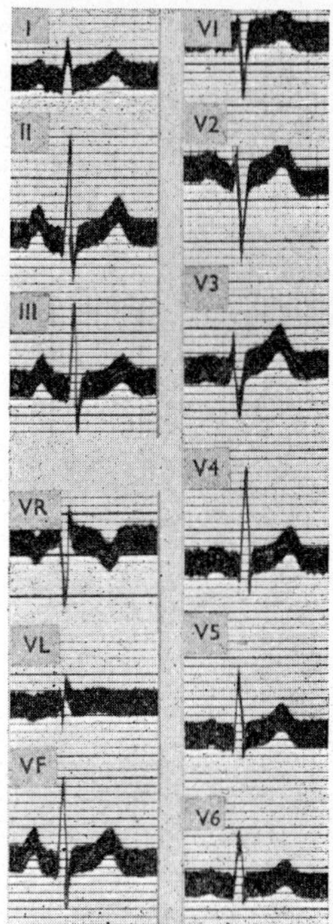

FIG. 29. Semi-vertical heart. The heart is semi-vertical because although there is a tall R wave in Lead VF the complexes of VL are small.

Rotation around the horizontal antero-posterior axis. Six positions have been described ; vertical, semi-vertical, intermediate, semi-horizontal, horizontal, and indeterminate.

With the vertical position the pattern of the ventricular complex in VL resembles that of V1 and V2, *i.e.* the right ventricular pattern. The ventricular complex of VF resembles that of V5 and V6, *i.e.* the left ventricular pattern (see Fig. 30). When the heart lies in the horizontal position the ventricular complex of VL resembles that of V5 and V6, and the ventricular complex of VF resembles that of V1 and V2 (see Fig. 31).

Rotation around the longitudinal axis. In recording the chest leads of a normal heart the transitional point, indicating the position of the interventricular septum, is, as described above, between V3 and V4 leads. If the heart rotates around the longitudinal axis in a clockwise direction the transitional point shifts to the left, as between V5 and V6. The VL lead may face the right ventricular cavity, when it will show a **RS** followed by a downward **T** wave (see Fig. 32). If the rotation is in an anti-

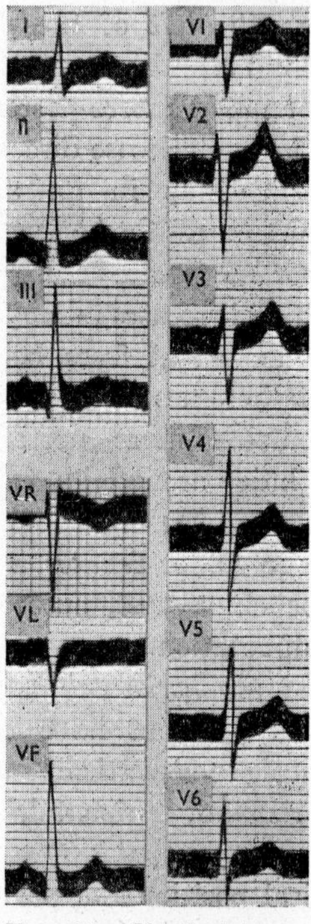

FIG. 30. Vertical heart. The heart is seen to be in the vertical position electrically because Lead VF shows a tall R wave and Lead VL a deep S wave.

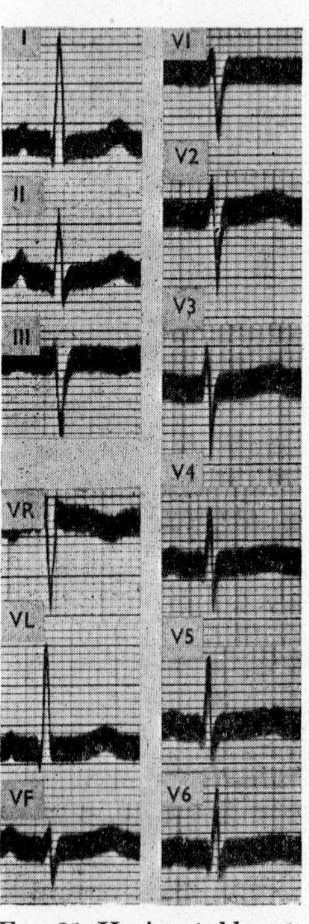

FIG. 31. Horizontal heart. The heart is horizontal because the R wave is tall in VL and the S wave is deep in VF. Also, the form of VL resembles that of V6.

clockwise direction the transitional point shifts to the right, between V1 and V2 or even farther to the right (see Fig. 33).

Rotation around the transverse axis. It is considered by some that the heart can rotate about a transverse axis, and that this may affect the limb lead records although it does not appreciably affect those of the chest leads. If the apex rotates backward

VF may face the right ventricle instead of the left ventricle as it usually does. The left leg lead will now show a **RS** instead of the normal **QR** deflection.

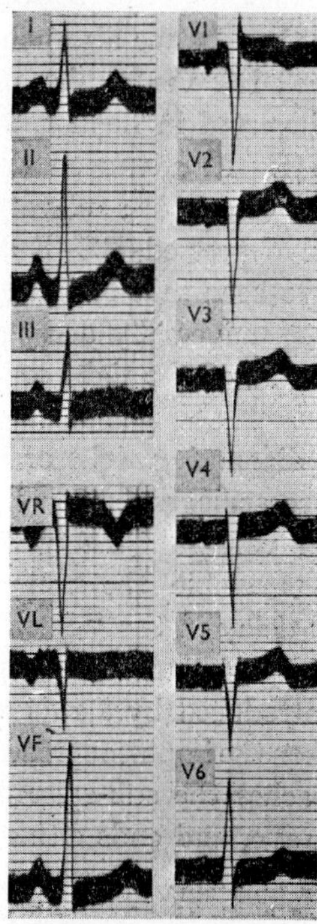

FIG. 32. Considerable amount of clockwise rotation around the longitudinal axis. The T.P. lies between V5 and V6. The heart is vertical.

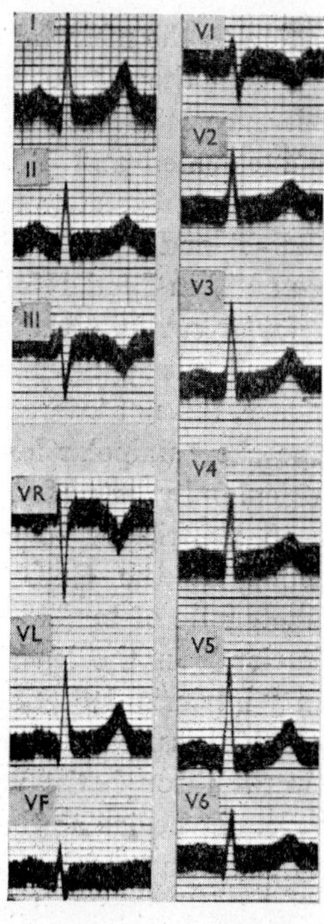

FIG. 33. Considerable amount of anti-clockwise rotation. The T.P. is seen to lie between V1 and V2.

Ventricular Hypertrophy

The diagnosis of hypertrophy of the ventricles from electrocardiograms still remains somewhat uncertain. The curves obtained in the standard limb leads, which were originally taken to indicate right or left ventricular preponderance, were found at autopsy to be misleading in some cases. The term axis deviation was then used instead of ventricular preponderance, for it was shown that with deep inspiration a tracing which was characteristic of left ventricular preponderance might become normal. In long-standing cases of ventricular hypertrophy changes occur in the standard limb lead curves, the **S–T** segment is displaced in the opposite direction to the main initial deflection and the **T** wave also points away from the **QRS**. Thus with advanced left ventricular preponderance **RS–T** is depressed and **T** is inverted in Lead I, and **RS–T** elevated and **T** upright in Lead III. In advanced right ventricular preponderance the reverse changes occur; elevation of **RS–T** and upright **T** in Lead I, and depressed **RS–T** and inverted **T** in Lead III. These curves have been said to indicate *ventricular strain*, although the term is not universally accepted. Curves of this type probably indicate ischæmia of the right or left ventricle, but not infarction.

The chest unipolar leads are helpful in diagnosing right or left ventricular hypertrophy. The chief electrocardiographic changes due to ventricular hypertrophy are high voltage **QRS** waves, widening of the **QRS** so that it may resemble the complex characteristic of bundle-branch block, and delay in the " intrinsic deflection " in the leads over the hypertrophied ventricle. The term " intrinsic deflection ", which was introduced by Lewis and Rothschild, is used to denote the moment when the impulse spreading outwards through the ventricular wall reaches the sub-epicardial muscle. It begins at the peak of the **R** wave, and ends either at the isoelectric level, or at the nadir of the **S** wave. However, in clinical cardiography it is usually measured from the beginning of the deflection to the peak of the upward deflection. In human cardiography it should more properly be called the intrinsicoid deflection, as the exploring electrode, even in chest leads, is comparatively far from the surface of the heart. The **R** waves are small and the **S** waves deep in the tracings taken from the leads over the ventricle which is not hypertrophied. Further, in left ventricular hypertrophy the transitional point may be displaced to the right, and in right ventricular hypertrophy to the left. The electrocardiogram of left ventricular hypertrophy is shown in Fig. 34. Tall **R** waves and inverted **T** waves are seen in V5 and V6, with depression of the **RS–T** interval. The **T** wave is inverted in VF. In right ventricular hypertrophy, as shown in Fig. 35, the **R** waves

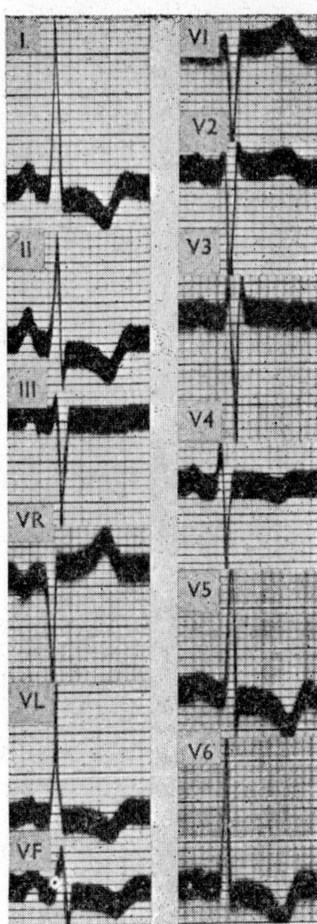

FIG. 34. Left ventricular hypertrophy. The R waves in V1 and V2 are even smaller than normal but the S waves are deeper than normal. In V5 and V6 the peak of R is abnormally late, R is too tall, the RS-T segment is depressed, and T is inverted.

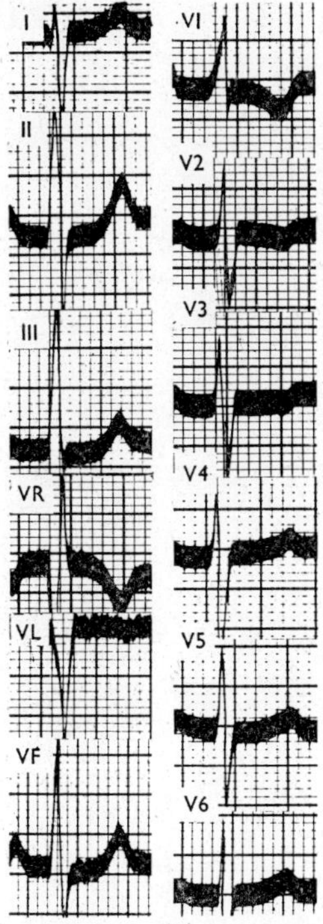

FIG. 35. Right ventricular hypertrophy. In V1, V2 and V3 R is abnormally large and its peak is late, QRS is a little widened and T is inverted.

are tall and **T** inverted in V1, V2, and V3. **QRS** is a little wide and the **T** wave is inverted in VR. Depression of the **RS–T** segment and inverted **T** waves in the chest leads facing the epicardial surface of the affected ventricle, with normal **QRS** complexes, is said to indicate ischæmia. It can be shown with the combination of the chest and limb leads that right axis deviation may be present with left ventricular hypertrophy.

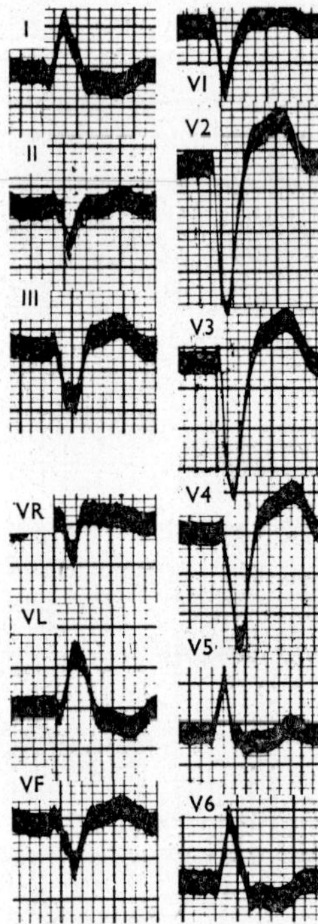

FIG. 36. Complete left bundle-branch block. QRS is at least of 0·12 sec. duration. In V1 and V2 R is small or absent and a deep broad S is present. In V5 and V6 a broad R occurs which may be notched or bifid.

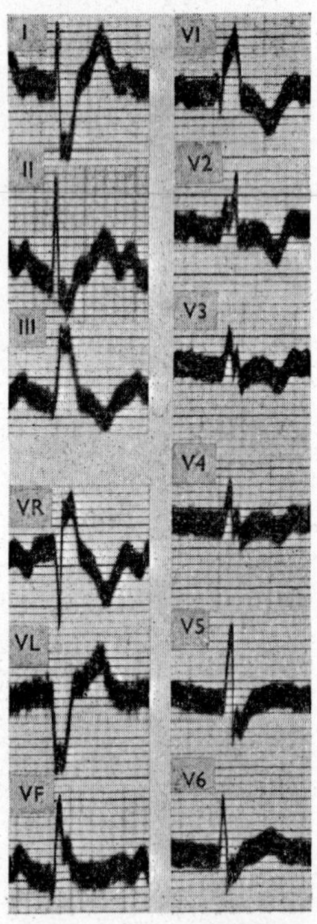

FIG. 37. Complete right bundle-branch block. The QRS complex is prolonged to 0·12 sec. or more. V1 and V2 show a broad notched R wave which is preceded by a very small primary R and S wave. In V5 and V6 the R wave is slender and followed by a broad S. It is seen that the pattern of right bundle-branch block can closely simulate that of right ventricular hypertrophy.

Bundle-Branch Block

The use of chest leads has confirmed the view that the common divergent, or Type I, bundle-branch block, as shown in the standard limb leads, is due to left bundle-branch block. The characteristic features of the unipolar chest leads in bundle-branch block are as follows ;—

Left Bundle-Branch Block. Leads V1 and V2, facing the right ventricle, show **r** small or absent, **S** deep and broad. Leads V5 and V6, facing the left ventricle, show **R** large, broad and notched (see Fig. 36). If a small **q** wave is present, there is probably left ventricular hypertrophy and not bundle-branch block.

Right Bundle-Branch Block. Leads V1 and V2 show a wide **RSR'**, or **RSR'S**, with usually a downward **T** wave. Leads V5 and V6 show a narrow **qR** wave followed by a wide **S**. **T** is usually upright (see Fig. 37). The pattern closely resembles that of right ventricular hypertrophy, but in the latter the **qRs** pattern is normal in Leads V5 and V6.

Goldberger (23) states that left bundle-branch block may be transient or permanent. As a transient condition it may occur for no apparent reason, or following infarction, congestive failure, during acute infections or it may result from quinidine. Permanent left bundle-branch block, because it is almost always due to organic heart disease, usually shortens life. Right bundle-branch block may also be transient or permanent. The transient variety may occur for no apparent reason, or follow pulmonary embolism or myocardial infarction. Permanent right bundle-branch block is associated with rheumatic, arteriosclerotic and hypertensive heart disease and coronary occlusion. When myocardial infarction and pulmonary embolism are absent right bundle-branch block is not of serious significance.

Myocardial Infarction

When a portion of the wall of the heart is the site of an infarct it becomes electrically inert, and an electrode placed opposite this area is described picturesquely as looking into the cavity of the ventricle through a window of inactive tissue. The **Q** wave may be abnormal in depth and width, signifying the presence of dead muscle tissue. The electrode registers the negative voltage of the ventricular cavity. The **R** wave is diminished in size over the damaged muscle. Whether or not it is present depends on whether there is muscle on the surface of the infarct. A tall **R** wave may occur at the edge of the infarct. The **RS–T** segment is displaced above or below the iso-electric level. An electrode facing the injured surface will show a rise in the **RS–T** segment, an electrode facing in the opposite direction will show a depressed **RS–T** segment.

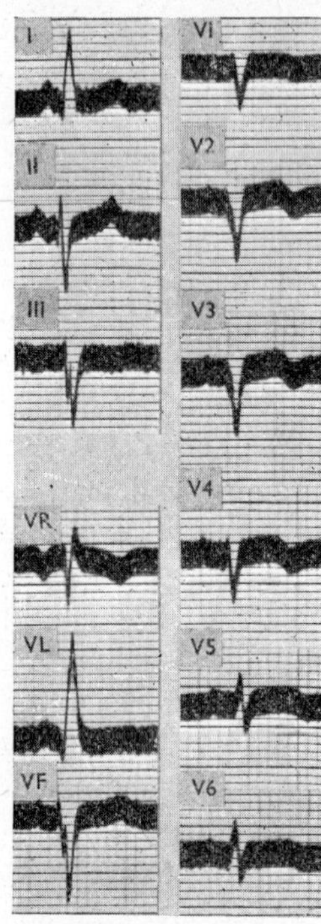

FIG. 38. Strictly anterior infarct. The infarct does not reveal itself in the standard leads. V1 to V4 are chiefly affected.

The **T** wave points in a direction opposite to that of the **RS–T** displacement.

The unipolar chest leads enable the site of the infarct to be determined with some degree of accuracy. The following types are described :—

Anterior infarction. The standard leads are often normal in this type of infarction. V1, 2 and 3, however, show the displaced **RS–T** segment and inverted **T** waves (see Fig. 38).

Antero-septal infarction. If in the above type of curves the **QRS** is widened and the **Q** waves are deep in V1, 2 and 3, the infarct has probably spread into the septum with involvement of the right bundle-branch.

Antero-lateral infarction. V4, 5 and 6 show the characteristic changes. They are also seen in the standard Lead **I** and unipolar Lead VL (see Fig. 39).

Extensive anterior infarction. Changes are seen in all the chest leads, and **T** is inverted in standard Lead **I** and in unipolar Lead VL.

Posterior infarction. The chest leads are often of no help in diagnosing posterior infarction, although occasionally the **T** waves are abnormally high. The important lead here is VF which shows elevation of the **RS–T** segment and sharply inverted **T** waves. Lead **III** shows similar changes (see Fig. 40). Similar changes in the standard Lead **III** may occur without infarction, in which case VF is normal. The unipolar lead VF will indicate whether a suspected $\mathbf{Q_3T_3}$ in the standard Lead **III** indicates infarction or not, or whether the pattern in Lead **III** is really $\mathbf{S_3T_3}$, indicating a transverse lie of the heart. When, in addition to the changes in VF, V6 or V5 and V6 show an abnormal **RST**, the infarct may be described as postero-lateral.

Septal infarction. Here the standard limb leads indicate a

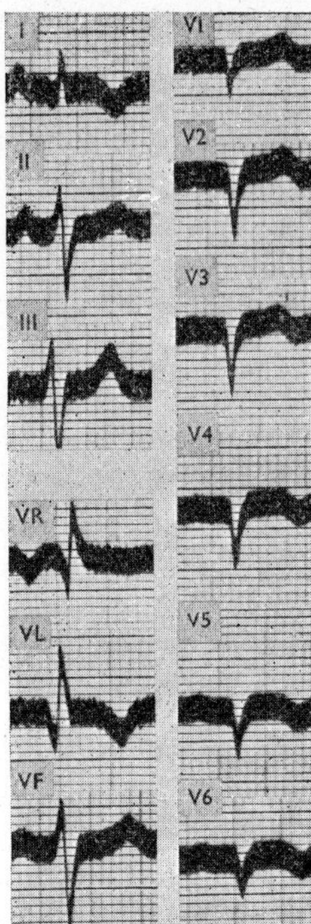

FIG. 39. Antero-lateral infarct. Maximal changes are seen in V4 to V6, but often all chest leads are involved. T is inverted always in VL and I.

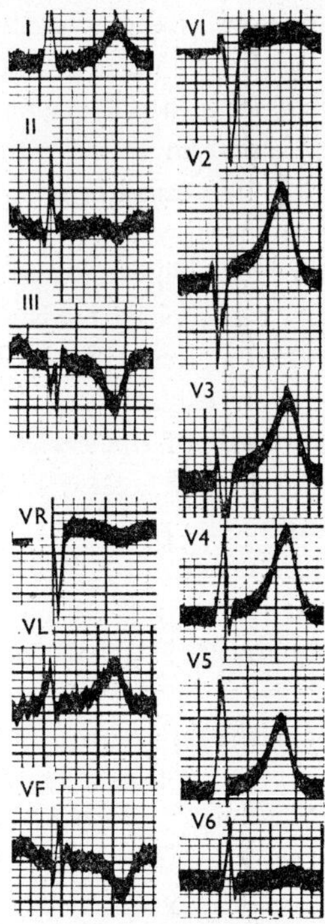

FIG. 40. Posterior infarction. The typical changes are seen in Leads VF and III. Although the V chest leads are often disappointing, they may show abnormally tall and symmetrical T waves, as in this case.

posterior infarction, and the chest leads indicate an antero-septal infarction.

Acute Pericarditis

When the epicardial surface of the heart is injured, the electrode facing the injured surface will show elevation of the **RS–T** segment. Thus both myocardial infarction, if it involves the epicardial surface of the heart, and pericarditis, if that also does so, will both show **RS–T** segment changes. With infarction a pathological **Q** wave is usually also present, but it is absent in pericarditis.

If we consider three leads, namely VL, VF and an anterior chest lead, it will be seen that in anterior infarction the **RS–T** segment is elevated in VL and also in the chest lead, but is depressed in VF. Conversely, in posterior infarction the **RS–T** segment is depressed in VL and in the chest lead (although commonly it is not very greatly depressed in chest leads) and elevated in lead VF.

In generalised pericarditis, leads facing both the front and back of the heart will show elevation of the **RS–T** segment. Therefore the VL, VF and chest leads all show elevation of the **RS–T** segment.

When pericarditis is complicating anterior infarction lead VL will show elevation of the **RS–T** segment, both as a result of the infarct and of the pericarditis, and a deep **Q** wave will be present in this lead. Lead VF will show elevation of the **RS–T** segment owing to the pericarditis at the back of the heart, but the **Q** wave will be normal. The chest leads will show elevation of the **RS–T** segment owing to the presence of the infarct and the pericarditis, and pathological **Q** waves will be present too.

When pericarditis complicates posterior infarction, lead VL will show elevation of the **RS–T** segment, owing to the pericarditis at the front of the heart, but no pathological **Q** wave will be present. Lead VF will show elevation of the **RS–T** segment, due both to the posterior infarct and the pericarditis at the back of the heart, and a pathological **Q** wave will be present as a result of the infarct. The chest leads will show elevation of the **RS–T** segment owing to the pericarditis, but no pathological **Q** wave will be present. Fig. 41 illustrates the five possibilities :—

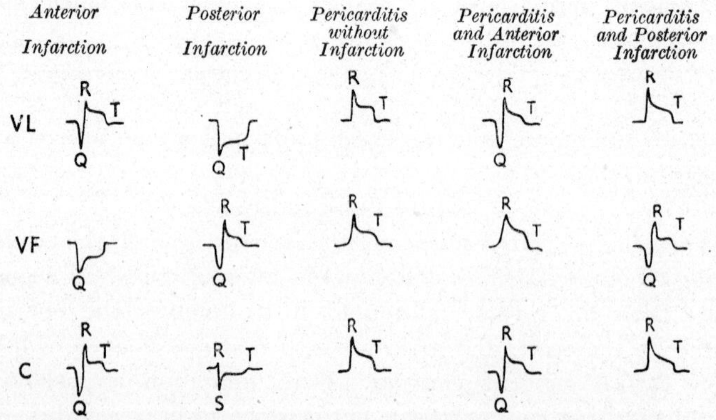

Anterior Infarction | *Posterior Infarction* | *Pericarditis without Infarction* | *Pericarditis and Anterior Infarction* | *Pericarditis and Posterior Infarction*

VL

VF

C

Fig. 41. Diagram showing electrocardiographic changes in Infarction and Pericarditis.

Massive Pulmonary Embolism

In acute cor pulmonale associated with an extensive pulmonary embolus electrocardiographic changes may be found. In the standard limb leads there is a deep **S** wave in Lead I, and a **Q** and inverted **T** wave in Lead III, together with an inverted **T** wave in the chest lead V1. These changes do not usually persist for any length of time, although rarely they may be seen for several months. Transient right bundle-branch block may also be associated with pulmonary embolism.

Conclusions. The use of the unipolar leads has enabled a more exact localisation of myocardial infarcts to be made, but this does not imply any alteration either in the treatment of the case, nor in our views as to prognosis. These leads have also allowed a more definite diagnosis to be made in cases of suspected posterior infarcts. Bundle-branch block, the presence of ventricular hypertrophy, and changes in the position of the heart, can also be diagnosed more accurately. The superiority of the unipolar over the bipolar chest leads is not universally accepted. Thus Evans (24) states: " Anyone who customarily used CR leads need not change to the unipolar chest leads in the hope that they would gain additional information in the clinical diagnosis ". Evans says that CR_1 portrays **P** waves better than does V1, and so is more useful in arrhythmias. Further, the **T** wave is often inverted in healthy adults in V1, rarely so in CR1, as the R wave is better portrayed in CR1 than in V1. It will be admitted by all that the reading of the unipolar leads is often difficult and uncertain and the theoretical basis for their interpretation is at times unconvincing. For more detailed information on unipolar leads the reader is referred to the book by Goldberger (23) and to articles by Hill (25) and Oram (26), on whose writings this section is largely based.

Cardiac Catheterisation

By the use of what is known as the Fick principle physiologists have determined the cardiac output in dogs. The method depends upon ascertaining the output of the right ventricle from the amount of blood passing through the lungs in a given unit of time. The output of the right ventricle equals that of the left. The volume of blood passing through the lungs can be calculated if the amount of carbon dioxide given off or the amount of oxygen taken up is determined, together with the arteriovenous difference of either of these gases. The oxygen utilised or the carbon dioxide produced can be ascertained by spirometric and gas analysis methods. The arterial blood is obtained by direct arterial puncture, and the mixed arteriovenous blood is withdrawn either by puncture of the right ventricle, or by passing a catheter down the external jugular vein into the right ventricle. The samples of blood are then analysed either for their O_2 or their CO_2 content. If the O_2 content is determined the cardiac output is determined from the formula :— Cardiac output in litres per minute = O_2 consumption in ml. per minute, divided by the arteriovenous O_2 difference in ml. per litre. Thus if the O_2 consumption is 250 ml/minute, the arterial O_2 content 200 ml./litre, and the venous O_2 content 150 ml./litre, then the

$$\text{cardiac output} = \frac{250}{200-150} = 5 \text{ litres per minute.}$$

Forssmann (27) in 1929 passed a ureteric catheter through a vein in his arm into his heart. His paper makes interesting reading, and the translation of the relevant section is as follows :—

"After successful experiments in passing a catheter on the cadaver, I undertook on myself the first experiment on living man. First, I submitted myself to an experiment by a colleague who kindly placed himself for this purpose at my disposal and punctured with a thick needle my right antecubital vein. I then passed, as in the experiment on the cadaver, a well-oiled ureteric catheter, size 4 Charrières, through the cannula in the vein. The catheter was passed quite easily for a distance of 35 cm. It then appeared to my colleague to be dangerous to go farther, so the experiment was stopped, although I was quite undisturbed.

"A week later I undertook another experiment on my own. As a vein puncture with a thick needle on one's own body presents certain technical difficulties, with a local anæsthetic I made a vein section in my left antecubital fossa and passed a catheter with little resistance for its whole length of 65 cm. This length appeared to me, after measuring the distance on the surface of the body, to correspond with the distance from the left elbow to the heart. All I felt during the passage of the catheter was a slightly warm sensation, such as results from an intravenous injection of calcium.

As the catheter passed through the subclavian vein I experienced an intense feeling of warmth behind the collar-bone under the insertion of the sternomastoid muscle, and at the same time, through irritation of the branches of the vagus, a dry cough. I proved the position of the catheter by an X-ray picture, and I observed the progress of the catheter myself on the screen in a mirror held by the sister."

A truly remarkable experiment!

Since then the method of cardiac catheterisation in man has become more and more extensively employed, and reference will be made to some of the publications during the succeeding years. In 1932 Grollman (28) employed catheterisation of the right auricle to determine the cardiac output in man. Further advances were made in 1941 by Cournand and Ranges (29). They allowed the catheter to remain in the heart for an hour or longer. They were thus enabled to determine the intra-auricular pressure, and by analysing the gas content of the auricular blood and of arterial blood, they determined the cardiac output according to the Fick principle. In 1944 McMichael and Sharpey-Schafer (30) published their observations on the effect of posture, venous pressure changes, and the administration of atropine and adrenaline on the cardiac output in man, as determined by cardiac catheterisation. Their investigations were made on normal male volunteers and took place two hours after the midday meal. A cardiac catheter was passed into the right auricle, and the oxygen unsaturation of the right auricular blood was determined by a Haldane gas analysis apparatus. The oxygen capacity was determined by hæmoglobinometry, and, with normal lungs, arterial puncture was not performed. It was assumed that arterial blood was 95% saturated, and in this way the arteriovenous oxygen difference was calculated. The mean figure for the arteriovenous oxygen difference was in the region of 45 ml./litre. The average resting cardiac output in the recumbent position was 5·3 litres a minute, and in the standing position 4 litres a minute. Raising the heart rate by the intravenous injection of 1 mg. of atropine increased the cardiac output and caused a fall in the intra-auricular pressure. Intravenous injection of adrenaline increased the cardiac output in doses that did not accelerate the heart or raise the blood pressure. Sharpey-Schafer (31) in 1944 made observations by means of cardiac catheterisation on the cardiac output in severe anæmias. He found that the resting minute oxygen consumption was not reduced in chronic and post-hæmorrhagic anæmia. The cardiac output was increased, up to 12 to 14 litres per minute, which helped to maintain the oxygen supply. There was also an increased removal of oxygen in the periphery, and a reduced blood volume which caused a greater total hæmoglobin concentration. McMichael and Sharpey-Schafer (32) in 1944 used the method of cardiac catheterisation to determine the effect of digoxin on the cardiac output of man, in normal persons and in patients suffering from cardiac failure. In all cases there was a fall in the right auricular pressure. It was found that if the initial cardiac output was normal or high, the fall in auricular pressure was accompanied by a fall in cardiac output. If, however, the cardiac output was low the fall in auricular pressure was accompanied by a rise in output. There may, therefore, be cardiac failure with high or with low output. Digitalis lowers the venous pressure and the cardiac output in normal persons and in patients suffering from some types of anæmia and cor pulmonale, and so they concluded that digitalis is unlikely to benefit the group of cases in which there is a high cardiac output. This view, however, is not universally accepted. In the low output cases of heart failure, which includes mose cases of congestive failure, lowering of the venous pressure by digitalis and other methods is often followed by a rise of cardiac output. The authors also concluded that as mechanical lowering of the right auricular pressure produces effects on cardiac output similar in degree to those produced by digoxin, the major beneficial effect of digoxin results from a peripheral action on venous pressure, and not from a tonic effect upon the heart. The slowing of the cardiac rate by digoxin in cases of auricular fibrillation did not appear to have a beneficial effect on cardiac output.

Cournand (33) in 1945 described his modified technique for sampling blood from the right auricle and the femoral artery, and Cournand et al. (34) in the same year, published further observations on measuring the cardiac output in man by catheterisation of the right auricle or ventricle. The catheter was left in the heart for up to twenty-four hours, and a special needle was devised for cannulisation of the femoral artery; the needle was strapped in position and a lock syringe attached for sampling. They found that the average difference between ventricular and auricular samples was for CO_2, 0·42 vols. %, and for O_2, 0·26 vols. %.

Work was now directed towards the investigation of congenital heart disease by means of cardiac catheterisation. Brannon et al. (35) demonstrated that in cases of atrial septal defects oxygenated blood passes from the left to the right atrium. In cases of hypertrophy of the right ventricle and prominent pulmonary arteries, due to other causes, cardiac catheterisation revealed no evidence of an atrial septal defect.

Dexter et al. (36) in 1946 showed that the cardiac catheter could be passed into the pulmonary artery and its branches. In 5 cases of patent ductus arteriosus they found a higher oxygen content in blood drawn from the pulmonary artery than in blood taken from the right ventricle. This was due to oxygenated blood passing from the aorta via the ductus to the pulmonary artery.

Johnson et al. (37) in 1947 introduced the method of heparinising the patient and not the saline. This is referred to later under the section Variations in Technique.

Howarth et al. (38) investigated cases of congenital heart disease. The magnitude of a left to right shunt through an auricular septal defect can be calculated from a comparison of the gas content of specimens removed from the superior and inferior venæ cavæ with that of specimens obtained from the right auricle and right ventricle. Blood obtained from the right auricle and right ventricle contained more oxygen than vena caval blood if the shunt is from left to right. A reduced arterial oxygen saturation when the lungs are functioning normally, suggests right to left shunt. In pulmonary hypertension with enlarged pulmonary arteries and a normal arterial oxygen saturation, the oxygen content of the blood obtained by cardiac catheterisation, showed no evidence of shunt, but the mean right ventricular pressure was greatly increased.

Holling and Zak (39) in 1950 published their observations on cardiac catheterisation of 70 cases of congenital heart disease, which are referred to later.

The Method

The requirements are as follows :—

Cardiac Catheters. These are of a modified ureteral type made of nylon, with a smooth unwettable plastic covering, flexible and radio-opaque. The catheters are obtainable from the U.S. Catheter and Instrument Co., Glens Falls, N.Y. They are 100 cm. or more in length and various sizes should be available, such as 6, 7, 8 and 9. For an infant a No. 6 will be required, while a No. 8 is used for the average adult. A short distance from the tip of the catheter there is a slight bend or angulation which enables the direction to be changed by rotation of the external end. A Luer fitting metal adaptor is fitted to the external end. The catheters are sterilised by means of formalin vapour.

A Saline Manometer. This is used to record the mean pressures in the chambers of the heart, and is sterilised by steam. It is mounted on a stand which rests on the floor adjacent to the table on which the patient lies. It can be adjusted in the vertical plane so that the zero mark can be set level with the sternal angle. Alternatively a metre rule with spirit level attached can be used to determine the zero level on the manometer, in which case the manometer is not moved up and down to the level of the sternal angle. The metre rule is placed horizontally from the angle of the sternum to the manometer and the marking on the manometer which corresponds with the zero reading is noted. To the lower end of the manometer is connected a sterile rubber tubing with an adjustable clip attached. The distal end of the rubber tubing is connected as required with the Luer fitting adaptor of the catheter. A short distance above the lower end of the manometer is a side tube to which is connected, by a sterile rubber tube fitted with an adjustable clip, a saline reservoir held by clips to the top of the manometer stand. The reservoir, previously sterilised by boiling, is nearly filled with sterile physiologic saline. The manometer is filled almost to the top from the reservoir before use, and it can be replenished by releasing the clip on the rubber tubing connecting the two (see Fig. 42).

Sterile Screw-capped Bottles. These contain a few ml. of sterile paraffin and one drop of heparin solution. These bottles are for the collection of blood samples for gas analysis.

" Cutting Down " set for skin incision and isolation of vein.

Sphygmomanometer or tourniquet.

Hypodermic syringes, 1 ml., 2 ml., 5 ml. and 20 ml.

Hypodermic needles, Nos. 20, 17, 15 and 1.

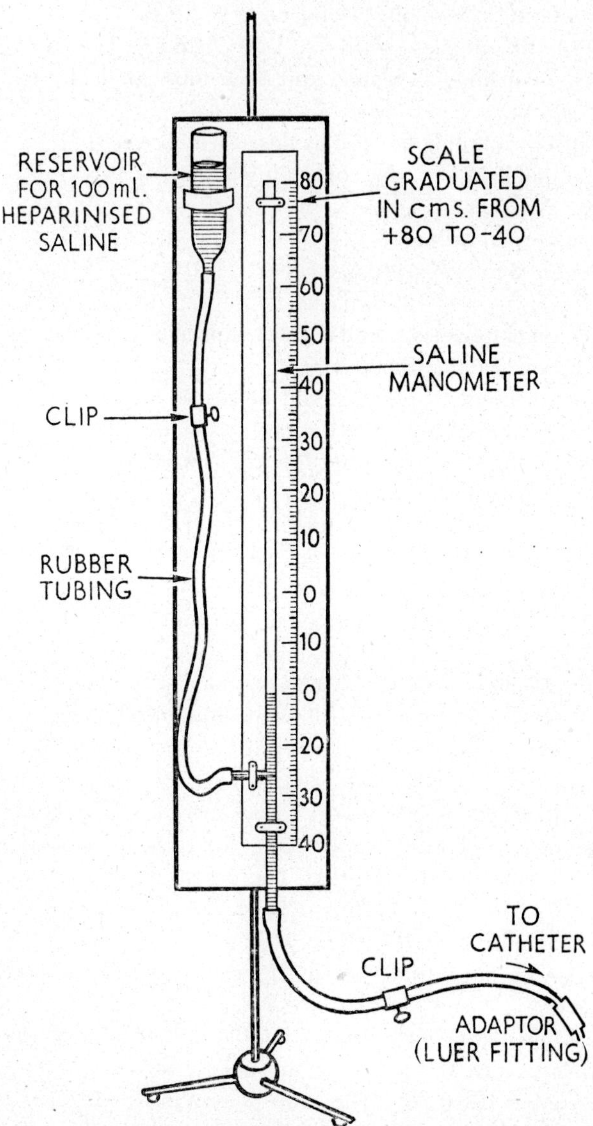

FIG. 42. Reservoir and Manometer for Cardiac Catheterisation.

Procaine hydrochloride solution, 2%.

Serum needles, 2½ inch, 17 gauge.

Ten 10 ml. all-glass syringes, Luer fitting. The syringes are sterilised by boiling in water, and then lubricated internally with sterile paraffin.

Ten blood sampling bottles, as described above.

One ampoule of heparin, containing 50 mg.

Catgut No. 0000.

Sterile normal saline.

Ether for skin preparation.

Sterile gowns, caps and masks.

Sterile mackintoshes, towels, towel clips and dressings.

Sterile bowls and gallipots.

On an emergency trolley should be placed an oxygen apparatus and B.L.B. mask. A mouth gag. Tongue forceps. Brandy, coramine, adrenaline and amyl nitrite. Two fine needles (4 inches long) for emergency cardiac puncture.

Preparation of the Patient. The patient's sensitivity to quinidine sulphate should be tested two days beforehand by giving 3 gr. If he shows no idiosyncrasy 5 gr. of quinidine sulphate and 3 gr. of Amytal are given by mouth one hour before the operation. The quinidine is given to try and prevent cardiac irregularities from developing during the catheterisation. It is a wise precaution to give 100,000 units of penicillin intramuscularly twice a day on the day of the operation, and to continue with this dosage for the next two days. Phenobarbitone, 1 to 3 gr., by mouth may be given to an adult and to children over ten years of age, two hours before the operation. Children under ten years of age require a general anæsthetic, and rectal Pentothal, 1 g. per 50 lb. of body weight, is satisfactory. If necessary this dose can be supplemented later by injection of more Pentothal through the cardiac catheter. Inhalation anæsthesia is unsuitable as it interferes with the blood gas analysis.

The Operation. The operation is carried out in the X-ray department, with the patient lying horizontal on a table covered with a rubber mattress. The table is provided with a horizontal fluoroscopic screen controlled by a foot switch. In addition to observing rigid surgical asepsis, operators must be well protected from scatter by means of lead aprons. Particular care should be taken to avoid exposure of the hands since it is not possible to wear leaden gloves. X-ray screening should be limited to about 25% of the erythema dose, which means about twenty minutes in all. Wood (40) states that the screening time should be limited to thirty minutes at 1 mA, or twenty minutes at 2 mA, or fifteen minutes at 3 mA. The same operator should not regularly perform more than two catheterisations a week It is desirable, but not essential, to have facilities for taking films to check the position of the catheter subsequently. The patient should be made as comfortable mentally and physically as possible before the operation starts and its nature should be explained to an adult. The cardiac output may be increased by anxiety, without a corresponding increase in the oxygen consumption. This will decrease the arteriovenous difference. A vein in either arm may be used for the catheterisation, but the left is preferable as the course of the veins to the right auricle is a more gradual curve than on the right side, and so a hold-up is less likely to occur. Whichever arm is selected the cephalic vein should not be used, as it joins the axillary vein almost at a right angle, which causes difficulty in passing the catheter beyond this point. The medial antecubital vein is best suited for the operation, and the point of insertion of the catheter should be a short distance distal to where two veins join. This will ensure a continuous flow of blood along the catheterised vein both during and after the operation, and will minimise the risks of thrombosis.

The selected arm is abducted to about 45°, and bound lightly to a well-padded arm splint. The sphygmomanometer cuff should be in place, and all but the antecubital fossa covered with sterile mackintoshes and towels. The exposed skin is cleaned with ether and the veins rendered prominent by inflation of the sphygmomanometer cuff. The skin and subcutaneous tissues around the site of the proposed incision and the perivenous tissues are now infiltrated with 2% procaine solution. Adequate intradermal anæsthesia, with the formation of a wheal at least the size of a half-crown, is important to prevent the subsequent occurrence of venospasm. An incision about 1 cm. long is then made through the skin in line with the vein, and the vein isolated by blunt dissection. Two fine catgut ligatures are passed round the vein, and the distal one is tied off, but not cut. The upper ligature is not tied, but its ends are secured with Spencer-Wells forceps. This ligature is used to apply gentle traction on the vein to steady it while it is opened and to control hæmorrhage. To the external end of the catheter, which has been well rinsed, inside and out, with sterile normal saline, is attached a 10 ml. all-glass syringe charged with sterile normal saline containing 25 mg. of heparin. All air is expelled from the catheter by depressing the plunger of the syringe, and both are laid on a sterile towel close to the operator's right hand. The other 25 mg. of heparin are added to the saline in the reservoir connected to the manometer, and the latter is filled to near the top with this solution.

Passing the Catheter. The segment of exposed vein is now raised by traction on the proximal loop of catgut and a small fish-mouth incision is made in its wall with pointed scissors. The tip of the catheter is immediately inserted into the vein, and gently pushed up its lumen for several centimetres. The heparin solution is then injected via the catheter and the syringe is left attached to its outer end. Further progress of the catheter is watched on the fluoroscopic screen with short exposures at frequent intervals. Force must be avoided and considerable patience is sometimes necessary. Entry of the catheter into the neck veins is prevented by turning the patient's head to the side of the operator, and if obstruction occurs at the thoracic inlet slight movement of the arm or shoulder, or a deep inspiration by the patient will usually permit it to pass easily. Should the catheter take a wrong direction it must be withdrawn some distance, and another attempt made after rotation of its external end. Once it has reached the superior vena cava it passes readily down into the right auricle. Manipulation of the outer end will direct it through the tricuspid valve into the cavity of the right ventricle. Premature systoles are commonly observed when the tip is in the vicinity of the tricuspid ring, and delay at this point should be avoided if possible. Having entered the right ventricle the catheter can be persuaded to turn upwards into the outflow tract, thence through the pulmonary valve into the main pulmonary artery, and if further advanced it will enter one or other pulmonary artery. It is wise to pass the catheter as far as the pulmonary artery before taking the first blood sample and pressure reading, for venospasm may occur and prevent further forward progress of the catheter, especially if the operation time is prolonged. Further, Warren (41) states that " samples of blood from the proximal pulmonary artery appear to be most representative of mixed venous blood, samples from the ventricle or atrium are more variable ".

Recording the Intracardiac Pressure. With the tip of the catheter in the pulmonary artery the manometer is connected by the rubber tubing to the outer end of the catheter in place of the syringe, care having been taken to exclude all air from the rubber tubing by allowing the heparinised saline in the reservoir to run freely through it, and then clipping the tubing between the manometer and catheter and the reservoir and manometer in this order. The clip between the manometer and catheter is now released and the saline level in the manometer will gradually fall until the pulmonary artery pressure is reached. It will then remain stationary or oscillate slightly. The reading is noted, the clip between the manometer and the catheter closed and that between the reservoir and manometer opened so that the manometer is again filled.

Removal of Blood Samples. The rubber tube from the manometer is disconnected from the catheter and 3 or 4 ml. of blood are drawn back into a saline-filled syringe. These are discarded, as they will be diluted with the saline in the catheter. A sterile 10 ml. syringe, previously lubricated with sterile paraffin, and containing about 1 ml. of paraffin, free from air bubbles, is now attached to the catheter, and 5 to 10 ml. of undiluted blood are withdrawn. The syringe is detached and the blood is injected through a serum needle under the liquid paraffin in one of the specimen bottles and stirred to mix with the heparin, to prevent clotting. In order to prevent air embolism the hilt of the catheter must be kept below the level of the right auricle when removing samples of blood. The outer end of the catheter must never be left open, so that when a syringe containing a blood sample is detached, either a fresh syringe filled with saline or the manometer tubing should be immediately attached in its place. A little heparinised saline is now allowed to run through the catheter to displace the blood contents.

The catheter is now gradually withdrawn, further pressure readings and blood samples being taken from the upper part of the right ventricle, the lower part of the right ventricle, the right mid-auricle and the superior vena cava. The normal mean pressures, referred to the sternal angle level, are:—Pulmonary artery, 13 to 20 cm. saline (10 to 15 mm. Hg.). Right ventricle, 11 to 16 cm. saline (8 to 12 mm. Hg.). Right auricle, −3 to +3 cm. saline (−2 to +2 mm. Hg.).

The catheter is then completely withdrawn, and the proximal catgut ligature tied to arrest bleeding. A skin suture may not be necessary, but should be available. After the operation movements of the arm should be encouraged to minimise risk of thrombosis. Immediately after withdrawal the catheter must be well washed through with water under pressure for several minutes, then hydrogen peroxide (10 vols.) is trickled slowly through until bubbling ceases, and it is finally washed again with tap water. The blood samples should be analysed immediately, and not allowed to stand overnight. Arterial puncture is only required when the cardiac output is being determined, and then some authorities do not perform it, their calculations being based on the assumption that the arterial blood is 95% saturated with oxygen. In cases in which there is a shunt between the two sides of the heart, the cardiac output cannot be determined by the Fick principle. If arterial blood is required, direct puncture is employed. It is thought by Cournand that the brachial rather than the femoral artery should be punctured. The tissues around the artery are first infiltrated with 2% procaine solution. For serial observations an indwelling needle is employed. A special Cournand needle is used, and is inserted with the sharp open-bore stilet in place. When the artery is pierced a small drop of blood appears through the fine bore. The sharp stilet is now removed when the blood spurts out. The sharp stilet is now replaced by a blunt one, and the needle is "threaded" up the artery a short distance and is then strapped in position. When the stilet is removed for blood sampling it should stand in peroxide solution, to prevent clotting when it is replaced. The blood samples are removed as is done for the intra-cardiac samples. When the cardiac output is being determined, the oxygen consumption is determined at the end of the operation, using the Benedict-Roth apparatus.

Variations in Technique. The catheter may be sterilised by boiling for ten minutes; it is then left to cool in the sterile towel, until it becomes sufficiently rigid for use.

Some workers employ a three-way stopcock to connect the fluid in the reservoir, the manometer, and the sampling syringe with the catheter. A Tycos manometer may be used instead of a saline one. In this case a few ml. of saline solution are introduced into the tubing in the part adjacent to the catheter attachment to minimise the risk of air embolism. There is thus an air lock between the manometer and the saline in the manometer tubing. Johnson et al. (37) take the zero level as one third of the distance from the sternum to the back, at the level of the third costal cartilage. The saline manometer readings average 11 mm. less than those recorded by the Tycos instrument. The saline manometer has the disadvantage of reacting slowly, especially when the catheter is full of blood. The Tycos manometer is brisk in its response. Electrical recording devices are now being more commonly employed. These give pulse tracings from which systolic, diastolic and mean pressures can be recorded, and the form of the pulse wave studied. In young children the catheter may be introduced into the saphenous vein, and passed up the inferior vena cava.

When a three-way stopcock is used the tap is placed so that the lumen of the catheter communicates with the fluid in the reservoir, and as the catheter is introduced into the vein a slow flow of fluid is maintained through the catheter at a rate of 20 to 30 drops a minute. As soon as the catheter is inside the heart shadow the saline flow is adjusted to 5 or 10 drops a minute.

Silk ligatures may be employed instead of catgut ones. At the end of the operation both ligatures are removed and bleeding is controlled by pressure. When the arterial needle is removed firm pressure must be maintained over the artery for at least five minutes and the pulses below carefully checked.

Some workers, such as Johnson et al. (37), prefer to heparinise the patient instead of the saline. In this case a heparin curve must be done the day before the operation, from which the necessary dose can be worked out to maintain the clotting t me during the operation, and for twenty-four hours afterwards, at ten to twenty minutes (normal three to seven minutes) by the capillary method.

Cournand et al. (42) advise that a direct vision electrocardiograph should be used during catheterisation to record the cardiac rhythm and enable abnormalities to be detected immediately.

Complications. Warren (41) says that several thousand human cardiac catheterisations have been done in various laboratories with no record of serious untoward effect. There are, however, certain risks attached to the procedure.

General Reactions. Fainting, sweating, nausea or vomiting may occur during catheterisation. Rigors are due to pyrogens in the catheter which has not been properly cleaned.

Veno-spasm. This is due, according to Wood (40), to the skin not being adequately anæsthetised, to the catheter not being washed free from disinfectant, or to the catheter being too large.

Air Embolism. Strict precautions are essential to prevent air entering the catheter, for in cases of congenital heart disease with right to left blood shunts, air emboli could pass into the systemic circulation. This has very rarely occurred, the air bubbles passing to the brain producing transient neurological signs.

Thrombosis. This may occur either in the veins or in the heart. If the saphenous vein is used it should be tied off as close to the femoral vein as possible at the end of the operation. Slight local thrombophlebitis at the site of the introduction of the catheter into the arm vein has been from time to time recorded. Johnson et al. (37) record the case of a markedly cyanotic infant, weight 19 lbs. A catheter was introduced into the right saphenous vein near the femoral junction and passed easily into the right auricle. The infant was heparinised during the operation. A month later death occurred, when " a clinically unsuspected, well-organised thrombus was found occluding the inferior vena cava, both common iliac veins and the right renal vein, and a large thrombus was attached to the right auricular wall at the base of one leaflet of the tricuspid valve ". Holling and Zak (39) found evidence either of systemic or pulmonary thrombosis or emboli in 6 of their 70 cases of congenital heart disease within fourteen days of catheterisation and one case died.

Disturbances of Cardiac Rhythm. Cournand et al. (42) consider these are the most important complications in cases of congenital heart disease. They include premature contractions, runs of ventricular tachycardia, ventricular fibrillation and auricular tachycardia. If cardiac catheterisation is done under electrocardiographic control, the disturbance of rhythm can be recognised early and the catheter withdrawn. These workers record sudden death in two adults, one with a long history of angina pectoris. In neither instance was the catheterisation performed with electrocardiographic control. Wood (40) records one fatal case of ventricular fibrillation in 233 catheterisations.

Conclusions. Cardiac catheterisation gives physiological information concerning the heart's action, as opposed to angiocardiography which reveals the anatomical condition of the heart and main vessels. The determination of cardiac output in health and disease is of value as a physiological experiment and in determining the types of heart failure. The chief value now is in the investigation of cases of congenital heart disease in which surgical procedures are contemplated. Catheterisation may also help in deciding whether a pulmonary-systemic anastomosis or a valvulotomy may give better results in certain types of congenital heart disease. A definite clinical diagnosis in any case of congenital heart disease is often very difficult, owing to the frequency with which multiple defects are present. Holling and Zak (39) state that cardiac catheterisation will enable certain malformations to be proved. Thus if the catheter passes through a septal defect it can be seen to do so on the X-ray screen. On the other hand, it must be understood that the passage of a catheter from the right to the left auricle does not prove that there is a functioning defect in the auricular septum. In about a quarter of normal subjects the foramen ovale may be patent, although functionless, allowing the passage of the catheter. In these cases the presence of a shunt from one chamber to another can only be proved by blood gas analysis. If the catheter tip is passed into the pulmonary artery the pulmonary stenosis can be recognised by the fall in pressure as the tip passes through it. An atrial septal defect with an arteriovenous shunt will result in blood in the right atrium being more oxygenated than is the blood in the venæ cavæ. Similarly, in uncomplicated ventricular septal defect blood samples from the right ventricle, especially from the region of the outflow tract, will usually show an increase in oxygen content as compared with vena caval and right atrial samples. This indicates a left to right shunt between the ventricles. With a patent ductus arteriosus the blood in the pulmonary artery is more oxygenated than is the blood in the right ventricle. By cardiac catheterisation Eisenmenger's complex may be distinguished from Fallot's tetralogy. The lesions in Fallot's tetralogy consist of stenosis or hypoplasia of the pulmonary artery, a defect in the interventricular septum, the aorta is displaced to the right and communicates with both ventricles, and the right ventricle is hypertrophied. In the Eisenmenger complex there is an increase in the size of the infundibulum, pulmonary valve and artery, together with an interventricular septal defect, enlarged right ventricle and dextroposition of the aorta. In Eisenmenger's complex therefore, the systolic pressure in the right ventricle equals that in the pulmonary artery, as there is no pulmonary stenosis. Systemic-pulmonary anastomosis, which is helpful in the Fallot's tetralogy, would not be likely to improve the patient suffering from Eisenmenger's complex.

Cardiac catheterisation will also establish the diagnosis of transposition of the great vessels, if it is found that the blood in the pulmonary artery is richer in oxygen than the aortic blood. In cases of "pure pulmonary stenosis", or as it is sometimes called "pulmonary stenosis with closed ventricular septum" cardiac catheterisation will decide whether pulmonary stenosis is present. Severe peripheral cyanosis may result from reduced cardiac output, without intra-cardiac shunt. In such a case the arterial blood would have a normal oxygen saturation. Cardiac catheterisation is also used to determine the increase in pressure in the pulmonary artery and right ventricle before the operation of valvulotomy in mitral stenosis. The fall in pressure after operation can be similarly demonstrated.

Thiocyanates and the Treatment of Hypertension

Potassium and sodium thiocyanate were originally recommended for the treatment of essential hypertension by Pauli (43) in 1903. The mode of action is obscure, but it has been suggested that they cause a relaxation of smooth muscle. They are readily absorbed from the gastro-intestinal tract and are distributed throughout body fluids in the same way as chlorides and bromides; they do not penetrate into the cells. They are excreted mainly through the kidneys, but this excretion can vary as much as 400% in different individuals.

Thiocyanates offer one of the few means of treatment of hypertension, but their use was limited, owing to toxic effects, until the dosage was controlled and rendered more safe by serum estimations. Barker and his colleagues (44, 45 and 46), who have treated many patients successfully over a number of years, emphasise the importance of frequent determination of serum levels of thiocyanates while treatment is in progress. They consider a concentration of 8 to 12 mg. per 100 ml. to be a safe level in the majority of cases. They recommend beginning the treatment by giving 0·3 g. per day and making blood cyanate determinations every week for four to six weeks, and subsequently every month. It is readily soluble, 0·1 g. in ½ oz. of water being given three times a day, or it may be prescribed as Elixir Sodium Thiocyanate (gr. 20 in fl. oz. 1), one teaspoonful twice a day. Enteric-sealed tablets, containing 0·2 g., or 0·065 g. of potassium thiocyanate are also sometimes given. If the blood pressure drops sharply, or if symptoms of fatigue or depression are marked, the dose can be decreased. If no blood pressure change or toxic symptoms occur after three to four weeks, and the blood concentration has not reached 6 mg. per 100 ml., the dose may be doubled. Barker and his colleagues, who reported on 246 cases, found that the systolic pressure may drop during the first two to four weeks, whereas the diastolic pressure may not be reduced for three to four months. The best clinical results were obtained with patients whose erythrocyte count was high and sedimentation rate low, and whose blood pressure was of the fluctuant type. Out of 246 patients, 76% showed some improvement. There were no toxic deaths, but patients showed toxic manifestations of one kind or another. Another series of 50 cases treated over eleven years, was reported by Kurtz, Shapiro and Selby Mills (47). These authors followed Barker's method of laboratory control. Subjective improvement was very definite in 63% of cases and fair in 17%. Satisfactory reduction of blood pressure was obtained in 78% of cases. There were no deaths that could be attributed directly or indirectly to thiocyanate. Fischmann (48) treated 40 cases with thiocyanate, 25 proving successful and 15 being failures. Of the successful cases, 3 showed no fall in blood pressure but improved symptomatically, especially as regards headache. Of the 15 failures the blood pressure fell in 6 cases without subjective improvement.

To set against these encouraging results, there have been some reports of fatalities and toxic effects following the use of thiocyanates. Foulger and Rose (49) in 1943 and Potter (50) in 1944 reported cases of acute goitre due to thiocyanate therapy. Other toxic effects include exfoliative dermatitis, weakness, dizziness, anorexia, thrombo-phlebitis, and hæmorrhagic encephalomalacia. The importance of a strict control of dosage based on weekly and later monthly serum determinations, and a careful watch for untoward symptoms cannot be over-emphasised. Further, thiocyanate should never be given if there is any evidence of renal failure. In our experience it may not lower the blood pressure, or the fall produced is only temporary.

Methonium Salts and the Treatment of Hypertension

Drugs of the methonium series have been introduced for the treatment of high blood pressure. Paton and Zaimis (51) pointed out the possible clinical value of hexamethonium iodide (C_6) in hypertension and vascular disease as it differs from tetraethylammonium iodide (T.E.A.) in its greater potency, slower action and more prolonged effect. Observations were next made by Organe, Paton and Zaimis (52) on the action of pentamethonium iodide (C_5) on man. On intravenous injection these drugs produce a fall in blood pressure, increase in pulse rate, vasodilatation which is more marked in the lower than in the upper limbs, diminution of sweating especially in the feet, dilatation of the pupils with possibly disturbance of accommodation. Nausea, headache and dryness of the mouth may be noted as side effects. The action of the drugs is on the ganglion cells of the autonomic nervous system, both sympathetic and parasympathetic, a blockage of impulses being produced there.

Campbell and Robertson (53) reported on the treatment of eight cases of hypertension and papillœdema with hexamethonium bromide. Treatment was commenced with the intramuscular injection of 100 mg. every four hours, and subsequently the drug was given by mouth by dissolving a 0·5 g. tablet in 20 ml. of water. The dosage adopted was 0·25 g. twice daily on the first day, 0·25 g. t.i.d. for the next two days, with a gradual increase up to 0·5 g. four to six times a day. The drug is most effective when taken before meals. Good results were obtained, the blood pressure falling, headache disappearing and papillœdema diminishing. Certain unpleasant reactions may occur, such as blurring of vision, dryness of the mouth, nausea, heartburn and constipation. More serious side effects include paralytic ileus, distension of the bladder, postural hypotension and fainting. In addition to the effect in lowering the blood pressure C_6 has a profound influence in diminishing gastric motility and gastric secretion. Kay and Smith (54) showed that the intramuscular injection of 100 mg. of hexamethonium iodide produced achlorhydria lasting for three hours. The action here is by vagal blockade, and the drug prevents the development of a true insulin response such as is noted with a complete vagotomy (see p. 172). When C_6 is given with insulin the gastric acidity first falls and then rises to little above the resting value. C_6 fails to prevent a histamine response of acid gastric secretion, for it is thought that histamine acts directly on the parietal gastric mucosal cells. Kay and Smith (55) also showed that the iodide and bromide of methonium were more powerful gastric depressants than is the chloride.

Pentamethonium iodide (Lytensium) is put up in ampoules for injection containing 100 mg./1 ml. Hexamethonium iodide (Hexathide) is also available in ampoules containing 50 mg./2·5 ml. The hexamethonium bromide (Vegolysin) tablets contain 250 mg. They are soluble in water.

In one of our cases of essential hypertension treated by C_6 we found that when hexamethonium iodide was given intravenously in a saline drip, the blood pressure fell from 220/130 mm. Hg. to 140/108 mm. Hg. after four doses of 10 mg. given at intervals of three minutes. The pressure began to rise again after one and a half hours. Hexamethonium bromide was subsequently given by mouth in doses of 250 mg. tablet crushed in water four times a day before meals, but the blood pressure was not so well controlled although there were no unpleasant side effects.

The dosage should be controlled by blood pressure readings taken weekly, as the drug may have a cumulative effect and bromism or iodism may ensue. Postural hypotension is one of the most dangerous of the side effects. It is especially liable to occur when the patient is standing still. Turner (56) records the case of a man who was " all right when walking from hospital to the bus stop, but the trouble came on when he was standing in the queue ". An abdominal belt or binder is a useful corrective and the patient should be instructed to contract his abdominal muscles, and, if possible, lie down if he feels faint. An injection of adrenaline should be given in severe hypotensive reactions.

Conclusions. It is too early to say whether the methonium compounds will prove as disappointing as the various other drugs recommended in the past for the treatmentof hypertension. They certainly should not be used indiscriminately and without proper control. They appear to be of most value in cases of threatened left ventricular failure, diminution of vision due to retinal changes, impaired renal function and when there appears to be a possibility of a stroke.

The absorption of the pentamethonium and hexamethonium salts, when given by mouth, appears, to be very uncertain, and in order to obtain an adequate fall in blood pressure as much as 3 to 4 g. per day may be necessary. Postural hypotension may result from these large doses. Further, the danger of bromism or iodism is enhanced when the patient is on a low salt diet. The drugs are excreted by the kidneys, and if there is renal failure much smaller doses must be employed.

The Rice Diet in Hypertension

Kempner (57) in 1944 introduced the rice diet for the treatment of patients suffering from renal and hypertensive vascular disease. He found improvement in the blood pressure and also in the size of the heart, retinal changes and electrocardiograms. A clinical trial of the diet was carried out for the Medical Research Council and the report was published in 1950 (58). Patients were encouraged to eat 250 to 350 g. of rice (dry weight) daily. It was boiled in water or steamed, with no added salt, milk or fat. It can be flavoured with sugar, lemon juice or fruit, and served dry or wet. The fluid was limited to 1 litre in twenty-four hours. The diet contained sodium 121 mg., potassium 1·91 g., chloride 195 mg., and nitrogen 3·14 g. (equivalent to 19·6 g. of protein).

A sample menu is as follows :—

Breakfast. Grape fruit (prepared), 5oz. ; boiled rice (dry weight), 2 oz ; sugar, 1 oz., and orange juice, 8 oz.

Mid-morning. Lemon juice, 1¼ oz., with water, 5 oz., and sugar ½ oz.

Lunch. Boiled rice (dry weight), 3 oz. ; golden syrup, ½ oz. ; blackcurrants (raw), 5 oz. ; sugar, ½ oz., and black grapes, 6 oz.

Tea. Boiled rice (dry weight), 1 oz.; sugar, 1 oz.; banana slices, 1½ oz.; orange juice, 2 oz., and lemon juice, 2½ oz.

Supper. Boiled rice (dry weight), 3 oz.; sugar, ¾ oz.; fresh peaches, 5 oz., and orange juice, 8 oz.

On retiring. Dessert cherries, 5 oz.

This diet contains C. 492 g., P. 26 g., and F. 3 g., sodium 83 mg., chloride 139 mg.

The Committee confirmed Kempner's findings of a fall in blood pressure. The average fall in 35 patients treated by the Committee over periods ranging from twenty to ninety-five days was 55 mm. Hg. systolic and 26 mm. Hg. diastolic.

It appears probable that the fall in blood pressure is due not to the low protein content, but to the low sodium in the diet. As soon as the sodium chloride intake is increased, even slightly, the blood pressure tends to rise. The diet is not without danger, as uræmia has been recorded during treatment by Schroeder (59) in 1948. If in non-œdematous patients the urinary sodium or chloride does not fall to a low level within a few days of starting the diet, the Committee emphasise that a careful watch must be kept on the blood urea and blood sodium content.

We have tried the diet on patients suffering from heart failure with high blood pressure and œdema, and in these cases we have found that the patient is usually too ill to take the diet.

Some Cardio-therapeutic Measures

The Use of Digitalis. Digitalis still remains supreme amongst the drugs used in the treatment of heart disease. Withering (60), in 1785, was one of the first to draw attention to the value of digitalis in producing diuresis in certain cases of heart failure. Since then the indications for its use have become more clearly defined, and it is recognised that its most beneficial effects are obtained in cases of cardiac irregularity due to auricular fibrillation. We no longer believe in the *circus* movement but the ventricle is slowed by increasing the degree of heart-block. It is also of value in auricular flutter, and, indeed, in heart failure from any cause. High blood pressure is not now considered a contra-indication, as it has been shown that in therapeutic doses digitalis does not cause a rise of systolic pressure, although the pulse pressure may be increased as the result of a fall in the diastolic level in cases of cardiac failure. Whether or not it acts as a direct *cardiac tonic* and should be employed in disorders associated with sinus rhythm has been a matter of dispute. It is usually held that digitalis in such cases is a cardiac tonic and slows the whole heart by its action on the vagus, thus prolonging diastole, increasing the force of systole and improving the coronary circulation and so the nutrition of the cardiac muscle.

In heart failure of a severe degree large doses are usually required. On account of the danger of producing severe toxic effects, the total quantity necessary is generally administered in divided doses at several hours' interval, but the beneficial effect is thereby inevitably postponed. This delay is partially due to the fact that digitalis takes about six hours before it is absorbed from the stomach ; it is also eliminated slowly by the intestines and kidneys, and so cumulative results may occur.

Digitalis may be administered either in the form of a good tincture or as a tablet of the dried leaves. One cat unit tablet corresponds approximately with 1 ml. (m. 17) of the tincture or 0·1 g. (gr. 1·5) of tab. digitalis pulv. (B.P. Add.). In order to obtain results as quickly as possible in cases of severe heart failure the maximum amount of digitalis, which can safely be administered to an individual, should be given within twenty-four hours. This may be taken to be m. 17 of the tincture or gr. 1·5 of the dried leaf for every 10 lbs. of body weight. Thus, for a man weighing 10 stones the amount required is m. 240 of the tincture or gr. 21 of the dried leaf tablet. When the weight of the patient is not known accurately, as will often be the case, three-quarters of the above amounts should be the maximum given. Digitalis should not be administered more often than every six hours. Thus, in an urgent case, in which no digitalis has been taken within the last ten days, m. 60 of the tincture may be given six-hourly for 4 doses, and then the dose reduced to m. 30, if digitalisation has not yet been effected. As soon as this occurs the drug should be discontinued for a day or so and then m. 20 of the tincture or less may be required three times a day to allow for daily elimination and to keep the patient under the influence of the drug. If digitalis has been administered within the last ten days the total calculated amount should be reduced to three-quarters if no signs of digitalis over-action are shown by the electrocardiogram, such as heart-block or premature ventricular systoles, and to one-half if they are present. In either case the total calculated amount is given in three equal doses at six-hourly intervals.

In conclusion, it may be said that massive doses should only be used in cases of heart failure of extreme urgency, and generally administration in smaller doses is the safest course to adopt.

The indications for discontinuing the drug are, according to Eggleston: Nausea or vomiting, unless this is due to venous congestion of the stomach, which is usually the case when it occurs shortly after the commencement of digitalis administration (Jensen (61)). The apex rate lower than 60. The occurrence of frequent ectopic systoles, heart-block, phasic arryhthmia or coupled beats. The latter are caused by a regular sequence of premature ventricular systoles following each normal ventricular contraction.

It is usually found if the digitalis is going to relieve the heart failure that diuresis takes place; if there is no diuresis, beneficial results are not likely to ensue, and diminution in the secretion of the urine is an additional sign of digitalis toxæmia. The diuresis is a manifestation of the effect of digitalis in filling the arteries and emptying the veins, and is due to an increased renal circulation and relief of renal congestion. Diuresis does not follow the administration of digitalis, even in massive doses, unless œdema is present.

Digitalis should not be administered more frequently than at six-hourly intervals, as this is the time taken for its absorption from the stomach, and in cases of auricular fibrillation it has been shown by Canby Robinson (62) that an effect is produced in two to five hours after oral administration. Sufficient warning of any toxic effects, which may be produced by its administration, is thereby given.

Digoxin. Wokes (63), in 1929, showed that the leaves of the foxglove *Digitalis lanata* are physiologically nearly four times as potent as are those of *Digitalis purpurea,* the species used in medicine. Smith (64), in 1930, isolated a pure crystalline alcohol-soluble glucoside, Digoxin, from the leaves of the *Digitalis lanata.* It possesses the advantage that it does not require biological standardisation. It is absorbed and excreted more quickly than is digitalis and can be given orally or intravenously. Intravenous injection is only advisable when an extremely rapid effect is required, or when the patient vomits anything taken by mouth. It must never be given intravenously if the patient has taken digitalis during the previous two weeks. In auricular fibrillation the average initial intravenous dose for an adult of 10 stones or over is 0·75 to 1 mg. A solution is obtainable in ampoules, each ampoule contains 0·5 mg. Digoxin in 1 ml. 70% alcohol. It must be diluted before use with 9 times the volume of freshly prepared sterile normal saline solution. The solution thus obtained is injected slowly into a vein, taking three to five minutes over the injection. The solution is very irritant and must not be injected outside the lumen of the vein. Wayne (65) has shown that the ventricular rate rapidly slows after such an injection, and that the maximum effect is obtained in one to two hours. Subsequently Digoxin is administered by mouth as described below.

For oral administration the initial dose is 1·5 mg. for patients weighing 10 stones or more, and 1 to 1·25 mg. for lighter patients. Digoxin must never be given by mouth if the patient has taken digitalis during the previous week. It is put up in "Tabloid" form, each containing 0·25 mg., to be taken in water, or in 30 ml. bottles containing 0·5 mg. in each millilitre of 80% alcohol. The solution is best given in chloroform water to disguise the bitter taste. After oral administration the ventricular rate begins to slow in about an hour and the maximum effect is obtained in about six hours. Six hours after the initial dose 0·25 mg. is given every six hours until the ventricular rate falls to 60 or 70. Subsequently a maintenance dose of 0·25 mg. twice a day may be required indefinitely.

Quinidine. This is a dextro-rotatory cinchona alkaloid, which was first used by Frey (66) in 1918 in cases of auricular fibrillation. Wenckebach (67) had previously, in 1914, obtained a temporary arrest of auricular fibrillation in one patient by giving 1 g. of quinine daily. Frey, in a series of 22 cases of fibrillation, obtained a restoration of normal rhythm in 50%. He gave the drug in doses of 0·4 g. (6 gr.) t.d.s. by mouth for three to eight days.

The administration of quinidine sulphate may be considered under the following headings :—

Selection of Case. Quinidine is of greatest value in cases of auricular fibrillation, especially when there is neither cardiac enlargement nor valvular disease (Cotton (68)). Best results are obtained in fibrillation of less than six months' duration, and in those cases in which the symptoms increase with the onset of fibrillation. The infective group of cases is more suitable than the degenerative. The drug can be tried in paroxysmal auricular fibrillation, as digitalis does not usually have any beneficial effect here (Parkinson and Nicholl (69)). It may be of value in auricular flutter, the normal rhythm being restored direct, without an intermediate stage of fibrillation. It is at times successful in those cases of flutter which have been converted to fibrillation by the use of digitalis, but which do not return to the normal sinus rhythm on discontinuing the drug. It does not appear to have any beneficial effect on premature systoles.

Contra-indications. There are certain definite contra-indications which apply, no matter what the nature of the cardiac disorder may be. Thus quinidine must not be given if the heart is greatly enlarged. When there is congestive failure the patient should first be treated with rest, digitalis and diuretics until compensation is restored. Then, after a week's cessation from the use of digitalis, quinidine may be given if thought advisable. Heart-block is also a contra-indication. It must not be given if there is a history of recent embolism. It is considered inadvisable to administer quinidine if fibrillation has lasted for six months, or to use quinidine and digitalis simultaneously.

Regimen. The patient must be kept in bed, and preferably at absolute rest, during the initial week of the treatment. This usually implies the necessity for skilled nurses. Attention must be paid to the bowels, and the diet should be such as will not give rise to flatulence.

Methods of Administration and Dosage. The drug is given by mouth in powder form in gelatine capsules. Probably the safest method is to give on the first day a test dose of 0·2 g. (3 gr.) to determine whether the patient has any idiosyncrasy to the drug. If no toxæmic symptoms appear, on the second day 0·4 g. (6 gr.) is given every three hours for four doses, and this is increased to five doses of 0·4 g. at three-hourly intervals on the third day. This dosage is then maintained until the end of the week, and if the normal rhythm has not been restored by this time the drug will probably not prove successful. The pulse should be taken before each dose is given, and if it is found to be regular the drug should be discontinued, at any rate temporarily, until a tracing has been taken. Further indications for discontinuing the administration of quinidine are a slowing of the auricular rate to about 250 per minute, or an increase of the ventricular rate to over 160. In the former case there is a danger of the ventricle following directly the auricular rate. The exact rate of the auricle and ventricle are best determined by an electrocardiogram.

Hay (70) recommends that quinidine should be given every two hours by day in ten equal doses, as its action soon passes off. Starting with a test dose of 0·2 g. (3 gr.) on the first day, 2 g. (30 gr.) are given on the second day in ten doses of 0·2 g. each. If necessary, the dose may be increased to 3 g. (45 gr.) a day in ten doses of 0·3 g. (4.5 gr.). The smallest beneficial dose appears to be one of 5 gr., which restored the normal rhythm in a case of auricular fibrillation of recent origin, under our care, which was associated with a toxic goitre. As much as a total of 375 gr. has, however, been required before a satisfactory result was obtained, and it may be necessary to continue indefinitely with small doses of 5 gr. daily, especially if a relapse occurs on omitting the drug.

Symptoms of Toxæmia and Dangers. Frey (66), in 1918, drew attention to the possibility of quinidine idiosyncrasy, resulting in such symptoms as respiratory failure and cerebral paralysis. Benjamin and V. Kapff (71), in 1921, recorded instances of embolus occurring during the administration of quinidine. This is especially liable to follow restoration of normal rhythm, and is, in all probability, due to the detachment of a clot from the wall of the auricle. Embolus formation is not necessarily fatal. The onset of ventricular fibrillation may cause sudden death.

Headache is nearly always experienced while quinidine is being taken. Other toxic symptoms include sweating, nausea, vomiting, diarrhœa, abdominal pain and a scarlatiniform rash. Dimness of vision, or the occurrence of frequent ectopic ventricular beats, is an indication for the immediate discontinuance of the drug.

Results of Quinidine Administration. Campbell and Gordon (72) found that quinidine restored normal rhythm in 64% of a series of 135 cases of auricular fibrillation. In 30% of these, however, fibrillation recurred after an average period of two years, but in the other 34% the normal rhythm was still maintained after an average period of nearly four years.

The Action of the Drug. The effect of quinidine upon heart muscle can be summarised thus: The auricular rate is slowed. The rate of conduction in the auricle, ventricle and A–V junctional tissues is reduced. The absolute refractory period of auricular muscle is prolonged.

Quinidine has also some effect upon the vagus nerve, causing a partial paralysis which tends to increase the ventricular rate.

The electrocardiographic changes which may occur during quinidine administration are, according to Hay (70): Slowing of auricular rate; the onset of auricular flutter and 2 : 1 heart-block; increase of ventricular rate; appearance of ectopic ventricular beats; restoration of normal rhythm in 50% of cases of fibrillation.

The Value of the Drug. The administration of quinidine has very definite dangers, and the cases in which it is worth a trial require careful selection, and very close watching during the treatment. Even if normal rhythm is established, the general condition of the patient is not always improved, while the underlying myocardial degeneration still remains.

Mercurial Diuretics and Ammonium Chloride. These drugs include mersalyl, Neptal, Mercupurin, Mercuhydrin, Novurit, and Esidrone. They are of great value in the treatment of congestive failure (right ventricular failure), and in acute œdema of the lungs (left ventricular failure). Mersalyl is an organic mercurial compound which was reported on clinically by Brunn (73) and by Bernheim (74) in 1924. It contains 36% of mercury, and is put up in 10% solution in 1 ml. and 2 ml. ampoules. Mersalyl has now replaced novasurol which was introduced by Saxl and Heilig (75) in 1920. Novasurol has been abandoned owing to its toxic effects, whereas mersalyl is not usually toxic. Andrews (76) reported a case of heart failure, without renal disease, in which the first intravenous injection of 0·5 ml. of mersalyl resulted in headache, epileptiform convulsions and unconsciousness, but the patient, a woman aged twenty-two, did not die. In the case described by Higgins (77) there was hypertensive heart disease with congestive failure. About 10 doses of mersalyl or Mercupurin had been given, when an intramuscular injection of 1 ml. of Mercupurin was followed an hour later by a severe chill, fever, dyspnœa, cyanosis, fall in blood pressure and prostration. Death seemed imminent. A month later the patient died and the kidneys showed some mild arteriolosclerosis, with very slight necrosis and calcification of the tubules, probably due to mercury. Volini et al. (78) reported 3 cases of very sudden death following the intravenous injection of mercurial diuretics, 1 from Mercupurin and 2 from Esidrone. In 2 of the cases electrocardiograms showed the development of ventricular fibrillation. Evans and Perry (79) have also published 6 cases of immediate death due to the same cause, and suggest that it may be advisable to give mercurial diuretics intramuscularly to patients with a low plasma protein. In other cases cramps may develop in the legs due to depletion of chlorides, and these can be relieved by the administration of sodium chloride. Mercurial diuretics should not be given in cases of acute nephritis, in lipoid nephrosis, or if the urine contains some granular or blood casts, or if there is hæmaturia. A test dose of 0·5 ml. mersalyl is first injected intramuscularly, and if there is no intolerance, as shown by hæmaturia, diarrhœa or irritation of the skin, a course of intravenous injections is begun. In order to render the urine acid, ammonium chloride in doses of gr. 30, is given by mouth every six hours. The ammonium chloride can be administered as a mixture : Ammon. chlor. gr. 30, ext. glycyrrhiz. liq. m. 20, sp. chlorof. m. 7, aquam ad 1 oz., or in the form of four 0·5 gram " stearettes ". On the third day of the administration of the ammonium chloride, 1 ml. of mersalyl diluted with 4 ml. of sterile normal saline is injected slowly into a vein in the arm. The arm is then raised to prevent venous thrombosis. The ammonium chloride is administered daily. On the fifth and ninth day 2 ml. of mersalyl, diluted with 8 ml. of sterile normal saline are injected intravenously. If a good diuretic response is obtained, such as 90 to 180 oz. of urine, the injections of mersalyl should be repeated at intervals of a week, the ammonium chloride being given by mouth for two days before, the day of, and the day after the injection, *i.e.* for four days each week. The total fluid intake during the twenty-four hours must be restricted to 35 oz. or less, and full digitalisation should be maintained to control the rate of the heart. The fluid intake and output should be recorded each twenty-four hours, and the patient weighed at first daily and later weekly. The degree of dehyration is reflected in the loss of weight. No salt should be used in the cooking of the food, and none added when it is eaten. In some cases we have found that the administration of ammonium chloride alone will produce a good diuretic response.

It is important that the weekly injections of mersalyl, with the corresponding administration of ammonium chloride, should be continued for an indefinite period providing a good diuresis ensues, and that the patient does not become unduly dehydrated. We have patients who have received this treatment for two years or longer, and who are still continuing with it, thereby being enabled to maintain a fair degree of health and activity. In other cases we have noticed that dehydration appears excessive after a prolonged course—the patient feeling weak and ill after each injection. Here the injections should be discontinued, and if required again later they should be given at longer intervals. Rechtschaffen and Gittler (80) record a case of acute dehydration following the subcutaneous administration of Meralluride (Mercuhydrin) Sodium. Within four hours of the initial dose the patient suffered from peripheral vascular collapse, bradycardia, elevation in temperature and a shaking chill. Recovery occurred within two hours. During the four hours after the injection there was a diuresis of 1,800 ml. It should be remembered that as much as 8 to 10 pints of excess fluid may be retained in the body tissues without pitting œdema being apparent. Such a condition may be termed latent œdema, and is associated with pulmonary congestion and œdema of the lungs, and with an engorged liver. It is much relieved by the administration of mersalyl or Novurit.

The Circulation Time

Various methods have been employed to estimate the circulation time in man. Bornstein (81) in 1912 made the patient breathe a mixture of air containing 5 to 7% CO_2. The time taken for the arterial blood to carry an increased amount of CO_2 to the respiratory centre was shown by an increased depth in the breathing. Since then various substances have been injected intravenously, such as fluorescin, histamine, calcium chloride, saccharin, ether, sodium dehydrocholate, calcium gluconate, and magnesium sulphate. Tarr, Oppenheimer and Sager (82) in 1933 gave an historical account of the methods which have been used, and reported their experiences with sodium dehydrocholate (Decholin Sodium). This measures the arm-to-tongue circulation time. The test is carried out before breakfast, with the patient lying as flat as possible, the right arm being supported at the level of the auricles. Five ml. of a 20% solution of Decholin are injected through a wide-bore needle into an antecubital vein, taking one to two seconds over the injection. The patient is told to raise his left hand directly he perceives a bitter taste under the tongue. The time is taken with a stop watch from the beginning of the injection of the Decholin to the signal that it has reached the tongue. The average normal time is thirteen seconds (extremes ten to sixteen seconds). Occassionally the patient complains of nausea after the injection, or of pain in the region of the gall-bladder. The circulation time is not affected by the weight, height, pulse rate or blood pressure of the patient. It is prolonged in congestive heart failure in the majority of cases, to between twenty and forty-seven seconds. The circulation time is also prolonged in myxœdema, and polycythæmia, but shortened in fevers, anæmia, and hyperthyroidism, when the latter is not complicated by heart failure. Bernstein and Simkins (83) in 1939 used magnesium sulphate to determine the arm-to-tongue circulation time. Six ml. of a 10% solution of magnesium sulphate are injected intravenously into an antecubital vein, and when it reaches the mouth the patient experiences a transient hot sensation in the pharynx and tongue, which spreads rapidly to the face, hands, perineum and legs. It is advisable to have at hand an ampoule of 10% calcium gluconate for immediate intravenous injection should an undue magnesium sulphate reaction occur With this method Bernstein and Simkins found the average arm-to-tongue circulation time 12·9 seconds (extremes 7 to 17·8 seconds). They classified cases of heart failure clinically into groups: (1) well-compensated; (2) with dyspnœa on exertion; (3) with dyspnœa and cyanosis; (4) with additional pulmonary congestion; (5) with ascites or œdema. In the majority of cases the circulation time was prolonged proportionately to the degree of heart failure, up to about thirty seconds. Lesions such as mitral stenosis or auricular fibrillation, if not accompanied by decompensation, did not affect the circulation time. The authors state, however, that the circulation time is not "the infallible diagnostic tool" it was once supposed to be, and it is not really uncommon to find a normal circulation time in a markedly decompensated patient. However, serial readings are of value, as the circulation time in an individual varies according to changes in his condition, being prolonged when he is worse and vice versa. They also found it of value in determining whether there is, or is not, cardiac failure in the presence of emphysema, *i.e.* whether the dyspnœa is predominantly pulmonary or cardiac. If the circulation rate is rapid, then the heart is well compensated. In 7 cases of bronchial asthma the arm-to-tongue circulation time was found to be shortened. The ether circulation (arm-to-lung time) is measured by injecting into an antecubital vein 5 m. of ether well shaken with 5 m. of normal saline, using a tuberculin syringe and a large needle. The time is recorded from the moment of injection to the moment when the patient or the observer smells the ether in the breath. The average normal time is 5·7 seconds (extremes 2·6 to 10 seconds). The arm-to-tongue time measures roughly the circulation rate as a whole, the arm-to-lung time indicates the functional capacity of the right ventricle. In right-sided failure, therefore, the ether time is prolonged, the lung-to-tongue time (the Decholin or the magnesium sulphate time minus the ether time) is a test for the functional capacity of the left ventricle. Thus Hitzig (84) showed that in isolated failure of the left ventricle the arm-to-tongue circulation time is almost always prolonged, sometimes up to three times its normal value, but the arm-to-lung time may be simultaneously normal. Occasionally, however, with severe left-sided failure the arm-to-tongue circulation time is normal, possibly owing to a very powerfully acting right ventricle. Cottrell and Cuddie (85) have used the Decoholin method to investigate the circulation time in 21 cases of bronchial asthma, and found it to be normal both during and between the attacks.

Conclusion. In our experience, using the Decholin method, the arm-to-tongue circulation time has proved of value in distinguishing between cardiac and pulmonary dyspnœa, especially in cases of emphysema or bronchial asthma complicated by auricular fibrillation, myocardial degeneration, or a valvular lesion.

REFERENCES

(1) Potain. *Mém d. l. soc. méd. d. Hôp. d. Paris*, 1867, 3.
(2) Mackenzie. *Journ. Path. and Bacteriol.*, 1892, **1**, 53.
(3) Waller. *Journ. Physiol.*, 1887, **8**, 229.
(4) Einthoven. *Annal. der Physik.*, 1903, **12**, 1059.

(5) Wilson, Johnston, Hill, MacLeod and Barnes. *Amer. Heart Journ.*, 1934, **9**, 459.
(6) Evans and Turnbull. *Lancet*, 1937, *ii*, 1127 and 1184.
(7) Barker, MacLeod and Alexander. *Amer. Heart Journ.*, 1930, **5**, 720.
(8) Gallavardin and Berard. *Arch. des Malad du Cœur*, 1924, **17**, 18.
(9) Smith. *Arch. Int. Med.*, 1918, **22**, 8.
(10) Herrick. *Journ. Amer. Med. Assocn.*, 1919, **72**, 387.
(11) Pardee. *Arch. Int. Med.*, 1920, **26**, 244.
(12) Rothschild, Mann and Oppenheimer. *Proc. Soc. Expt. Biol. and Med.*, 1926, **23**, 253.
(13) Parkinson and Bedford. *Heart*, 1928, **14**, 195.
(14) Barnes and Whitten. *Amer. Heart Journ.*, 1929, **5**, 142.
(15) Pardee. *Arch. Int. Med.*, 1930, **46**, 470.
(16) Fernichel and Kugell. *Amer. Heart Journ.*, 1931, **7**, 235.
(17) Wolferth and Wood. *Amer. Journ. Med. Sci.*, 1932, **183**, 30.
(18) Wood and Wolferth. *Amer. Heart Journ.*, 1934, **9**, 706.
(19) *Amer. Heart Journ.*, 1938, **15**, 235.
(20) Wilson, Johnston, MacLeod and Barker. *Amer. Heart Journ.*, 1934, **9**, 447.
(21) Goldberger. *Amer. Heart Journ.*, 1942, **23**, 483.
(22) *Brit. Heart Journ.*, 1949, **11**, 103.
(23) Goldberger. "*Unipolar Lead Electrocardiography*", 1949, 2nd Edit. Henry Kimpton, London.
(24) Evans. *Brit. Heart Journ.*, 1949, **11**, 92.
(25) Hill. *Lancet*, 1950, *i*, 985.
(26) Oram. *Post-grad. med. Journ.*, 1949, **25**, 151.
(27) Forssman. *Klin. Woch.*, 1929, **8**, 2085.
(28) Grollman. "*The Cardiac Output of Man in Health and Disease*", 1932, Williams & Wilkins Co., Baltimore.
(29) Cournand and Ranges. *Proc. Soc. Exp. Biol.*, 1941, **46**, 462.
(30) McMichael and Sharpey-Schafer. *Brit. Heart Journ.*, 1944, **6**, 33.
(31) Sharpey-Schafer. *Clin. Sci.*, 1944, **5**, 125.
(32) McMichael and Sharpey-Schafer. *Quart. Journ. Med.*, 1944, N.S., **13**, 123.
(33) Cournand. *Federation Proc.*, 1945, **4**, 207.
(34) Cournand, Riley, Breed, Baldwin and Richards. *Journ. Clin. Invest.*, 1945, **24**, 106.
(35) Brannon, Weens and Warren. *Amer. Journ. Med. Sci.*, 1945, **210**, 480.
(36) Dexter, Burwell, Haines and Seibel. *Bull. New Eng. Med. Center*, 1946, **8**, 113.
(37) Johnson, Wollin and Ross. *Canad. Med. Assocn. Journ.*, 1947, **56**, 249.
(38) Howarth, McMichael and Sharpey-Schafer. *Brit. Heart Journ.*, 1947, **9**, 292.
(39) Holling and Zak. *Brit. Heart Journ.*, 1950, **12**, 153.
(40) Wood. *Brit. Med. Journ.*, 1950, *ii*, 639.
(41) Warren. "*Methods in Medical Research*", 1948, **1**, 224. The Year Book Publishers, Inc., Chicago.
(42) Cournand, Baldwin and Himmelstein. "*Cardiac Catheterization in Congenital Heart Disease*". The Commonwealth Fund, New York, 1949. London, Geoffrey Cumberlege, Oxf. Univ. Press.
(43) Pauli. *Münch. med. Woch.*, 1903, **50**, 153.
(44) Barker. *Journ. Amer. Med. Assocn.*, 1936, **106**, 762.

(45) Wald, Lindberg and Barker. *Journ. Amer. Med. Assocn.*, 1939, **112**, 1120.
(46) Barker, Lindberg and Wald. *Journ. Amer. Med. Assocn.*, 1941, **117**, 1591.
(47) Kurtz, Shapiro and Selby Mills. *Amer. Journ. Med. Sci.*, 1941, **202**, 378.
(48) Fischmann. *N. Zealand Med. Journ.*, 1944, **43**, 267.
(49) Foulger and Rose. *Journ. Amer. Med. Assocn.*, 1943, **122**, 1072.
(50) Potter. *Journ Amer. Med. Assocn.*, 1944, **124**, 568.
(51) Paton and Zaimis. *Nature*, 1948, **162**, 810.
(52) Organe, Paton and Zaimis. *Lancet*, 1949, *i*, 21.
(53) Campbell and Robertson. *Brit. Med. Journ.*, 1950, *ii*, 804.
(54) Kay and Smith. *Brit. Med. Journ.*, 1950, *i*, 460.
(55) Kay and Smith. *Brit. Med. Journ.*, 1950, *ii*, 807.
(56) Turner. *Lancet*, 1950, *ii*, 353.
(57) Kempner. *Med. Journ. N. Carolina*, 1944, **5**, 125.
(58) Med. Res. Council Rep. *Lancet*, 1950, *ii*, 509.
(59) Schroeder. *Amer. Journ. Med.*, 1948, **4**, 578.
(60) Withering. " *An Account of the Foxglove* ", 1785, Birmingham.
(61) Jensen. *Lancet*, 1924, *i*, 747.
(62) Canby Robinson. *Amer. Journ. Med. Sci.*, 1920, **159**, 121.
(63) Wokes. *Quart. Journ. Pharm. Pharmacol.*, 1929, **2**, 292.
(64) Smith. *Journ. Chem. Soc., London*, 1930, 508.
(65) Wayne. *Clin. Sci.*, 1931, **1**, 63.
(66) Frey. *Berl. klin. Woch.*, 1918, **55**, 417 and 849.
(67) Wenckebach. *Die unregelmässige Hertzätigkeit, und ihre klinische Bedeutung*, 1914, 125.
(68) Cotton. *Proc. Roy. Soc. Med.*, 1922–23, **16**, 3.
(69) Parkinson and Nicholl. *Lancet*, 1922, *ii*, 1267.
(70) Hay. *Quart. Journ. Med.*, 1922, **15**, 313.
(71) Benjamin and V. Kapff. *Deutsch. med. Woch.*, 1921, **47**, 10.
(72) Campbell and Gordon. *Quart. Journ. Med.*, 1936, **29**, 205.
(73) Brunn. *Wien. klin. Woch.*, 1924, **37**, 901.
(74) Bernheim. *Therap. d. Gegenw.*, 1924, **65**, 538.
(75) Saxl and Heilig. *Wien. klin. Woch.*, 1920, **33**, 943.
(76) Andrews. *Brit. Med. Journ.*, 1942, *i*, 24.
(77) Higgins. *Journ. Amer. Med. Assocn.*, 1942, **119**, 1182.
(78) Volini, Levitt and Martin. *Journ. Amer. Med. Assocn.*, 1945, **128**, 12.
(79) Evans and Perry. *Lancet*, 1943, *i*, 576.
(80) Rechtschaffen and Gittler. *Journ. Amer. Med. Assocn.*, 1950, **144**, 237.
(81) Bornstein. *Kongr. f. inn. Med.*, 1919, **29**, 457.
(82) Tarr, Oppenheimer and Sagar. *Amer. Heart Journ.*, 1933, **8**, 766.
(83) Bernstein and Simkins. *Amer. Heart Journ.*, 1939, **17**, 218.
(84) Hitzig. *Proc. Soc. Exper. Biol. and Med.*, 1934, **31**, 935.
(85) Cottrell and Cuddie. *Brit. Med. Journ.*, 1942, *i*, 70.

CHAPTER IX

THE LUNGS

Primary Atypical Pneumonia

(Virus Pneumonia)

Owing perhaps to the greater facilities for, and importance attached to, radiographic examination of the lungs, attention has been increasingly directed during recent years to certain catarrhal pulmonary conditions, usually of a benign character, in which the X-ray films show soft shadows in the lung fields. The term primary atypical pneumonia has been used to cover a group of allied diseases, such as virus pneumonia, pneumonitis, influenzal pneumonia, broncho-pneumonia of unusual or undetermined ætiology, acute diffuse bronchiolitis, acute bronchiolitis with atelectasis, and atypical pneumonia with leucopenia. When we have excluded conditions of which the cause is thought to be known, such as influenza due to Pfeiffer's bacillus or to the viruses A, B or X associated with staphylococci or streptococci, the pneumonic consolidation of psittacosis, Rickettsia infections such as the Q fever of Australia, American Q fever and ornithosis, we are left with a group of cases in which the cause is unknown, but is probably a virus, and which may be designated as primary atypical pneumonia, virus pneumonia, or virus pneumonitis.

Primary atypical pneumonia tends to appear in small epidemics and probably also exists endemically. It is not highly contagious but may infect doctors and nurses looking after cases in hospital wards. Young adults are chiefly affected and there is no particular seasonal incidence. The disease has not been transmitted to animals, but Bragg (1) in 1945 successfully conveyed it to human volunteers by spraying the nose and throat with a bacterium-free filtrate obtained from the throat washings and sputum collected from patients suffering from atypical pneumonia. Thus 3 out of 12 men receiving this inoculum developed the disease twelve to fourteen days later, and cold agglutinins for group O human red cells were found in their serum in titres varying from 1/128 to 1/1,024, twenty to twenty-seven days after infection.

The mortality rate of the disease is low, about 0·2%, and few observations have been published on the post-mortem findings.

Longcope (2) observed areas of deep-red moist solidification in the lungs, with purulent material in the bronchi. The alveoli in the affected areas were filled with coagulated serum containing red corpuscles and mononuclear cells, polymorphonuclears being rarely seen. Campbell et al. (3) consider that the primary process is a peribronchitis, peribronchiolitis, bronchitis and bronchiolitis, with swelling of the bronchial epithelium and exudation into the bronchi and bronchioles, resulting in œdema, absorption of the contained air and localised areas of collapse. The alveolar walls become thickened and the alveoli contain mononuclears. Areas of encephalitis were also seen. Perrone and Wright (4) reported a fatal case of primary atypical pneumonia complicated by encephalitis, the patient dying on the fourteenth day of the illness. Foci of increased cellularity were seen in the cerebrum, cerebellum, basal ganglia and paraventricular tissue. The cells forming these foci were astrocytes and microcytes. There were also areas of lymphocytic perivascular infiltration in the meninges.

Clinical and Laboratory Findings. The incubation period varies from two to twenty-one days or longer. The onset is frequently insidious with malaise, severe headache, a racking dry cough and muscular pains in the limbs and abdomen. Anorexia may be a marked feature, and at times the patient complains of pain in the chest and dyspnœa ; or the illness may begin with an upper respiratory tract catarrh. Some cases are apyrexial, the patient having a persistent cough with catarrhal symptoms, and the nature of the disease is only recognised when the lungs are examined radiographically. The temperature usually rises to 100° or 103° F., and after remaining at about this level for eight to ten days, falls by lysis, although secondary rises of temperature are sometimes met with.

The sputum is usually mucoid and at times contains a few streaks of blood, or small hæmoptyses of a teaspoonful or so occur, but the expectoration is never " rusty " or of a " prune juice " appearance. It contains no predominating or characteristic organisms, but mononuclear cells may be seen. The physical signs in the lungs are indefinite and variable, small areas of collapse, indicated by slight dullness and weak air entry, may appear from day to day. The most characteristic finding is the presence of showers of sticky râles, heard especially after cough, over the affected portions of the lungs. In some instances there is dry pleurisy and rarely a pleural effusion develops. The pulse rate is often lower than would be expected from the temperature. In more severe cases there is marked dyspnœa and cyanosis, the temperature is high and irregular, the patient being severely prostrated. The white cell count is usually normal but there may be a slight leucopenia. The presence of a leucocytosis would indicate the advisability of reconsidering the diagnosis. The blood Wassermann reaction may be positive for a short period, and during the acute stage of the illness the sedimentation rate of the red cells is increased to between 20 and 40 mm. % plasma at one hour.

Peterson, Ham and Finland (5) described the presence of cold agglutinins in high titre in the serum of patients suffering from primary atypical pneumonia, and this observation has been confirmed by Horstmann and Tatlock (6), and others. In the majority of cases the reaction is positive between the second and fourth weeks of the illness. Dilutions of the patient's serum are made from 1/4 to 1/4,096 in 1 ml. volume, and to each tube is added 0·1 ml. of a 2% suspension of washed group O human erythrocytes. The tubes are kept at 0° C. overnight, and readings made immediately on removing them from the ice box, and again after they have stood at room temperature for several hours, to see whether the reaction is reversible at room temperature, and so indicative of the presence of a true cold agglutinin. The test is not entirely specific as it has been observed in African trypanosomiasis.

Although there are no typical X-ray findings, the diagnosis cannot be made in the absence of abnormal shadows in the skiagram of the lungs. There is often a marked discrepancy between the extent of the clinical and radiological findings, the latter being more extensive; further the shadows in the film frequently persist for some time after convalescence is established and the patient is afebrile. Patchy opacities may be seen, somewhat resembling those cast by areas of bronchopneumonia. They are often irregular in shape and vague in outline and may have a hazy or ground-glass appearance, migrating in position from day to day. At times the affected areas present a reticulated appearance. Campbell et al. (3) found that 81% of the lesions were situated at the base, each side being equally affected. Drew et al. (7) observed that the costo-phrenic angle, especially on the left side, is a common site for the shadow, and, owing to areas of atelectasis, the diaphragm may be raised on one side and the mediastinum correspondingly displaced. Complications are rare, the violent cough has been thought to give rise to multiple fracture of ribs, and encephalitis is a dread development. Venous thrombosis in the legs, and polyarthritis have been occasionally described.

Cases may be mistaken for pulmonary tuberculosis, especially when the X-ray shadows are situated near the apex, and in other instances an erroneous diagnosis of primary atypical pneumonia has been made on radiographic evidence, when the patient was in reality suffering from lung abscess or bronchial carcinoma. At times the prolonged continuous type of fever with a relatively slow pulse rate and low white cells count suggests enteric fever. In influenza no abnormal shadows are likely to be seen on X-ray examination of the lungs. Difficulty may also arise with cases of pneumonia which have been treated with sulphonamides, when the signs in the lungs persist, there is no leucocytosis, and the X-ray shadow has a reticulated appearance. Further, an area of basal bronchiectasis with surrounding inflammatory changes may lead to diagnostic difficulty. The lesions of primary atypical pneumonia do not give rise to subsequent pulmonary fibrosis.

Treatment. It is most important to keep the patient in bed until the temperature has been normal for a week, and he should not resume work until the sedimentation rate of the red cells is normal and the X-ray shadows have disappeared. Penicillin, streptomycin and the sulphonamides are useless, and the latter may be dangerous giving rise to a hæmolytic crisis. Dramatic results are obtained with the use of aureomycin. We have seen the temperature fall to normal within thirty-six hours of commencing treatment, with a rapid improvement in the patient's condition. The dosage recommended is given below in the article on Q fever. Steam inhalations may relieve the distressing cough, but it is wise to avoid the use of opiates, except in small doses. For severe cyanosis and dyspnœa oxygen should be administered by nasal catheter or the B.L.B. mask.

Q Fever in Great Britain

Derrick (8), in 1937, first described Q fever in Queensland, Australia, and, by injecting infected blood and urine into guinea-pigs, Burnet and Freeman (9) found the causative agent to be a rickettsia, the *Rickettsia burneti*. Derrick described 9 cases occurring among employees in a large meat works and said the name " Q fever was chosen until a fuller knowledge should allow a better name ". Q fever has subsequently been recognised in Europe, Africa and America. Specific agglutination or complement-fixation reactions are given by the rickettsia with serum from Q fever convalescents, the antibodies persisting for several years. The *R. burneti* has been found in the bandicoot, a small bush animal, and in various ticks. It was first thought that infection occurred in man by inhaling dust containing dried tick excreta. It was subsequently shown that occupational exposure to dairy cattle and drinking raw milk from infected cows were the most likely sources of human infection. The cows do not appear ill, but have a chronic infection of the udder from which the milk becomes contaminated.

Stoker (10) in 1949, working in Cambridge, tested specimens of serum from patients diagnosed as suffering from atypical pneumonia, and found Q fever complement-fixing antibodies in 3 specimens out of 24 examined. Two of these patients had never been overseas, and this was regarded as evidence that Q fever occurs in the British Isles. Later in 1949 Harman (11) described 8 cases of Q fever treated at the Royal Cancer Hospital, London. The diagnosis was confirmed by serological tests, and by isolating the *R. burneti* in one case.

Clinical and Laboratory Findings. The disease is characterised by a sudden onset. The temperature often rises rapidly to 103° or 104° F. It may fall to normal once or twice in the twenty-four hours and this is thought not to be due entirely to taking anti-pyretics. The pulse is slow, and there are often heavy sweats, with rigors in severe cases. Prostration, delirium and even coma have been described. Headache, both retro-orbital and occipital, is severe, together with generalised muscular aching. Within a few days a dry irritating cough appears, which aggravates the headache. Occasionally a little blood-stained sputum is expectorated. Chest signs, although slight, can be found on careful examination ; there are small areas in the lungs of high-pitched bronchial breathing with fine râles, suggestive of localised alveolar exudation with lobular collapse or consolidation. A few cases have been described with lobar consolidation, pleural friction or pleural exudation. The spleen may be palpable. Derrick described conjunctival congestion in 2 of his original 9 cases. X-ray examination of the lungs shows patchy rather uniform shadows, which may persist after the patient is apparently recovered. Rickettsial affections in man are usually accompanied by skin rashes, but this is not so in Q fever. There is no naso-pharyngeal catarrh. The temperature often falls by lysis after a week, but the febrile period may be prolonged to three or four weeks. There is usually no anæmia, and the white cell count is generally within normal limits, although there may be a relative or absolute lymphocytosis. The virus was found in the blood of 8 of Derrick's cases, but in only 3 cases in the urine. The serum taken by Derrick on the twelfth and twentieth days of the disease showed an increase in agglutination titre with a rickettsial emulsion from 1 in 4 to 1 in 20. The death rate is low, some authorities placing it at 1 in 500 cases, and the prognosis is worse in patients after the age of fifty.

MacCallum and his co-workers (12), who investigated the cases described by Harman, concluded that the nurse, two pathologists and the post-mortem attendant, who were victims of the disease, were all infected from the same patient. The incubation period in the case of the post-mortem attendant was fifteen days, which agrees with Derrick's figure of fifteen days or less. They further found an endemic focus of Q fever at a town in the South-East of England, *R. burneti* being isolated from the raw milk from some of the farms in the neighbouring area, although the cows appeared to be healthy. Whittick (13) reported on the post-mortem findings in the fatal case in Harman's series. Rickettsiæ were found in the lungs, spleen, testis, brain and kidneys. The microscopical appearances of the lungs resembled those found in psittacosis and virus pneumonia.

Manderson (14) described a case in Bristol in 1949 which presented the clinical features of Q fever, and in which specimens of serum taken on the twenty-sixth and thirty-ninth days of illness gave a positive agglutination in a titre of 1 in 80. This was considered to be diagnostic, and as the first specimen was obtained over three weeks after the onset of the illness a rise in titre was not to be expected. Further observations on the strains of *R. burneti* isolated in Great Britain have been made by Marmion and Stoker (15).

Differential Diagnosis. Derrick considered the possibility of the following conditions when he was investigating his cases:—Typhus fever, undulant fever, typhoid and paratyphoid fevers, leptospirosis and influenza. It is probable that cases in this country have been mistaken for virus pneumonia.

Treatment. Apart from symptomatic treatment for relief of headache the drug of choice is aureomycin. It should be given in capsules by mouth, each capsule containing 250 mg. Smaller capsules of 50 mg. are made which can be used for children. The daily dose recommended is 15 to 20 mg. per kg. body weight. For an adult 250 mg. is given every six hours for the first twenty-four hours, then 500 mg. every six hours for two days, and then 1,000 mg. every six hours until the temperature has been normal for forty-eight hours. The response to aureomycin is often dramatic, the temperature rapidly falling to normal, the headache vanishing, the sweating ceasing and the patient feeling well and asking to get up. In very severe cases the temperature may not fall to normal for over ten days. Toxic reactions are rare, but nausea and vomiting may occur, which can usually be relieved by alkalis.

The Prevention of Tuberculosis

The large number of cases of tuberculosis in this country and abroad constitutes a challenge to the public health authorities and invites us to consider what steps can be taken to control and eradicate the disease. There are two types of tubercle bacillus which affect man, the bovine and the human. Bovine tuberculosis is a disease of cattle, and children are its chief victims, the source of the infection being milk or butter containing living bovine bacilli.

Bovine Tuberculosis

Childhood tuberculosis due to bovine infection, involves especially the glands, bones and intestines, although sometimes the lungs are affected both in children and in adults. Bovine tuberculosis could be completely eradicated by the application of efficient public health measures to ensure a pure milk supply, and, in certain countries, such as America and Scandinavia, this has been very largely effected. This desirable result can be achieved in two ways, either by stamping out the disease from the dairy herds or by killing the tubercle bacilli in infected milk by pasteurisation. In

Norway, Finland, Guernsey and America the former method has been adopted. The cattle are tested by the injection of tuberculin, and the positive reactors, including those infected with tuberculosis, are disposed of either by slaughtering or by removal from the herd. The animals are retested with tuberculin every six months. In this way " attested herds " are formed, which are free from tuberculosis and yield a pure milk supply. Area eradication is the most effective method of stamping out the disease in cattle. All the herds in regions, large and small, must be "attested". In this country a certificate of attestation is issued by the Ministry of Agriculture and Fisheries, and according to the quarterly statement of the Ministry of March 1950 the numbers of " attested " herds were, England 20,568, Wales 14,204, and Scotland 12,527. It is probable that in Great Britain about 20% of milk comes from " attested " herds, whereas the average incidence of tuberculosis in dairy cows not so attested is 20 to 25%.

The designations in force in connection with the sale of milk in this country are as follows :—*Tuberculin tested milk.* This is milk from cows which pass a periodical veterinary examination and tuberculin test. If the milk is bottled on the farm it may be described as *Tuberculin tested milk* (certified). This milk may also be pasteurised. *Accredited milk.* This is raw milk from cows which pass a periodical veterinary examination, but not a tuberculin test. It must satisfy the same bacteriological tests for cleanliness as raw tuberculin tested milk. *Pasteurised milk.* This is milk which has been retained at a temperature of 145° to 150° F. for at least thirty minutes, or which has been retained at a temperature of not less than 162° F. for at least fifteen seconds. It must pass a methylene blue reduction test for cleanliness and keeping quality, and a phosphatase test to indicate whether the heat treatment has been adequately carried out.

In order to stamp out, in addition to tuberculosis, brucella and other infections conveyed by milk, the only safe way is that of universal pasteurisation, to which, unfortunately, there is a good deal of opposition at the present.

Infection by Human Tubercle Bacilli

It used to be taught that nurses and doctors and others in contact with open cases of pulmonary tuberculosis were not in danger of contracting the disease, and that adult pulmonary tuberculosis was, in the large majority of cases, due to a reactivation of a childhood infection. Such a view has fortunately been discredited; as it engendered a false sense of security and led to a neglect of adequate precautions. It is now universally recognised that pulmonary tuberculosis is a herd disease, transmitted usually by the inhalation of tubercle bacilli. Those closely associated with tuberculous patients may become infected from the patients' cough, by droplet infection, or by contamination of the fingers by touching objects infected with drying sputum. Nurses, when making beds, may inhale dust containing tubercle bacilli, disturbed and scattered in the air when the blankets and sheets are shaken. Children in homes where one or both parents suffer from "open" tuberculosis are almost certain to become infected. The same applies to children taught by a schoolmaster or schoolmistress who has "open" disease, or who are looked after by a nurse similarly affected. By an "open" case is meant one in which tubercle bacilli are found in the sputum.

The Mantoux Test

This test enables us to determine when children and young adults become infected with tuberculosis. It is performed by injecting into the skin of the forearm 0·1 ml. of old tuberculin (O.T.) diluted to 1/10,000. The arm is observed forty-eight hours later, and a positive reaction consists of a central zone of oedema, not less than 5 mm. in diameter, surrounded by a zone of erythema. If the test is negative it is repeated twenty-four hours later using now 0·1 ml. of 1/1,000 O.T. If this is negative a third test is made with 0·1 ml. of 1/100 O.T. The first test should be made in the lower part of the forearm, the succeeding ones at higher levels. At birth all children are Mantoux negative. In children of the hospital class at the age of two to three years, 70% are Mantoux positive when they have been in contact with "open" cases of pulmonary tuberculosis, whereas only 12% are positive when they are non-contact cases. During school life 40% of these non-reactors become infected with tuberculosis. This is known as the primary infection with tuberculosis, and in many cases gives rise to no symptoms of ill health. Later, when the primary focus has calcified, it may be revealed by X-ray examination. About 20 to 30% of medical students and nurses who begin work at hospitals are Mantoux negative, indicating that they have not been infected with tuberculosis, and during their work in hospital the majority of the negative reactors become positive, showing that infection has occurred. At the time of conversion from Mantoux negative to Mantoux positive the individual may notice symptoms of ill-health. He or she may lose weight, become easily tired, run a slight temperature, or erythema nodosum may appear. Others show more definite evidence of pulmonary tuberculosis. A shadow may be seen in the lungs on X-ray examination or a pleural effusion may form. It has been found in Great Britain by Daniels (16) that of 2,120 nurses who were Mantoux positive when first examined 43, or 2%, developed tuberculosis while working in hospital, and of 452 negative reactors 27, or 6%, developed the disease.

No nurse who is a negative reactor should be allowed to work in a sanatorium or look after cases of tuberculosis elsewhere. Special care should be taken in general hospitals of nurses or students at the conversion period. The chest should be X-rayed, and the nurse taken off duty for three months. A second X-ray should be taken at the end of six weeks. Extra milk and eggs should be ordered. If at any time during this observation period any of the symptoms of ill-health mentioned above are noted, the nurse or student should be warded, a record of the temperature taken, the sedimentation rate of the red cells determined, and the sputum, if any, and stomach washings examined and cultured for tubercle bacilli.

The following precautions should be taken by nurses looking after open cases of tuberculosis in a hospital or sanatorium :—

1. Nurses must wear masks and gowns when carrying out any nursing treatment. Masks are to be worn once only, and after use placed in a special container for sterilisation. Gowns must be changed daily.

2. Sputum pots must contain 2% lysol and must be changed twice a day. They are to be soaked in 2% lysol for twelve hours before emptying. Gloves must be worn when handling sputum pots.

3. All crockery and cutlery used by patients must be boiled in a special crockery boiler and then washed.

4. All sheets, pillow cases, blankets, pillows and mattresses must be put into a special container prior to sterilisation. Nurses must wear masks and gowns when handling the bedding.

5. Patients must wear a mask during examinations of the chest.

6. Patients must use paper handkerchiefs. These are to be placed in a special paper bag after use and burnt. Handkerchiefs must not be kept under the pillow.

7. All newspapers and books are to be placed after use in a dressing bin and then burnt.

8. Any food not eaten by the patient must be put in the rubbish bin and burnt.

9. On admission the patient's day and night clothes must be sterilised and then sent to the relatives, or kept until the patient's discharge. The patient shall wear hospital clothes which are subsequently sterilised with the bedding.

In hospital unsuspected cases of pulmonary tuberculosis, especially in surgical wards, are a source of danger to nurses. This has been shown by Stammers (17). The incidence is probably about 4 per 1,000. All patients admitted to hospital should have a chest examination by miniature radiography as soon after admission as possible.

B.C.G. Vaccination

For many years after the discovery of the tubercle bacillus by Koch in 1882 attempts were made to raise the resistance of the individual against the disease by means of a vaccine.

The Bacille Calmette Guérin vaccine (B.C.G.) is a stable living culture of bovine tubercle bacilli produced by Calmette and Guérin (18) in France in 1906 from an organism isolated from the milk of a tuberculous cow. By subcultures over a period of thirteen years its virulence was reduced so that the bovine bacilli became avirulent to animals and man. On injection into an animal the vaccine produced a localised nodular lesion, with no dissemination of the disease. It was found that virulent tubercle bacilli could be injected into the vaccinated animal without harmful results. In 1921 Weill-Hallé (19) first used B.C.G. to vaccinate children in Paris, and Irvine (20) states that by 1934 over a million children throughout the world had been so vaccinated. In 1930 B.C.G. fell into disrepute, owing to a tragedy at Lübeck, in Germany, when after inoculating by mouth 271 infants, 77 died of tuberculosis. It was later proved that the vaccine used was a mixture of B.C.G. and a virulent strain of living tubercle bacilli kept in the same incubator.

Those responsible for this malpractice were imprisoned (21). Since then it is probable that no fatalities have followed the use of the vaccine.

Attention has been directed to possible difficulties and disadvantages in the use of B.C.G. by Wilson (22). Thus the vaccine should be used within fourteen days of its preparation. It should be kept at a temperature of 3° to 6° C. The virulence of the vaccine is not fixed, so that if it is too virulent there may be harmful local reactions, and if the virulence is too feeble, inadequate protection will be afforded. The vaccine must be injected into the superficial layer of the skin, if it is given deeper long-standing ulcers may form. When used to vaccinate infants born of tuberculous mothers, the infant must be taken away from the mother at birth, or, if taken away later, the infant must be observed for six weeks after separation, to make sure that it has not contracted tuberculosis. After vaccination the infant must be kept away from a tuberculous parent for two to three months, to allow immunity to develop. The fact that the vaccination has taken is shown by the conversion of the Mantoux reaction from negative to positive, and this occurs in over 85% of cases vaccinated intradermally.

Very satisfactory statistics have been published from Scandinavia. Heimbeck (23), in Scandinavia, found that a large proportion of student nurses became infected with tuberculosis early in their hospital training, 50% of the nurses being negative reactors on entering hospital. Of the negative reactors 29·6% developed tuberculosis, but only 2·6% of the positive reactors. With the use of B.C.G. to convert the negative to positive reactors, the incidence of tuberculosis fell to 2·3% in this group.

Nordwall (24) in a training school for nurses in Stockholm, found that before the use of B.C.G. 40% of the negative reactors developed tuberculosis during their training. After vaccination with B.C.G. only one nurse developed tuberculosis, and that in a mild form. Malmros (25) writing from Oerebro, Sweden, points out that "conscientious tuberculin-testing has perhaps been used to a greater extent in Scandinavia than elsewhere", and it has been observed continuously that previously Mantoux-negative adolescents fall ill with tuberculosis.

Wallgren (26), who is largely responsible for the widespread use of B.C.G. vaccination in Sweden, says that revaccination is not commonly done in that country. The tuberculin sensitivity persists for three to ten years, or more, and affords protection during the most susceptible childhood ages.

Hertzberg (27), of Oslo, gives authoritative statistics of the results of B.C.G. vaccination in Norway, where such vaccination is now compulsory. All those vaccinated were negative reactors, and the majority became positive reactors two months later. In many cases the tuberculin reactions became stronger as time went on, and this is considered to be due to the supervention of a reaction due to the human type of bacillus, *i.e.* to the "vaccination allergy" induced by the B.C.G. is added a "superinfection allergy", due to contact with human tubercle bacilli, as bovine tuberculosis has been eradicated from Norway. Hertzberg found that protection is greatest when superinfection follows B.C.G. vaccination at an interval of about four years.

Rosenthal (28) and his colleagues in America record their experiences of thirteen years' study of B.C.G. They found that the application of the vaccine to all age groups is a safe and effective procedure. They used the method of multiple puncture scarification.

B.C.G. vaccination is now being used in certain hospitals in England to give protection to the staff. It should be offered to nurses or students who are negative on two consecutive tests, made at an interval of two weeks, to O.T. 1/100. The second test should be made with a different batch of O.T. from that used on the first occasion. No vaccination must be given to an individual suffering from measles, whooping cough, eczema, furunculosis, or to one being inoculated against another infection, such as diphtheria. The B.C.G. vaccination must be done immediately after the second negative Mantoux test. The vaccine must be shaken well before use, if there is more than a faint haziness, or if clumps are observed in the fluid after shaking, the ampoule should be discarded. A glass tuberculin syringe, fitted with a Luer needle, No. 25 or 26 (B.W.G.), $\frac{1}{4}$ or $\frac{1}{2}$ inch long is used for the injection. The skin over the left deltoid is cleaned with spirit and 0·1 ml. of the vaccine containing 0·5 mg. per ml. is injected strictly intradermally. A wheal about 5 mm. in diameter is produced. No dressing need be applied. In infants the injection may be made into the skin of the outer surface of the buttock. Vaccination may also be performed by multiple puncture or by scarification. A stronger vaccine is then required, containing 20 mg. per ml. This vaccine is not obtainable in this country. For further information the reader is referred to the Ministry of Health Memo (29). After vaccination the nurse must be segregated from exposure to tuberculosis for six weeks. The Mantoux test is then repeated and should now be positive to 1/100 O.T. If the test is negative, vaccination should be repeated immediately, and segregation again enforced for six weeks. A local reaction with a small, shallow ulcer about 10 mm. in diameter may develop after three to six weeks, which may take two months to heal. The Mantoux test must be repeated every twelve months after successful vaccination, and if it becomes negative, re-vaccination should be carried out.

It is hoped that the results obtained in England will be as good as those in other countries, but in every case of exposure to " open " tuberculosis there should be no relaxation of other safeguards against infection, such as disinfection of sputum and avoidance of contact with droplet infection and with infected articles. Pulmonary tuberculosis developing in adults over the age of forty accounts for a large number of cases in all countries. The incidence in this group will not be affected by vaccination limited to children and young adults. Further, as stated above, these infected adults are largely responsible for the development of pulmonary tuberculosis in young children. In the programme already planned for the control of tuberculosis little attention has yet been paid to the problem of the re-infection of adults over the age of forty.

Mass Miniature Radiography

The use of mass miniature radiography for selected groups of adults, such as factory workers, and those in the services, has revealed an incidence of about 4 per 1,000 unsuspected cases of pulmonary tuberculosis. In some cases a shadow is seen, in others a cavity. The discovery of a shadow often causes unnecessary alarm and despondency as frequently the disease is not active. When such a shadow is seen, the patient should be admitted to hospital in order to try to decide whether or not the disease is active. The practical difficulty is the long waiting period before a bed is available, and what the unfortunate individual is to do in the meanwhile. Those cases with a cavity are almost certainly active. Until adequate accommodation can be provided for the isolation and treatment of the active and " open " cases, mass radiography appears of little value either as a preventive or curative measure.

Artificial Pneumothorax

Historical. Carson (30), of Liverpool, in 1822, first suggested that air might be admitted into the pleural cavity as a therapeutic measure in certain diseases of the lungs. Cayley (31), in 1885, at the Middlesex Hospital, London, was responsible for the establishment of a pneumothorax by pleural incision in a case of intractable hæmoptysis. Forlanini (32), in Italy, must undoubtedly be regarded as the originator of the modern pneumothorax treatment by puncture for pulmonary tuberculosis, his work dating back to 1882. Lillingston (33), in 1910, was one of the first to adopt this method in England.

The Indications

Collapse of the lung, by the introduction of air into the pleural space, is chiefly of value in the treatment of pulmonary tuberculosis. It is sometimes used for the relief of pain in dry pleurisy associated with pneumonia or with a peripherally situated bronchial carcinoma. A diagnostic artificial pneumothorax may be helpful in determining whether a shadow shown by X-ray examination is intrapulmonary, in the chest wall, or associated with the diaphragm or mediastinum.

Pulmonary Tuberculosis. There is a tendency now not to hasten to establish an artificial pneumothorax immediately pulmonary tuberculosis is diagnosed, but to see first how the patient responds to bed rest combined with streptomycin and P.A.S. therapy. Artificial pneumothorax is of value in unilateral disease, with or without thin walled cavities, when dense fibrosis is not present. It may also be employed in similar types of bilateral lesions, either as a bilateral pneumothorax, or as a unilateral pneumothorax combined with a phrenic crush operation on the other side and an artificial pneumoperitoneum. In cases of hæmoptysis which do not respond to other methods of treatment, the introduction of about 800 ml. of air into the pleural space may sometimes control the bleeding. It should only be attempted if it is reasonably certain which lung is the source of the hæmoptysis.

The Contra-indications

An artificial pneumothorax should not be induced in miliary pulmonary tuberculosis, nor in very toxic exudative lesions of the pneumonic or broncho-pneumonic type. In such cases the dyspnœa is increased by an artificial pneumothorax and the general condition of the patient rapidly deteriorates. There is also a serious risk of the formation of a tuberculous empyema. A satisfactory collapse is not usually obtained in chronic fibrotic lesions or with thick walled cavities. Active tuberculous tracheo-bronchitis, especially when there is bronchial stenosis, as shown by bronchoscopy, is another contra-indication. Here again there is a risk of tuberculous empyema. Tension cavities in the lungs, resulting from partial bronchial obstruction so that air enters on inspiration and does not come out on expiration, often become larger when the lung is collapsed by artificial pneumothorax.

A cavity at the apex of the dorsal lobe is difficult to collapse by an artificial pneumothorax alone, but an additional phrenic crush on the same side together with an artificial pneumoperitoneum has in our experience at times been successful. In some cases a fair degree of collapse is obtained by the pneumothorax, but the diseased portion of the lung is not adequately relaxed owing to adhesions. Under these circumstances a thoracoscopic examination should not be made for four to six weeks, as the adhesions, if fine, often stretch. The thoracoscopist should always err on the side of caution in attempting to divide thick or awkwardly situated adhesions, as serious sequelæ may result from hæmorrhage or empyema. Despite what is said to the contrary, those who have carried out practically every refill themselves on patients for many years will agree that many of their most satisfactory cases, engaged in full work, have what is known as a bad pneumothorax, with dense adhesions and much pleural thickening. Cavities with fluid levels, however, which do not close, are an indication that the pneumothorax should be abandoned and some other form of collapse treatment attempted.

As pointed out by Young (34) the greatest cause of failure of an artificial pneumothorax is lack of continuity in personnel. " The trouble has been that the technique seems so easy that it is carried out by inexperienced workers who do not understand either the proper selection of cases or the finer points in its conduct." The patient should always be screened immediately before the refill, and the whole treatment, lasting for several years, should be carried out by one individual.

The Method

The requirements are as follows :—

Pneumothorax Apparatus. There are several types in use. The Lillingston and Pearson apparatus is that which we usually employ. It has the advantage of simplicity, and can be used both for inserting air and also for removing it in cases of spontaneous pneumothorax.

The arrangement of the pneumothorax apparatus can be seen by a reference to the diagram, and a detailed description is not necessary (see Fig. 43). A and B are glass bottles, B being graduated in ml. from 0 to 1,100. C is a glass manometer. D is a four-way glass connection. E is a glass connection. F and G are glass filters containing sterile wool. H, I, J and K are glass tubes. L, M, N, O and P are rubber tubes. Q is the needle. 1, 2, 3 and 4 are clips on the rubber tubes.

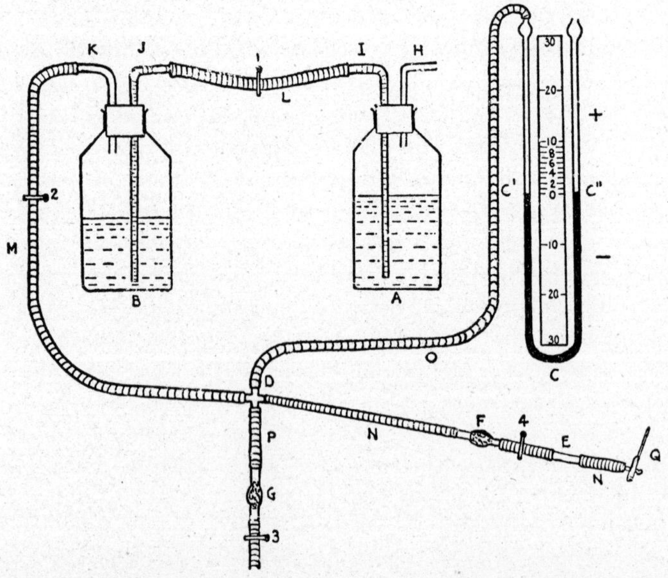

Fig. 43. Diagrammatic representation of Modified Lillingston and Pearson Pneumothorax Apparatus. The bottle B is graduated in ml. from 0 to 1,100.

Pneumothorax Needles. The needle used for the primary induction is often referred to as the No. 1 needle. The form devised by Clive Riviere is commonly employed. It consists of a blunt-ended cannula with a thin edge for penerating the pleura, and a

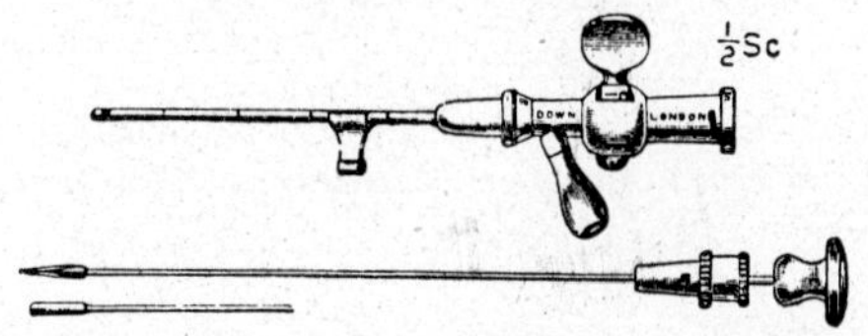

FIG. 44. Clive Riviere Needle (No. 1 Needle).

trocar for piercing the tissues of the chest wall. The needle used for refills is of a different pattern ; it may be referred to as the No. 2 needle. The Saugman pattern is the one we prefer. This is shorter than the No. 1 needle and has a bevelled cutting edge like an ordinary hypodermic needle. It is provided with a stilette for clearing purposes. These needles are illustrated in the text (see Figs. 44 and 45). The Morland needle has a solid point, with a lateral opening near the tip. It must be dry sterilised as a drop of moisture is very liable to cause blocking.

A 2 ml. syringe and hypodermic needle of sufficient length to reach through the chest wall to the pleura. (This distance is rarely more than 3 cm.)

Sterile 2% procaine hydrochloride solution.

Iodine, spirit lamp and sterile towels.

Some restorative, such as brandy or adrenaline should be at hand.

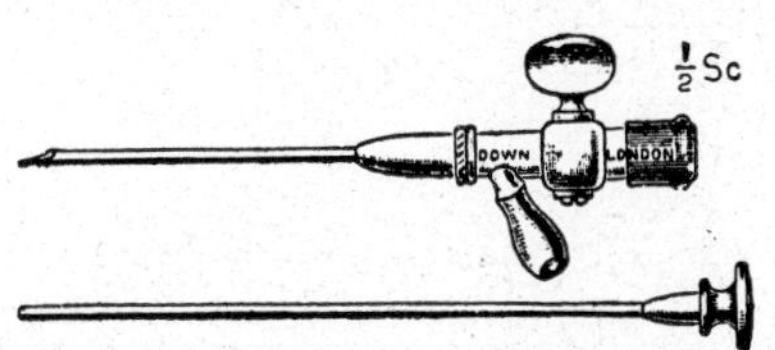

FIG. 45. Saugman Needle (No. 2 Needle), with Rubber Cap to act as a Stuffing-box.

Preparation of the Apparatus. The glass bottles, rubber tubes, glass tubes and glass filters are all sterilised by boiling. The needles are sterilised by placing them in spirit and subsequently flaming. The manometer is filled to the zero point with water coloured with a little red ink. This does not stain the glass and makes readings easy.

The glass filters are filled with sterile cotton wool. The tubes are placed in position. Bottle A is filled with coloured solution of perchloride of mercury (1/1000), or with 1/100 carbolic acid. The fluid is passed over to Bottle B, by blowing a little air into bottle A with a Higginson syringe attached to the tube H, which starts the siphon action. With the clips 1, 2 and 3 open the fluid in the bottles can now be run from one to the other by raising or lowering one of them. Half the fluid should be left in bottle B and half in A. The apparatus should be examined to see that there are no leaks before use. This can be done by closing clips 3 and 4 and opening clips 1 and 2. If, now, bottle A is raised, air will be driven from bottle B into the manometer and the fluid in limb C′ depressed. The level in the manometer should remain constant as long as the bottle A is kept in the same position. In the same way, if bottle A is lowered the fluid in limb C′ will rise. It can easily be ascertained that air can be driven through the pneumothorax needle by opening clips 1, 2 and 4 and closing 3. If the end of the needle is now put under methylated spirit, having withdrawn the trocar and closed the side tap, air will be seen bubbling from the end of the needle on raising bottle A.

Preparation of the Patient. The patient is in bed. He should be given an aperient the night before the operation, and the induction should not be made immediately after a meal. Half an hour before the operation an injection of $\frac{1}{4}$ gr. morphin. sulph. should be given, in order to calm the patient and diminish any tendency to pleural shock. If the pneumothorax is to be induced on the right side of the chest the patient lies on his back turned towards his left side, with the right arm forward above the head, which is kept low, and a pillow is placed under the chest and left shoulder, so as to widen the intercostal spaces. The site of election for the first puncture is in the sixth space in the anterior axillary region. The skin over this area is painted with iodine, and sterile towels placed on the bed-clothes and against the chest.

The Operation. The procaine solution is injected, about 2 ml. being used. The skin over the intercostal space is held taut with two fingers of the left hand. The needle is then inserted obliquely, just in front of the fingers, and a little procaine injected intradermally to cause a bleb. After a short pause the needle is moved into a position at right angles to the chest wall, and gradually pushed through the intercostal space. Procaine is slowly injected as the needle moves downwards to the pleura. Care should be taken to inject the solution right down to the pleura, as this probably plays a part in the prevention of pleural shock which may cause a fatal result.

The patient must now be warned against coughing during the operation. If the desire to cough is irresistible, due warning must be given, otherwise the sudden increase in the pleural pressure when the patient coughs, with the pneumothorax needle in the pleural cavity, would drive the fluid out of the manometer. This can be prevented, if warning is given, by squeezing the tube N, leading from the needle to the manometer, or by closing the clip 4.

The rubber tube N leading to the manometer is attached to the side arm of the No. 1 needle. Clips 1, 2 and 3 are closed and clip 4 opened. With the trocar in position the needle is pushed through the skin at the anæsthetised spot, and through the intercostal muscles, for about 1 cm. or less if the patient is very thin. It must be held firmly in the hand, with the top of the trocar in the palm, and not in the position of a pen between the fingers. The trocar is now withdrawn and the stopcock turned, so that the lumen of the needle is in communication with the tube leading to the manometer. The cannula is now pushed on through the remainder of the intercostal muscle down to the pleura.

When it is in contact with the pleura, but not through it, an oscillation will probably be observed in the manometer, not directly synchronous with respiration and of small extent. The cannula is now pushed through the pleura, which can often be felt to give way with a snap. Great care must be taken here not to penetrate the lung. When the cannula is in the pleural cavity the fluid in the limb C″ of the manometer falls below zero and oscillates with respiration. These oscillations correspond accurately with the respiratory movements, falling with inspiration in the limb C″ of the manometer and rising with expiration. A reading is now taken, each centimetre of fall of fluid in the limb C″ corresponding with a change of pressure in the pleural cavity of 2 cm. of water. The oscillations should be at least 3 to 6 cm., and are often as much as 10 cm. Thus a reading of − 10, − 2 may be obtained, giving a mean negative intrathoracic pressure of − 6 cm. water. The respiratory fluctuations are greater when the patient takes a very deep breath, but the reading should be taken with ordinary moderately deep breathing. The needle may become blocked during its passage through the deeper parts of the chest wall, in which case it can be cleared with the stilette which is supplied with the No. 1 needle. The visceral layer of the pleura may also come in contact with the end of the cannula and cause obstruction. Letting in a small quantity of air by opening clips 1 and 2 is the best means of dealing with such a condition. When it is certain that the end of the cannula lies free in the pleural cavity, air may be admitted. This is accomplished by opening the clips 1 and 2, when the air is sucked from the bottle B into the chest, and fluid passes over from bottle A into bottle B to take its place. When about 100 ml. have thus passed in by suction, the bottle A can be raised slightly and another 200 ml. of air admitted. The clips 1 and 2 are then closed, and the manometric readings taken for inspiration and expiration, with the patient breathing quietly and moderately deeply as before. They will still be negative, unless the air has been injected into a small loculated pleural space. These readings may be — 8, — 1. The mean pressure would in this case be — 4·5. The pressure changes, and the amount of air injected, would then be recorded as follows : — 6, 300 ml., — 4·5. It is to be noted that with this pneumothorax apparatus readings of intrapleural pressure cannot be taken while air is flowing in. The clips 1, 2 and 3 must be closed in order to obtain a reading. The needle is now withdrawn from the chest and a little iodine again applied to the site of the puncture. A collodion dressing is not usually required. If there is a tendency to cough, a large pad and a firm chest binder should be used in order to minimise extravasation of air. The patient is kept in bed at rest for the first month of pneumothorax treatment.

Refills. The same apparatus is required as for the initial pneumothorax operation, but a No. 2 needle (Saugman) is used. The patient is prepared as before, but it is not usually necessary to give a preliminary injection of morphine unless he is very nervous. It is wise, however, not to omit the anæsthetisation of the pleura with procaine, as death may follow from pleural shock in refills as well as during the primary induction. A spot close to that used for the induction is chosen. The rubber tube leading to the manometer is attached to the side arm of the No. 2 needle with the stilette slightly withdrawn, so that it does not protrude beyond the point. The pneumothorax apparatus has already been prepared with the fluid in bottle B up to the 100 mark, the remainder being in bottle A. The clips 1, 2 and 3 are closed. The needle is now pushed straight through the chest wall at the anæsthetised spot into the pleural cavity. Directly it is felt to enter, the stilette is withdrawn and the stopcock closed, so that the lumen of the needle is in communication with the manometer. The fluid in the manometer will now oscillate. The pointed needle is used, as the air introduced at the primary induction (on the previous day) will prevent the lung being injured.

The reading is then taken. This will be found to be lower than the final reading at the previous injection, as some of the air introduced has been absorbed. Clips 1 and 2 are now opened and air allowed to enter the pleural cavity. After about 200 ml. have passed in, the clips should be closed and a reading taken to make sure that the needle is in the pleural cavity and that the pressure is not rising too quickly. About 400 or 500 ml. will probably be enough for the first refill, in order to reduce the negative pressure in the pleural cavity by about 2 or 3 cm. of water. Thus the readings at the first refill may be − 5·5, 400 ml., − 2. If there are many adhesions, and the lung is not collapsing well, a smaller quantity of air should be required to reduce the negative pressure to a similar degree. The needle is then withdrawn.

The spacing of refills and the determination of the correct amount of air to be injected are matters of extreme importance, and are comparable with the administration of a vaccine. In neither case is it a matter of routine ; in each the personal factor of the patient is of paramount importance. Usually the second refill is given two days after the first, and the third three days after the second. The interval can then be gradually lengthened to a week, ten days, a fortnight, three weeks and a month. High intrapleural pressures should be avoided, as they cause mediastinal displacement, possibly tend to promote pleural effusion, and seem to have a direct relation to loss of weight on the part of the patient.

If there is a rise of temperature after the initial induction, the first refill should not be given the next day. The temperature should be allowed to subside first. A rise of temperature just before a refill is due probably indicates that the refills are being given at too long intervals, and that the lung is starting to re-expand. A rise of temperature after a refill is sometimes an indication that too much air has been injected. An X-ray should be taken at the end of the second week to determine the degree of pulmonary collapse, and the subsequent treatment should be subjected to X-ray control in order to determine what degree of collapse is necessary to produce the optimum effect, as judged by temperature, pulse and body weight, and also so that the range of intrapleural pressure which produces such collapse can be ascertained. It is not usually necessary to use a positive pressure to produce satisfactory collapse.

Some Difficulties and Complications. The manometer has been described as the heart of the pneumothorax apparatus. It is certainly of vital importance, not for the actual introduction of the air, but for its safe introduction.

The character of its oscillations affords the only reliable guide as to whether the end of the needle lies free in the intrapleural space. These typical movements have already been described.

Certain abnormal events may occur, in which case no air must be admitted into the chest:—

A negative pressure may be obtained on inserting the needle into the chest, but the fluid in the manometer may show this as a stationary negative pressure, without any respiratory excursions. This indicates that the needle has been in the pleural cavity, but is now either blocked or in the lung. The negative pressure may increase for a little with each inspiration, without any oscillations occurring if the needle is in the lung. The pressure may be slightly positive during expiration at the primary induction and negative during inspiration, indicating that the needle is in a bronchus or small cavity in the lung. The manometer may show a positive pressure which rises slowly or rapidly, indicating that the needle is in a blood vessel. Blood may then be seen passing through the glass connection E in the rubber tube attached to the needle. The pressure may be negative, but show irregular respiratory oscillations if the needle is in a pleural cavity much loculated by adhesions. From such examples as these, it will be realised how important it is to be certain that the manometer indicates that the needle is in the pleural cavity before any air is admitted. A refill may be very difficult if the lung has expanded and is touching the chest wall. In such a case the patient should expire deeply and hold the breath in expiration as the needle is inserted through the pleura. In this way the pleural space can often be found.

Complications. *Pleural shock* may occur, especially if the patient is very nervous and if the pleura is inflamed and not anæsthetised. Some authorities deny the existence of pleural shock, but their evidence is not conclusive.

Surgical emphysema may develop within a few hours of the injection of air, either as the result of coughing or of injury to the lung, or because the air has been injected extrapleurally between the pleura and the intrathoracic fascia. If a lung, which is bound down to the chest wall by adherent pleura, is punctured, surgical emphysema may develop without the introduction of any air.

Air Embolus. This may occur from introduction of air into a vessel, especially a pulmonary vein, in which the pressure is negative.

Effusion. This is especially liable to occur if adhesions are present and if high positive intrapleural pressures are used. About 50% of pneumothorax cases develop an effusion in the pleura during some time of their treatment. This may be: *Small,* giving rise to little constitutional disturbance, and often unrecognised except by X-rays. *Large,* causing constitutional disturbance with pyrexia. The fluid is serous, rich in cells and frequently contains tubercle bacilli. It indicates an active tuberculous pleurisy. *Infective,* often accompanied by rigors. This is pyogenic in origin.

In any case pleural adhesions are likely to occur both at the apex and the base, and it is improbable that a satisfactory collapse will be obtained afterwards, unless the fluid is repeatedly removed as soon as it forms and is replaced by air. The apical adhesions form because the fluid runs up to the top of the pleural space when the patient lies down.

Atelectasis. In some cases of artificial pneumothorax, especially after division of adhesions, a portion of the collapsed lung becomes atelectatic. Maher-Loughnan (35) has drawn attention to this complication and its frequent association with pleural effusion, and considers it an important cause of relapse in cases of pulmonary tuberculosis treated by unilateral artificial pneumothorax. We have treated several cases of this type and found that by alternately allowing the lung nearly to expand and subsequently collapsing it again, it is often possible to effect re-aeration of the atelectatic portion of lung. It is also helpful to tilt the foot of the bed on 8-inch blocks.

Duration of Treatment

It is always difficult to decide when the pneumothorax should be abandoned in cases which are maintaining good health. A refill every three to six weeks, or at longer intervals, is a small price to pay for health, and there is no means of knowing whether the disease will become active again when the lung is allowed to expand. Further, when the pneumothorax has been maintained for several years, there is a possibility that as the lung expands it will displace the mediastinum to the affected side and cause respiratory difficulties. As a working rule it may be said that the pneumothorax should never be abandoned in less than two years, that five years is an average life for a pneumothorax, and if it is continued for over seven years it is probably wiser to go on with it indefinitely.

A pneumothorax had been maintained for six years in one of our patients in whom there had originally been a cavity in the right upper zone. The right lung appeared well controlled and the patient was in good health. She wished to abandon the pneumothorax. She came into hospital and the lung was allowed to expand with diminishing refills under streptomycin-cover. Three and a half months later she did not feel well and on X-ray examination we found an oval shadow (5·5 × 2·5 cm.) of uniform density in the right upper zone just above the right interlobar fissure. The disease was once more active.

Artificial Pneumoperitoneum

Historical. By introducing air into the peritoneal space, the diaphragm, if free from adhesions, can be raised 3 or 4 or more inches with a corresponding diminution in the volume of the lungs (see Fig. 46). The rise is usually greater on one side than the other, especially when the pneumoperitoneum is combined with a phrenic crush. A lateral view of the chest, however, may show that only a portion of the diaphragm is elevated.

The method was introduced by Vajda (36) in Hungary in 1933 for the treatment of bilateral pulmonary tuberculosis, and, in 1934, Banyai (37) combined pneumoperitoneum with phrenic paralysis to obtain a more effective pulmonary collapse. During the last decade this method has been more extensively employed and representative articles published on the subject in America

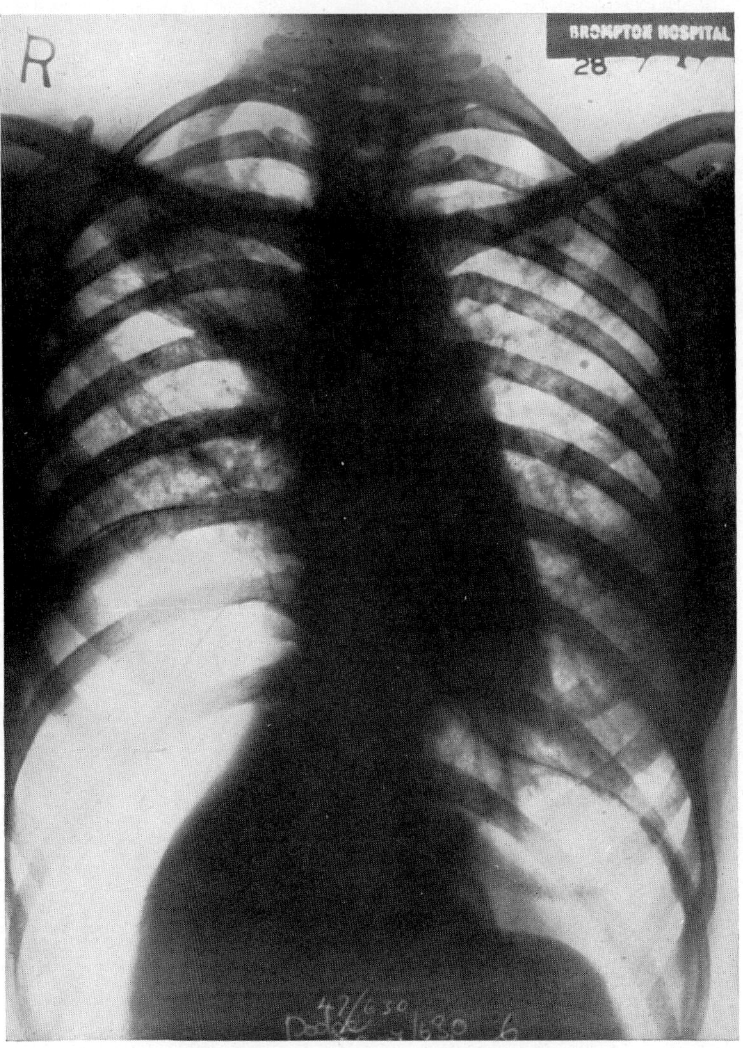

Fig. 46. Pneumoperitoneum and left phrenic crush.

[*To face p.* 262.

include those by Rilance and Warring (38), Anderson and Winn (39), Crow and Whelchel (40), Mitchell and his colleagues (41), Gilmore (42) and Murphy (43). In Great Britain reference may be made to the writings of Keers (44) and Edwards and Logan (45).

The Indications. Pneumoperitoneum is of value in the treatment of basal, mid-zone and apical lesions. Anderson and Winn (39) found that in a series of 113 cavities, 58·6% of apical, 57·7% of mid-zone, and 58·8% of basal ones were closed by pneumoperitoneum treatment. In 91 cases with a positive sputum 56% became negative with the treatment. We have employed it with satisfactory results in various types of pulmonary tuberculosis, including apical lesions in which an artificial pneumothorax was impossible owing to adhesions, in cases of pneumothorax in which adhesions were present, to try and divide which would have been dangerous, and in bilateral lesions. In the majority of cases a phrenic crush should be performed on the side on which the disease is most advanced, and streptomycin, or streptomycin combined with P.A.S. (para-aminosalicylic acid) can with advantage be administered simultaneously. Pneumoperitoneum is helpful in controlling small areas of disease in one lung, in preparation for a thoracoplastic operation on the more affected side. A dorsal lobe cavity, which does not collapse in response to an artificial pneumothorax combined with a phrenic crush, may sometimes be successfully closed by a pneumoperitoneum. Pneumoperitoneum is also of help in the emergency treatment of a severe hæmoptysis, in which case it is not necessary to know from which side the bleeding is occurring. We usually prefer to establish the pneumoperitoneum three to four weeks prior to the phrenic crush, but with an apical dorsal lobe cavity the pneumoperitoneum and phrenic crush should be instituted at about the same time.

As Mitchell and his co-workers (41) state, with almost no exceptions pneumoperitoneum can be abandoned and re-established at will, as the space does not become lost owing to an adhesive peritonitis.

The Method. The requirements are the same as those for artificial pneumothorax, but a Saugman refill needle is used both for the induction and for refills. The fluid in the bottles of the pneumothorax apparatus is adjusted for the induction and for refills, with the fluid in bottle B at the 100 mark, the remainder being in bottle

A. If the patient is nervous phenobarbitone gr. 2 should be given by mouth three-quarters of an hour before the induction. The patient lies on his back in bed, with his head resting on a pillow. The initial puncture should be made on the left side, 1½ inches below the subcostal margin, at the outer edge of the rectus muscle. Some authorities, such as Gilmore (42), prefer a point 2 to 3 inches to the left about an inch below the umbilicus. If the puncture is made on the right side there is danger of injuring the liver or gall bladder. Proximity to an abdominal scar must always be avoided, owing to the risk of abdominal adhesions beneath the scar. The skin is painted with iodine, and 2 ml. of 2% procaine are injected through the skin and subcutaneous tissues down to the peritoneum. The Saugman needle, with stilette inserted but not passed through to the needle point, is attached to the rubber tube N of the pneumothorax apparatus, and slowly pushed through the abdominal wall, the clips 1, 2 and 3 on the rubber tubes of the apparatus being closed. The patient must raise his head and shoulders off the pillow, not resting on his elbows, while the needle is being inserted, in order to render the abdominal muscles tense. The peritoneum can usually be felt, and there may be some pain as the needle penetrates it. The patient now rests his head again on the pillow. When the end of the needle is in the peritoneal space it will be found that the stilette can be passed through to the hilt, the end of the stilette now projecting just beyond the needle tip. This is not possible when the end of the needle is in the tissues of the abdominal wall. The common mistake is not to insert the needle far enough. The stilette is now withdrawn, the stopcock on the needle closed so that the lumen communicates with the manometer. Usually no swing is seen on the manometer as the patient breathes. About 40 ml. of air are run in by opening the clips 1 and 2. The initial pressure is now taken by closing clip 2. This is usually 0, and on breathing a slight manometric swing can be seen, the pressure rising with inspiration and falling with expiration. In some cases there is a negative pressure if the needle is inserted just underneath the diaphragm. After running in about 800 ml. of air the pressure may rise to +6 +2 cm. water, or it may still remain at zero. The liver dulness usually disappears as the air is introduced, often before a pressure reading can be obtained. Flicking the abdominal wall in the right iliac region may cause a manometric swing, and this is a confirmatory sign that the needle is in the peritoneal space. The needle is now withdrawn and the puncture sealed with gauze and collodion. The patient should lie flat for twenty-four hours after the induction.

The first refill is given the next day, the second refill four days later, and the third refill five days after that. Subsequently refills are given every seven days. The amount of air required is usually 800 to 1,000 ml., and the pressures are found to be positive, such as +6, 1,000 ml., +12 cm. water. It is unwise to raise the final pressure above a mean of +12. At each refill a few bubbles of air should be sucked back into the syringe on injecting the local anæsthetic, to indicate that the needle is in the peritoneal space. Some writers advice the patient to wear an abdominal belt after the establishment of the pneumoperitoneum, but we have not found this necessary unless the abdominal muscles are very lax. The electrocardiogram shows changes due to rotation of the heart with displacement of the apex upwards and outwards. T_2 becomes flattened, T_3 inverted and Q_3 is apparent.

Some Difficulties and Complications. The chief difficulty is to be sure that the needle is in the peritoneal space. It is probably not uncommon for the intestine to be perforated, but usually no harm results, and if the air is injected into the colon it is quickly passed per rectum. Perforation of the stomach may give rise to more serious symptoms. In one of our cases a pneumoperitoneum was induced at 11 a.m. The readings recorded were 0, 500 ml., +4. At 7.45 p.m. there was a sudden attack of dyspnœa with severe collapse. The patient was pale, sweating, the pulse rapid and frequent, and severe pain was complained of in the left subcostal region, and top of the left shoulder. The temperature rose to 100·4° F., falling to normal during the next three days. There was no vomiting and no abdominal rigidity. The next day the patient was improving, although he still looked pale and ill. An X-ray examination showed air below each diaphragm. It was thought that there had been a small perforation of the stomach which rapidly sealed over. Other severe complications include intra-abdominal hæmorrhage from perforation of mesenteric vessels, which may cause death. Air embolism with the rapid onset of convulsions is not necessarily fatal. Peritoneal effusion forms in about 4% of cases, and is probably present in a larger proportion, although in insufficient amount to be detected clinically. Cohen (46) has pointed out that a tuberculous ascites may develop in cases of pneumoperitoneum, even when the pulmonary lesion is probably arrested or healed. This is very liable to be followed by adhesive peritonitis. Pneumoperitoneum should be abandoned immediately ascites is detected. In cases of myocardial weakness the establishment of a pneumoperitoneum may precipitate an attack of congestive heart failure.

In some cases the digestion and appetite are seriously impaired, and nausea, vomiting or pain may necessitate the abandonment of the pneumoperitoneum. Pain may be referred to one or other shoulder, if there are diaphragmatic adhesions, and we have noted such pain to disappear after the phrenic crush has paralysed the affected side of the diaphragm. Air may pass from the peritoneum into the mediastinum, into the pleura, into the subcutaneous tissues, or along the inguinal canal into the scrotum, forming there a pneumocele. In other cases a small umbilical hernia may appear. Rilance and Warring (38) in 1944 noted 7 cases of acute appendicitis in 101 cases undergoing pneumoperitoneum treatment, an incidence eleven times greater than in other sanatorium patients.

Streptomycin and Para-aminosalicylic Acid in the Treatment of Pulmonary Tuberculosis

Streptomycin is still being used in the treatment of pulmonary tuberculosis. The two main drawbacks are the possibility of vestibular nerve involvement, with giddiness which often persists for long periods and may be permanent, and the appearance of drug-resistant tubercle bacilli which renders further administration of streptomycin useless. With smaller doses of streptomycin, and possibly owing to greater purification of the substance, giddiness is a less frequent complication. We have treated a considerable number of patients suffering from pulmonary tuberculosis with streptomycin and have only had two cases of severe giddiness. The drug should always be discontinued directly any evidence of vestibular involvement appears. It was shown in a report to the Medical Research Council in 1948 (47) that resistant organisms are generally found within two months of beginning treatment. Even before treatment a minute number of streptomycin-resistant tubercle bacilli can be found in the sputum. Bignall and his colleagues (48) in a report to the Medical Research Council in 1950 tried the effect of varying the administration of streptomycin in four ways. In one group of cases 0·5 g. of streptomycin was injected six-hourly in alternate weeks; in the second group 0·5 g. was given six-hourly in alternate months; in the third group 0·25 g. was administered six-hourly without intermission; and in the last group 1 g. of streptomycin was injected once a day, without intermission. The total course in each group lasted for six months. The cases chosen were those of acute, progressive, bilateral lesions of presumably recent origin, in the age group 15 to 30 years. No delay in the emergence of streptomycin-resistant bacilli was found in any group, and from the clinical point of view there did not appear to be any difference between the continuous or intermittent forms of treatment. The method of choice appears to be to give 1 g. of dihydrostreptomycin in a single dose daily, and this causes least inconvenience to the patient.

Para-aminosalicylic Acid (P.A.S.)

Bernheim (49), in 1940, showed that the addition of sodium salicylate to a phosphate buffer solution of *p*H 6·7 containing living tubercle bacilli stimulated the rate of oxygen consumption. Lehmann (50), in 1946, found that only pathogenic tubercle bacilli showed an increased oxygen consumption in the presence of salicylates or benzoates. After testing over 60 allied compounds Lehmann (51) subsequently found that para-aminosalicylic acid was the most active in producing a bacteriostatic effect upon the tubercle bacillus. Favourable results were soon obtained with the use of P.A.S. on animals infected with tubercle bacilli, and Lehmann (51), in 1946, first employed the drug clinically to treat tuberculous abscesses following thoracoplasty, which had remained unchanged for several months before being so treated. Daily local injections of a 10% neutral solution of P.A.S. were given, with favourable results. He also administered the drug orally in doses of 10 to 15 g. daily in courses of eight days. There was a rapid improvement in the patient's condition, with fall in temperature and decrease in the sedimentation rate of the red cells. Vallentin (52), in 1946, used P.A.S. in the treatment of pulmonary tuberculosis, tuberculous empyema, miliary tuberculosis and tuberculous meningitis. No favourable effect was noted in the case of miliary tuberculosis or tuberculous meningitis. In exudative pulmonary tuberculosis there was a rapid clinical and radiological improvement, with loss of tubercle bacilli from the sputum, but on discontinuing the treatment relapse frequently occurred. In 1947 Dempsey and Logg (53) reported similar encouraging results in cases of pulmonary tuberculosis in Britain, and they noted a reduction in the size of cavities during treatment. Erdei (54), in 1948, commented on the very great improvement in the patients' general condition, which was usually noted about the third day of P.A.S. treatment. In 1949 Joules and Nassau (55) treated 10 cases of extensive bilateral pulmonary tuberculosis, and, although some benefit was noted in half the cases, they concluded that in none of the patients was the prognosis materially altered for the better, as the effect of the drug was only temporary. Nagley and Logg (56) considered that the main value of P.A.S. is in the treatment of the acute exudative type of pulmonary lesion, especially in rendering such patients fit for collapse therapy. It has the advantage over streptomycin that it does not produce P.A.S.-resistant strains of tubercle bacilli, except possibly after prolonged treatment. Thus Carstensen and Andersen (57) reported from Sweden that resistance to P.A.S. develops in over 50% of cases treated for four–five months. Graessle and Pietrowski (58) in America produced evidence that the combined use of P.A.S., in relatively low concentration, with streptomycin (approximately 0·5 micrograms to 1 unit) prevents or greatly retards the *in vitro* development of streptomycin-resistant tubercle bacilli. It was shown in a report to the Medical Research Council in 1949 (59) that the incidence of streptomycin-resistant bacilli can be considerably lowered by the combined use of streptomycin and para-aminosalicylic acid. This is the method which is being used more extensively at the present time.

Method of Administration. P.A.S. is given as the sodium salt by mouth in doses varying from 12–24 g. every twenty-four hours. It can be administered as sugar-coated tablets (Paramisan sodium), each containing 0·33 or 0·5 g. of the sodium salt, as sugar-coated granules (Paramisan sodium) containing $33\frac{1}{3}\%$ by weight of the sodium salt, as enteric coated tablets (Bactylan) containing 0·69 g. of the sodium salt or as cachets (Paramisan sodium) each containing 1·5 g. Alternatively it can be prescribed in a mixture, which, however flavoured, has a bitter and unpleasant taste. The prescription which we use as an alternative to the tablets is Sod. para-aminosalicyl. gr. 84, (3 g.), saccharin. gr. $\frac{1}{5}$, emulsio. cassiæ m. 5, emulsio. chloroform. m. 15, syrup. simplic. m. 60, aq. ad fl. oz. 1. This is taken after a little food every two and a half hours from 9 a.m. to 9.30 p.m. (= 18 g.) for six days a week. It should be freshly prepared each week. In some patients P.A.S. causes nausea, vomiting, or diarrhœa, but this often passes off in a few days. An alkali taken just before each dose will often relieve the gastric symptoms, and the diarrhœa may be checked by a bismuth, chalk and opium mixture. If these measures fail the dose of P.A.S. should be halved. Some of our patients have been unable to take the drug, the sight of the bottle or of the tablets, or the thought of the next dose provoking intolerable nausea.

Other side effects are uncommon, but they include a skin irritation or rash, drug fever, hæmaturia or albuminuria, and hypoprothrombinæmia. In cases in which there is albuminuria or hæmaturia the drug should be stopped and the urine rendered alkaline. By keeping the urine alkaline it may then be possible to continue the course as soon as the urine is clear.

Madigan and his co-workers (60) showed that hypoprothrombinæmia can be prevented or cured by the daily oral administration of 10 mg. of synthetic vitamin K. Cayley (61) drew attention to the depression in the serum potassium level which may occur during P.A.S. treatment. This leads to paralytic limb lesions and disturbances of cardiac rhythm. It seems probable that the fall in blood potassium is due to the sodium in the salt administered, as suggested by Nagley (62). A calcium salt (Paramisan calcium) is also available in powder form for preparing solutions and in cachets. This would probably avoid this complication.

P.A.S. is rapidly excreted in the urine, and, in order to obtain the best results, a blood concentration of 5 to 10 mg. per 100 ml. should be maintained. The P.A.S. treatment may be continued effectively for periods up to 5 or 6 months.

Conclusion. Neither streptomycin nor P.A.S. can be regarded as the long awaited cure of pulmonary tuberculosis, although striking and notable results are achieved in many instances, especially in the recent exudative types of lesion, and in tracheobronchial tuberculosis. We have not seen tuberculous cavities of any size close during the treatment. P.A.S. has the advantage that it can be safely administered at home while the patient is awaiting admission to hospital or sanatorium.

Bronchography

It is not possible to visualise clearly the outline either of the bronchi and their ramifications or of pulmonary cavities by means of a direct X-ray examination. If, however, some substance opaque to the rays is introduced into the bronchi, their configuration is clearly revealed.

Lipiodol or Neo-Hydriol (ol. iodisat. B.P. Add.) is a compound of iodine in poppyseed oil, which contains 40% iodine. It is a transparent oil of a light brown colour, which is opaque to the X-rays, and so heavy that it sinks in water. On prolonged exposure to air it darkens and should not then be used for injection. Sicard and Forestier (63), in 1922, injected Lipiodol into the trachea in man, using a cannula introduced into the glottis with the aid of a laryngoscope, or else passing it through a curved needle inserted through the crico-thyroid membrane.

The Indications. X-ray photographs of the lungs after intra-tracheal injection of Lipiodol afford a graphic representation of the position of the trachea and main bronchi, of cavities in the lung connected with patent bronchi, of bronchial and pleural fistulæ, and of the relative permeability of the bronchial fields in different portions of the lungs.

Thus, it will show displacement of the trachea and bronchi due to pulmonary fibrosis or other causes, the presence of bronchiectasis in its various stages, and whether or not the lumen of the bronchi is obliterated by obstruction within or without, such as that caused by a foreign body, new growth or fibrosis. Lipiodol injections are of value in suspected cases of bronchiectasis, to determine whether there is a cavity present, and, if so, the extent of lung involved. They also show the condition of the apparently sound lung. A lobectomy for bronchiectasis would generally be contra-indicated if the Lipiodol injection showed that the opposite lung was also the seat of bronchiectatic changes.

The X-ray appearance of the lung in bronchiectasis after Lipiodol injection is shown in the accompanying plate (see Fig. 47).

Methods. Iodised oil (Neo-Hydriol, Lipiodol, etc.) may be introduced into the bronchial tree to render it radio-opaque by

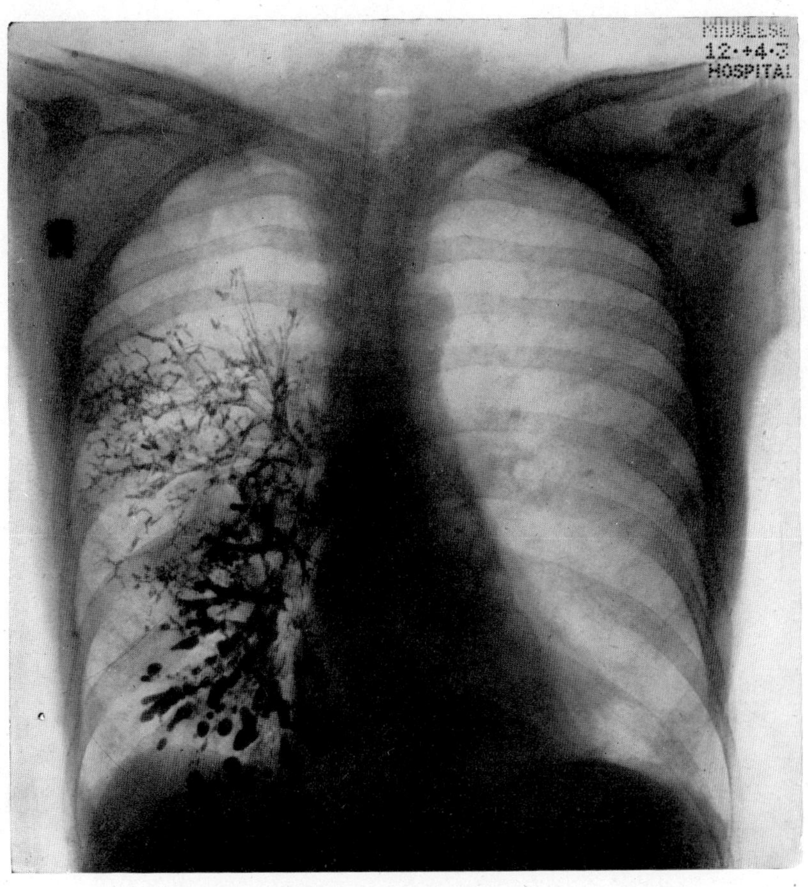

Fig. 47. Radiogram of lung after injection of Lipiodol, showing normal and dilated bronchi.

[*To face p.* 270.

one of the three following routes :— (1) Through the crico-thyroid membrane. (2) Over the back of the tongue. (3) Via the nose.

With practice any of these methods can give satisfactory results in a high proportion of cases, but the most consistently reliable is the crico-thyroid route. It is easier to fill the upper lobes by this method, a minimum of surface anæsthetic is required, and the whole procedure can be completed in fifteen minutes. It should be avoided, however, in patients having large quantities of purulent sputum owing to the risk of subsequent cellulitis of the neck. Whichever method is to be used, a few days' preliminary postural drainage is advisable to empty the bronchi of sputum as far as possible. In addition, the patient should be tested for sensitivity to iodine and cocaine derivatives. Ten grains of potassium iodide by mouth t.d.s. should be given for three days to see if iodism results as judged by lachrymation, nasal catarrh and a skin rash. In patients who are iodine-sensitive, an erythematous rash may appear one to three days after the operation, or an urticarial rash about the tenth day, and fatalities have been reported. If, therefore, the patient is sensitive, it is wiser not to proceed with the investigation.

After a satisfactory iodide test, two minims of 2% amethocaine hydrochloride or 5% cocaine solution are injected subcutaneously, idiosyncrasy to the drug being shown by faintness, pallor, dyspnœa, tachycardia and tremors. Unfortunately a negative test is not a guarantee of insensitivity but if such symptoms do arise, the investigation should not be continued except under a general anæsthetic.

Premedication is seldom required, but an apprehensive subject should be given morphine sulphate gr. ¼ by injection. or gr. 4 of hexobarbitone orally, half an hour beforehand.

The operation should be carried out in the X-ray department with the patient lying on a table capable of being tilted in either direction.

Crico-thyroid Route

Apparatus. Minim syringe with fine needle (No. 17 hypodermic).

Minim syringe with stouter needle (No. 12 hypodermic).

Lipiodol syringe. This should be strong, as considerable pressure is required to force the oil through the needle. We use a 25 ml. syringe with three finger rings, the needle being straight (No. 15 S.W.G., ¾ inch long), short-bevelled, with a bayonet fitting to the syringe.

Sterile $\frac{1}{2}\%$ procaine hydrochloride solution.

Sterile 2% amethocaine hydrochloride solution.

Neo-Hydriol.

Iodine and wool.

Sodium thiopentone or other rapidly acting intravenous barbiturate should always be immediately available along with oxygen and carbon dioxide, in the event of idiosyncrasy to the surface anæsthetic manifesting itself.

The Operation. The patient lies in a semi-recumbent position on the adjustable table, supported by three or four pillows beneath the shoulders, the head and neck being straight and extended as far as possible over a sandbag. The skin of the neck is painted with iodine, the crico-thyroid membrane identified and the skin, subcutaneous tissues and crico-thyroid membrane anæsthetised by injecting $\frac{1}{2}$ to 1 ml. of $\frac{1}{2}\%$ procaine through the fine needle. Next, using the stouter needle, m. 7 to 10 of 2% amethocaine hydrochloride are injected rapidly into the larynx through the same puncture wound. A few bubbles of air should be sucked back into the syringe before the injection is made to ensure that the point of the needle is in the lumen of the larynx, and the injection should be made at the end of expiration. The needle is withdrawn immediately after the injection, which will produce a bout of coughing. The patient is now told to sit up and cough until he no longer feels a desire to do so. He should spit out and not swallow the excess of local anæsthetic. When the coughing has subsided, he is warned that any cough after injection of the iodised oil will spoil the subsequent X-ray films. He now resumes the semi-recumbent position with the head well extended as before. The Neo-Hydriol is poured into the special syringe and the needle introduced through the crico-thyroid membrane while the larynx is steadied with the operator's free hand. On withdrawing the piston a bubble of air will indicate that the needle is in the correct position and this should be checked at frequent intervals during the injection, especially after a change in the patient's position. He is now turned slightly to the right side and instructed to breathe quietly through the mouth. Four or five ml. of iodised oil are then injected and about half a minute is allowed for this to run down to the bronchi of the lower and dorsal lobes. With the needle still *in situ* the patient is carefully sat up and inclined forwards and to the right, the head being kept extended. A further 3 to 4 ml. of oil are injected and another half-minute allowed for this to fill the middle lobe. He is then replaced in the semi-recumbent position but lying completely on his right side; a further 4 to 5 ml. of oil are introduced and the needle is then withdrawn. A few seconds are allowed for the oil to reach the upper lobe bronchus. All pillows except one for the head are now removed. The patient's feet are raised and the head lowered by tilting the adjustable table in order to fill the upper lobe. The pectoral branch is best filled by turning him for a few seconds into the prone position. X-ray films in inspiration are now taken in antero-posterior and lateral positions with the patient recumbent and then repeated with him erect. The needle is then reintroduced through the crico-thyroid membrane and the left lung filled in exactly the same way, but with the patient turned always slightly to the left. It should be remembered that on the left side, as the upper lobe bronchus comes off rather more anteriorly, the patient should be inclined somewhat more to the prone position during its filling. Films are then taken in the antero-posterior and left posterior oblique positions. If only the left side has been filled a left lateral film can also be taken. The procedure is a simple application of a knowledge of the anatomy of the bronchial tree as depicted in Fig. 48.

After completion of the operation postural drainage is advisable to remove most of the injected oil, and the patient is not allowed to eat or drink until the anæsthetic effect has worn off.

Oral Route

Apparatus. 2 ml. syringe.
Curved metal cannula (Record fitting).
Lipiodol syringe.
Curved metal cannula with bayonet fitting.
Conical measuring cylinder graduated in ml.
Sterile 2% amethocaine hydrochloride solution.
Adrenaline hydrochloride solution, 1 in 1,000.
Neo-Hydriol.
Gauze swabs.
Sodium thiopentone, oxygen and carbon dioxide for emergency use.

The Operation. The patient sits on an armless chair facing the

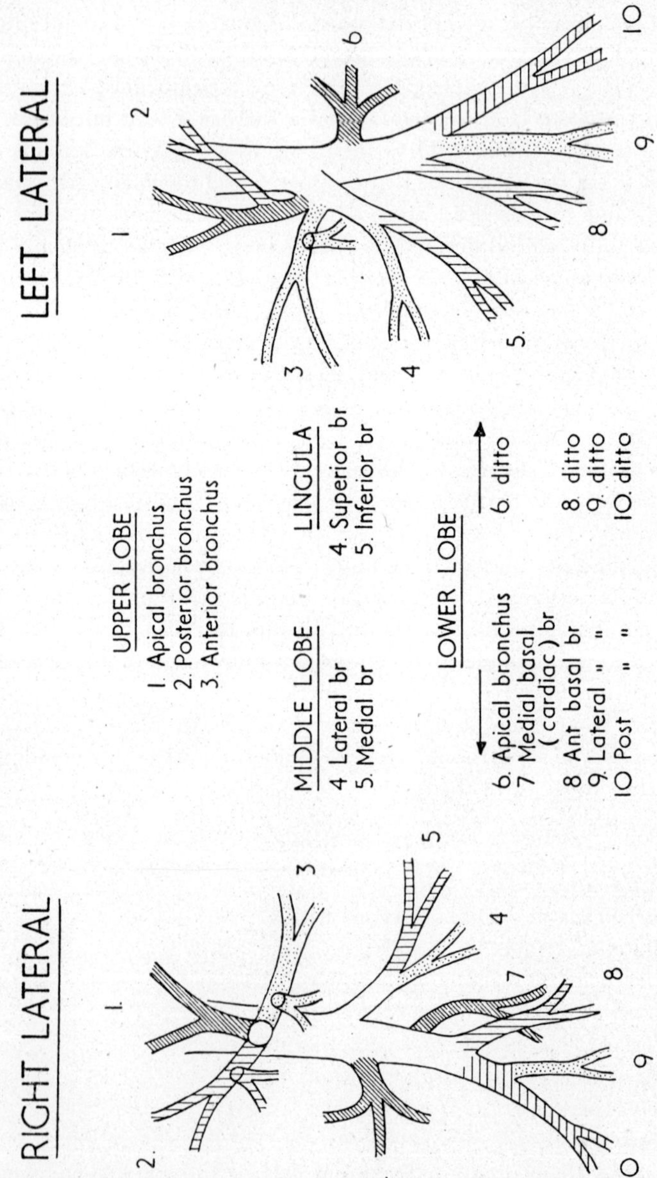

FIG. 48. Diagram of scheme of nomenclature of the segmental bronchi. (Brock, *Thorax*, 1950, 5, 222.)

operator, with his tongue protruded and protected from the lower incisors by means of a gauze swab. Four ml. of 2% amethocaine and 1 ml. of 1 in 1,000 adrenaline are now poured into the conical measuring cylinder and this total amount should not be exceeded. One ml. of this mixture is drawn into the 2 ml. syringe and injected rapidly over the back of the tongue by means of the curved cannula. This will cause the patient to cough and so disseminate the local anæsthetic. He should spit out any excess and avoid swallowing it. A further 1 ml. is then injected into each pyriform fossa in turn in the same way. Alternatively, a pledget of wool twisted on the end of a malleable probe and soaked in the anæsthetic solution may be held gently in each pyriform fossa until the desire to cough and retch has subsided. Some minutes are allowed for the anæsthetic to take full effect and the index finger of the left hand is then hooked gently over the back of the epiglottis and base of the tongue. If surface analgesia is adequate this should cause no distress and the superior aperture of the larynx can be identified. A further 1 ml. of the anæsthetic solution is then injected down the trachea between the vocal cords by guiding the curved cannula along the side of the left index finger and into the upper part of the larynx. Some operators prefer to use a laryngeal mirror in order to see the exact position of the cannula rather than to rely on palpation. When coughing has subsided the patient's tongue is held well forward by means of a gauze swab wrapped round its anterior third, as in this position it is almost impossible to swallow. The patient is instructed to breathe quietly through his mouth and to lean towards the right, but keeping his head upright. By means of the Lipiodol syringe and its attached cannula the iodised oil is then dripped steadily on to the back of the tongue. Provided the patient does not swallow, it will flow round either side of the epiglottis and down the larynx. While the first 5 ml. are being injected the patient is inclined backwards and to the right to fill the right lower lobe; during the injection of the next 4 or 5 ml. he should lean forward and to the right to fill the middle lobe and as soon as the third 5 ml. have been injected he should lie on the adjustable X-ray table and be postured for filling the branches of the upper lobe as described for the crico-thyroid method. When films have been taken of the right side, the procedure is repeated for the left lung but with the patient inclined towards the left side throughout.

Nasal Route

The Operation. The patient sits facing the operator with his head fully extended, his tongue protruded and held by means of a gauze swab. A short piece of sterile thin rubber tubing, $1\frac{1}{2}$ to 2 inches long, is attached to the 2 ml. syringe and inserted for a distance of 1 to $1\frac{1}{2}$ inches into the more patent nostril beneath the inferior turbinate. The same anæsthetic solution is used as for the oral route. He is then told to inhale deeply through the nose and at the beginning of inspiration 1 ml. of the surface anæsthetic is injected through the rubber tubing. As the solution reaches the pharynx and larynx he will cough and should spit out the excess. A further 1 ml. is then injected in the same way and this will usually be found to produce satisfactory anæsthesia after waiting for some minutes. The piece of thin rubber tubing, or another similar piece, is then attached to the nozzle of the lipiodol syringe and the iodised oil is injected steadily through this into the anæsthetised nostril. With the patient breathing through his nose, head extended, and tongue held well forward to prevent swallowing, the oil will flow down the pillars of the fauces, fill up the pyriform fossæ and then overflow and spill down the larynx. During the injection of the oil, posturing is the same as already described for the oral route.

Bronchography in Children

Children under the age of ten will usually require a general anæsthetic of sufficient depth to abolish the cough reflex. Premedication is advisable and Omnopon gr. 1/30 per stone of body weight together with atropine sulphate gr. 1/150 to 1/100 is very satisfactory. Anæsthesia is induced with cyclopropane and an endotracheal tube is inserted via the mouth with the aid of a laryngoscope. The anæsthetic is then continued with gas, oxygen and ether. Ether can be recommended because of its bronchodilator action. A T-piece is attached to the outer end of the endotracheal tube and one orifice is corked during the induction. When anæsthesia is fully established this cork is removed and the bronchial tubes are aspirated through a gum-elastic catheter connected to a sucker. To the Lipiodol syringe is attached a soft nasal catheter which has a mark on it indicating the length of the endotracheal tube. After aspiration of the bronchi this catheter is inserted down the endotracheal tube up to the mark, the anæsthetic being continued via the other limb of the T-piece. Posturing during injection of the oil is exactly the same as for the crico-thyroid route but two assistants should be available to support the child in the correct positions. The amount of oil injected into each side should not exceed 1 ml. per year of apparent age. As soon as the oil has been injected, the anæsthetist may cause the child to hyperventilate for a short time by the addition of a little carbon dioxide and the X-ray films are taken during the period of apnœa which follows. When the films of both sides have been taken, most of the oil is removed by means of the gum-elastic catheter and sucker as before.

The anatomical distribution of the bronchial tree should be borne in mind in all these operations, as depicted by Brock (64) (see Fig. 48).

REFERENCES

(1) Bragg. *Journ. Amer. Med. Assocn.*, 1945, **127**, 146.
(2) Longcope. *Practitioner*, 1942, **148**, 1.
(3) Campbell, Strong, Grier and Lutz. *Journ. Amer. Med. Assocn.*, 1943, **122**, 723.
(4) Perrone and Wright. *Brit. Med. Journ.*, 1943, *ii*, 63.
(5) Peterson, Ham and Finland. *Science*, 1943, **97**, 167.
(6) Horstmann and Tatlock. *Journ. Amer. Med. Assocn.*, 1943, **122**, 369.
(7) Drew, Samuel and Ball. *Lancet*, 1943, *i*, 761.
(8) Derrick. *Med. Journ. Austral.*, 1937, *ii*, 281.
(9) Burnet and Freeman. *Med. Journ. Austral.*, 1937, *ii*, 299.
(10) Stoker. *Lancet*, 1949, *i*, 178.
(11) Harman. *Lancet*, 1949, *ii*, 1028.
(12) MacCallum, Marmion and Stoker. *Lancet*, 1949, *ii*, 1026.
(13) Whittick. *Brit. Med. Journ.*, 1950, *i*, 979.
(14) Manderson. *Lancet*, 1949, *ii*, 1085.
(15) Marmion and Stoker. *Lancet*, 1950, *ii*, 611.
(16) Daniels. *Lancet*, 1944, *ii*, 165, 201, 244.
(17) Stammers. *Lancet*, 1949, *ii*, 1011.
(18) Calmette, Guérin, Boquet and Nègre. "*La vaccination préventive contre la tuberculose par le B.C.G.*". Paris, Masson & Cie, 1927.
(19) Weill-Hallé and Turpin. *Bull. et mém. Soc. d. hôp. de Paris*, 1925, **49**, 1589.
(20) Irvine. *Practitioner*, 1947, **159**, 50.
(21) Lange and Pescatore. "*Die Sänglinstuberkulose in Lübeck*". Berlin, Julius Springer, 1935.
(22) Wilson. *Brit. Med. Journ.*, 1947, *ii*, 855.
(23) Heimbeck. *Ann. Inst. Pasteur*, 1929, **43**, 1229.
(24) Nordwall. *Acta tuberc. Scand.*, 1944, **18**, 45.
(25) Malmross. *Brit. Med. Journ.*, 1948, *i*, 1129.
(26) Wallgren. *Brit. Med. Journ.*, 1948, *i*, 1126.

(27) HERTZBERG. "*The Achievements of B.C.G. vaccination*". Oslo, I. Kommisjon Hos. Johan Grundt Tanum Forlag. 1948.
(28) ROSENTHAL, LESLIE and LOEWINSOHN. *Journ. Amer. Med. Assocn.*, 1948, **136**, 73.
(29) Ministry of Health Memo, 322/B.C.G. July 1949.
(30) CARSON. "*Essays, Physiological and Practical*", 1822. Wright, Liverpool.
(31) CAYLEY. *Clin. Soc. Trans.*, 1885, **18**, 278.
(32) FORLANINI. *Gazz. d. Osp.*, 1882, **3**, 537, etc.
(33) LILLINGSTON. *Practitioner*, 1913, **90**, 129.
(34) YOUNG. *Brompton Hosp. Rep.*, 1949, **18**, 56.
(35) MAHER-LOUGHNAN. *Tubercle*, 1950, **31**, 74.
(36) VAJDA. *Ztschr. f. Tuberk.*, 1933, **67**, 371.
(37) BANYAI. *Amer. Rev. Tuberc.*, 1934, **29**, 603.
(38) RILANCE and WARRING. *Amer. Rev. Tuberc.*, 1941, **44**, 323 ; *ibid.*, 1944, **49**, 353.
(39) ANDERSON and WINN. *Amer. Rev. Tuberc.*, 1945, **52**, 380.
(40) CROW and WHELCHEL. *Amer. Rev. Tuberc.*, 1945, **52**, 367.
(41) MITCHELL, HIATT, MCCAIN, EASOM and THOMAS. *Amer. Rev. Tuberc.*, 1947, **55**, 306.
(42) GILMORE, *Diseases of the Chest*, 1947, **13**, 153.
(43) MURPHY. *Diseases of the Chest*, 1947, **13**, 631.
(44) KEERS. *Edin. Med. Journ.*, 1947, **54**, 30 ; *Brit. Journ. Tuberc.*, 1948, **42**, 58.
(45) EDWARDS and LOGAN. *Tubercle*, 1945, **26**, 11.
(46) COHEN. *Lancet*, 1948, *ii*, 1006.
(47) Medical Research Council. *Brit. Med. Journ.*, 1948, *ii*, 769.
(48) BIGNALL, CLEGG, CROFTON, SMITH, HOLT, MITCHISON and ARMITAGE. *Brit. Med. Journ.*, 1950, *i*, 1224.
(49) BERNHEIM. *Science*, 1940, **92**, 204.
(50) LEHMANN. *Lancet*, 1946, *i*, 14.
(51) LEHMANN. *Lancet*, 1946, *i*, 15 ; *Svenska Lakartidnigen*, 1946, **43**, 2029.
(52) VALLENTIN. *Svenska Lakartidnigen*, 1946, **43**, 2047.
(53) DEMPSEY and LOGG. *Lancet*, 1947, *ii*, 871.
(54) ERDEI. *Lancet*, 1948, *i*, 791 ; *ibid*, 1948, *ii*, 118.
(55) JOULES and NASSAU. *Tubercle*, 1949, **30**, 98.
(56) NAGLEY and LOGG. *Lancet*, 1949, *i*, 913.
(57) CARSTENSEN and ANDERSEN. *Lancet*, 1950, *i*, 878.
(58) GRAESSLE and PIETROWSKI. *Journ. Bacteriol.*, 1949, **57**, 459.
(59) Medical Research Council. *Lancet*, 1949, *ii*, 1237 ; *Brit. Med. Journ.*, 1949, *ii*, 1521. See also *Brit. Med. Journ.*, 1950, *ii*, 1073.
(60) MADIGAN, GRIFFITHS, LYNCH, BRUCE, KAY and BROWNLEE. *Lancet*, 1950, *i*, 239.
(61) CAYLEY. *Lancet*, 1950, *i*, 447.
(62) NAGLEY. *Lancet*, 1950, *i*, 592.
(63) SICARD and FORESTIER. *Bull. et Mém. d. l. Soc. méd. d. Hôp. d. Paris*, 1922, **46**, 463.
(64) BROCK. *Thorax*, 1950, **5**, 222.

CHAPTER X

ANTITHYROID SUBSTANCES

Iodine

Previous to the publications of Plummer and Boothby (1) in 1924 there was considerable difference of opinion concerning the advisability of administering iodine to patients suffering from Graves' disease. In this year, Plummer showed in a series of 400 cases that large doses of Lugol's solution, 10 to 15 m. once or twice daily, given as a pre-operative measure, caused a lowering of the basal metabolic rate and an improvement in the patient's condition. It has been found that if the iodine is continued for a longer period the B.M.R. rises again and the patient's condition deteriorates, although the final state is often better than before the treatment was begun. The use of iodine as a pre-operative treatment has rendered thyroidectomy a comparatively safe operation and has resulted in enormous benefit to the sufferers from thyrotoxicosis.

Goitrogenous Substances

Closely linked with the discovery of other antithyroid agents, was the observation that certain substances, when administered by mouth, produce hyperplasia of the thyroid gland. Thus Chesney et al. (2) found that cabbage and other plants of the Brassica family, when fed to rabbits cause thyroid hypertrophy. The active agents appears to be nitrile derivatives, and Marine et al. (3) observed that acetonitrile, when added to the food of rabbits, produces enlargement of the thyroid gland.

In 1941 the MacKenzies and McCollum (4), while engaged in a purely scientific enquiry, chanced upon a discovery of considerable clinical importance. They were investigating the possibility that sulphaguanidine " when fed to rats on a purified diet containing synthetic B vitamins, would prevent the synthesis of additional essential nutrients by the intestinal flora." They observed that after periods varying from six to sixteen weeks a hypertrophy and hyperæmia of the thyroid gland with loss of colloid was invariably produced. It was later found that this effect was not abolished by adding iodide to the diet, but could be neutralised by adequate doses of thyroxine.

Kennedy and Purves (5), in the same year, showed that rape seed and allyl-thiourea were powerful goitrogenic substances, and in 1943 the MacKenzies (6) found that thiourea and thiourea derivatives, especially 2-thiouracil, produced thyroid hyperplasia with inhibition of hormone production. Astwood (7) used thiourea and thiouracil in the treatment of patients suffering from thyrotoxicosis, and showed that the daily administration of 1 to 2 g. of thiourea, or of 0·2 to 1 g. of thiouracil, resulted in the relief of the patient's symptoms, and a return to normal of the serum cholesterol and basal metabolic rate, usually after a latent period of two to three weeks. These results were rapidly confirmed by Williams and Bissell (8) and by Himsworth (9). Both thiourea and thiouracil have a similar action in cases of thyrotoxicosis, but, because of the action of side effects, such as nausea, vomiting, and an unpleasant smell in the breath, which may accompany the use of thiourea, thiouracil, methyl-thiouracil or propyl-thiouracil are the drugs now usually employed.

Modes of Action. Iodine, sulphonamides and thiourea derivatives are believed to exert their antithyroid properties in different ways. There is a balance between the activities of the pituitary and the thyroid, for the thyrotropic hormone, known also as the thyroid stimulating hormone or T.S.H., liberated from the anterior lobe of the pituitary, stimulates the thyroid to form thyroxine, by increasing its power of taking up iodine and also by increasing the rate of the release of iodine, probably as thyroxine. This was shown by Stanley and Astwood (10) by means of radioiodine. Thyroxine, on the other hand, inhibits the pituitary production of T.S.H. The T.S.H., in addition to increasing the output of thyroxine, is thought to cause hyperplasia and increased vascularity of the thyroid gland, and, in some cases, to accentuate the degree of exophthalmos.

Radioiodine experiments also support the view that thyroxine is formed from tyrosine combined with iodine. The synthesis is effected in certain stages. Iodine is liberated from iodides in the presence of peroxidase, manganese and oxygen. Thiourea and its derivatives prevent the liberation of iodine from iodide by interfering with this peroxidase system, and so block the formation of thyroxine. Iodine, thus liberated, combines with tyrosine in the presence of a cytochrome enzyme to form first monoiodotyrosine and then diiodotyrosine. Sulphonamides effect their antithyroid action at this stage by competing with tyrosine for the iodine and so they inhibit the formation of diiodotyrosine. Diiodotyrosine is next converted, in the presence of a cytochrome enzyme, into thyroxine. This is stored in the thyroid as thyroglobulin, a substance with a large molecular weight of 700,000. Thyroglobulin is acted on by a proteolytic enzyme, and thyroxine, with a molecular weight of 69,000, is now liberated. Iodine is believed to produce its antithyroid effect, partly by inactivating the proteolytic enzyme, and partly by inactivating the T.S.H. of the anterior pituitary.

Clinical Applications. All types of thyrotoxicosis respond to thiouracil treatment, and, as has been described by Himsworth (11), Nussey (12), Reveno (13) and others, equally good results have been obtained in cases of primary and secondary Graves' disease, although the response may be slower with a toxic adenoma. Grainger, Gregson and Pemberton (14), on the other hand, found that primary cases responded much more favourably than do secondary ones, in fact, the longer the duration of the goitre, the less favourable the response to thiouracil. All observers agree that patients who have recently received iodine show a delayed response when treated with thiouracil. Thiouracil is equally efficacious in the treatment of thyrotoxicosis resulting from recurrence after thyroidectomy. King and Rosellini (15) successfully treated a case of acute thyroiditis, administering 200 mg. of thiouracil three times daily. The patient was free from symptoms in a week, and was cured after a further two weeks' treatment, taking 200 mg. daily. Thiouracil has also been used by Raab (16) in angina pectoris, and he found that 4 out of 10 cases were entirely free from symptoms during the treatment. Thiouracil is considered by some to be more efficacious than iodine in the pre-operative treatment of thyrotoxicosis, for by its use the surgeon can operate on a non-toxic goitre. Bartels (17) reports that it is especially of advantage in very severe cases of Graves' disease, especially those of long standing, which either do not tolerate, or fail to respond to, iodine therapy. Further, by giving Lugol's solution after the B.M.R. has been reduced to normal by thiouracil, the operation may be rendered easier, the gland being less vascular, less hyperplastic and less friable. Neither pregnancy nor diabetes are contraindications to the use of thiouracil. In pregnancy it is wiser not to continue the thiouracil during the last month, but to substitute it then by iodine, for in one case treated with thiouracil by Eaton (18) up to the confinement, the child at birth had an enlarged thyroid. Diabetes mellitus associated with thyrotoxicosis may be improved by thiouracil treatment, less insulin being subsequently required, but this is not so in every case, for Rose and McConnell (19) treated a thirteen-year-old girl with thiouracil, the result being that there was no increase in carbohydrate tolerance, and no diminution in insulin requirement.

Contra-indications. Thiouracil should be used with great caution if the goitre is causing sufficient pressure symptoms to warrant surgical intervention, as a rapid enlargement of the gland might result in a catastrophe. Thiouracil is contra-indicated if the patient has to go abroad after the stabilising treatment is completed, where adequate supervision with blood counts and basal metabolic readings are not available.

Stabilising Treatment. Some authorities do not keep their patients in bed during the initial period of treatment, allowing them to continue at work, providing adequate laboratory controls are carried out. We prefer the patient to be in hospital during the stabilising treatment, and in bed for the first three or four weeks. Before the thiouracil treatment is begun the following observations should be made: The weight of the patient, the pulse rate, the blood pressure, the circumference of the neck, the basal metabolic rate, the total white cell count and percentage of polymorphonuclear cells, and the blood cholesterol. The drug is given in tablet form by mouth, 200 mg. b.i.d. In some cases a satisfactory response is not obtained until the dose is raised to 200 mg. t.i.d. The white count is repeated twice a week during the early stages of treatment; the other observations, apart from the daily temperatures and pulse record, being carried out weekly. Dried yeast tablets (D.C.L.) two t.i.d., may be given during the treatment, with the idea of preventing the development of agranulocytosis, but they are of doubtful value. The first effects of the thiouracil treatment are usually seen within one or two weeks, the lag being due to the time taken to use up the stores of thyroid hormone and prevent the formation of more. In some cases no improvement is noted for four to twelve weeks, especially if iodine has been recently given. As soon as the B.M.R. is falling satisfactorily, which is usually in about four weeks, the thiouracil dosage is reduced to 100 mg. three times or twice a day. When the B.M.R. has fallen to between 0 and — 10 (Aub du Bois) a maintenance dose of between 100 to 200 mg. daily should be given. The dose must be sufficient to keep the B.M.R. at this low level. The progress chart of one of our patients, a woman aged forty-six years with a small hyperplastic goitre is given below :—

THIOURACIL CASE SHEET

Date 1945	B.M.R. (Aub du Bois)	Blood Cholesterol mg./100 ml.	Leucocytes per c.mm.	Polymorphs	Pulse per min.	Blood Pressure mm. Hg.	Wt. lbs.	Thiouracil mg.
Oct. 25	+44	158	7,800	68%	102	140/70	83	200 t.i.d.
Nov. 1	+32	192	6,300	numerous	100	128/68	87	200 t.i.d.
Nov. 15	+20	190	8,700	,,	78	132/72	96	200 t.i.d.
Nov. 21	+19	218	9,200	,,	84	110/80	99	200 t.i.d.
Nov. 29	+14	246	6,300	,,	88	112/60	103	200 t.i.d.
Dec. 6	+ 7	236	8,800	,,	84	120/65	108	100 b.i.d.
Dec. 13	+ 9	276	5,600	,,	76	118/66	111	100 b.i.d.
Dec. 20	0	250	10,000	,,	76	125/62	117	100 b.i.d.

A low white cell count before the commencement of thiouracil does not appear to be a contra-indication to its use. Thus in one of our cases the white cell count was 3,700 per c.mm. with 55% polymorphonuclears before treatment, and during treatment the count rose to 5,100 per c.mm. with 60% polymorphonuclears. This point has also been noted by Nussey (12). Auricular fibrillation may require simultaneous administration of quinidine, although some cases are restored to normal rhythm by the use of thiouracil alone, as recorded by McGavack et al. (20) in 12 out of 18 cases. If there is congestive failure it is wise to administer digitalis.

Overdosage of thiouracil is shown by marked increase in the size of the thyroid gland, or by symptoms of hypothyroidism such as a bloated appearance, a feeling of heaviness, lassitude and depression. If there is any increase of exophthalmos during any stage of the treatment or if the goitre enlarges considerably, gr. 1 of dried thyroid should be given daily by mouth to diminish the output of thyrotropic hormone from the pituitary.

Maintenance Treatment. It is quite probable that the dosage of thiouracil will have to be frequently adjusted during the early stages of the maintenance treatment. The B.M.R. and leucocyte count should be determined every month until the condition is firmly stabilised, subsequently three-monthly readings should suffice. As a routine measure every case should be treated continuously for ten months.

Toxic Reactions. These have been met with in from 10 to 20% of cases treated, but with the general use of smaller doses than were originally prescribed, they appear to be less frequent. The most dangerous complication is agranulocytosis, and unfortunately it may appear without any warning and rapidly prove fatal, despite regular control of the dosage of thiouracil by B.M.R. and white cell readings. In a survey of 1,091 cases treated at eleven clinics in America and at University College Hospital, London, Moore (21) reported that 19 patients developed agranulocytosis, of which 5 proved fatal. It is therefore probable that the mortality from agranulocytosis is about ½% or less, and its importance must not be over-exaggerated. Wosika and Braun (22) reported a fatal case in a woman aged fifty years who had taken a total amount of 29·4 g. of thiouracil during eleven weeks, in average-sized doses. The response of the thyrotoxicosis to the thiouracil had been good. The symptoms of the agranulocytosis consisted of fever, sore throat with redness and a dirty white exudate, and restlessness. The patient died in coma in six days, the white cells falling to 500 per c.mm. with a complete absence of neutrophils. The usually accepted forms of treatment were of no avail; pentnucleotide, yellow bone marrow, ascorbic acid, thiamine hydrochloride, whole blood, liver, folic acid and penicillin. Cargill and Lesses (23) had a fatal case just a year after the initiation of treatment, which had been most carefully controlled throughout. The development of agranulocytosis appears to be a matter of idiosyncrasy, unpredictable and probably unpreventable, but fortunately rare. The patient should always be warned to discontinue the thiouracil directly he feels a sore throat, enlarged cervical glands, or malaise, or if he develops a cold or skin rash. He should then immediately report to his doctor for a blood count. Moore (21) found that there is a period of maximal danger of agranulocytosis between the fourth and eighth weeks of treatment, so that at this stage particular vigilance is necessary, and it is also at this period that there is the greatest likelihood of leucopenia, by which is meant a white cell count below 3,000 per c.cm. without evidence of infection. Penicillin should be given in any case of leucopenia, to prevent the secondary infection which so often proves fatal. Thus Rothendler and Vorhaus (24) successfully treated a case by injections of 20,000 units of penicillin every three hours for four days, together with daily injections of 2 ml. of crude liver, and a whole blood transfusion of 500 ml.

Other toxic reactions make a formidable list, but fortunately are not often seen. They include drug fever, usually about the eighth day, morbilliform or urticarial rashes, allergic arthritis, nausea, vomiting, abdominal pains, diarrhœa, headache, enlargement of lymph glands or of the submaxillary glands, œdema of the legs, jaundice of an obstructive type, increase of exophthalmos, thrombocytopenic purpura, acute hæmolytic anæmia, heart-block, mental stupor, confusion and delusional insanity.

Methyl-thiouracil and Propyl-thiouracil

These substances were introduced as being less toxic and more potent than thiouracil. Radioiodine and clinical tests indicate that methyl-thiouracil is from two to one and a half times as effective as thiouracil, whereas propyl-thiouracil is probably no more effective than thiouracil, dose for dose. The initial dose for methyl-thiouracil is usually 100 mg. b.i.d., and for propyl-thiouracil 100 mg. t.i.d. The dosage is subsequently reduced when the B.M.R. has fallen to maintain it at a figure between 0 and — 10. Himsworth (25) considers there is little to choose between the toxicity of these three drugs. The American workers, such as Beierwaltes and Sturgis (26) prefer propyl-thiouracil, but methyl-thiouracil is often employed in England, and is the preparation we use. Propyl-thiouracil is certainly not free from toxic effects. Agranulocytosis developed in the first two cases in which we used it, in doses of 50 mg. t.i.d., but neither proved fatal. Bartels (27) in America, also reported three cases of agranulocytosis and eleven of leucopenia during propyl-thiouracil treatment. Juliar and Harris (28) have further described a fatal case of agranulocytosis due to propyl-thiouracil.

The Combined Use of Iodine and Thiouracil Derivatives. Whether iodine should be simultaneously administered with a thiouracil derivative in the routine treatment of thyrotoxicosis is a matter of opinion. We do not do so. Beierwaltes and Sturgis (26) recommend that 5 minims of Lugol's solution should be given daily together with propyl-thiouracil. They claim that if an operation is subsequently performed the thyroid is less friable and bleeds less easily, and, further, as the iodine acts at a different point in the formation of thyroxine than does thiouracil, the restoration to health of the patient is accelerated. Astwood (29), however, believes that iodine should not be used with a thiouracil derivative in the treatment of thyrotoxicosis, as there is a high frequency of recrudescence of thyrotoxicosis during prolonged treatment with the two substances.

Pre-Operative Treatment. There is here also a difference of opinion. Should iodine be used alone or combined with a thiouracil derivative ? Beierwaltes and Sturgis (26) recommend that 100 mg. of propyl-thiouracil should be given t.i.d. a.c., together with 4 drops of iodine solution daily, until the B.M.R. has fallen to zero. The operation should be performed provided also that the clinical features of thyrotoxicosis have been controlled. No antithyroid drugs are required after the operation. This treatment is suitable both for cases of exophthalmic goitre and of toxic adenoma. Bartels (30) says that the pre-operative use of propyl-thiouracil has reduced the operative mortality in surgical thyroid clinics from 3 % to 0·1 %, and it should always be used in severe cases. We are accustomed to prepare our patients for operation by the use of iodine alone, except in very severe cases in which a satisfactory response cannot be obtained. In such instances we believe that methyl-thiouracil should first be used, and if a satisfactory response results, iodine is also prescribed during the last two weeks of the pre-operative treatment.

Results of Treatment with Thiouracil Derivatives. A satisfactory assessment of the results of thiouracil treatment can only be made after the patient has discontinued the drug for several years. In the majority of the reports the figures are based on periods of one or two years' observation or less, and there is considerable variation in the results observed. Danowski et al. (31) used thiourea and iodine, as they consider that thiourea " is not only at least as effective as thiouracil but also less toxic." One hundred and eighteen patients were so treated, and of these 89 were followed for periods of six months to more than two years. Eight patients were observed for five to sixteen months following a course of thiourea which had lasted from 6·2 to 24 months. The B.M.R. remained satisfactory in all of these cases, but there was recurrence of clinical symptoms of hyperthyroidism in one of them. Poate (32) believes that methyl-thiouracil is superior to other thiouracil preparations, and in a series of 200 cases considered there is an 80% chance of "cure" without operation. The average period of treatment was nine months, and with a large thyroid a year or longer might be required. If thyroideum siccum has also been used the maintenance treatment should be prolonged for another two to four months. Verel (33) observed a series of 62 patients treated with thiouracil or methyl-thiouracil for periods between six months and four and a half years. In all cases the thyrotoxicosis was successfully controlled and the majority were back in full employment within six weeks of starting treatment. Thyroidectomy was performed in two cases, in one instance on account of persistent granulopenia, in the other because of excessive thyroid enlargement. In 33 cases the result was satisfactory after the thiouracil had been discontinued for three months or longer. One patient developed myxœdema after being off thiouracil for nineteen months. In 5 cases in which no thiouracil was taken for thirty-three to thirty-nine months no relapse occurred. Ravdin et al. (34) believe that sustained remissions after treatment for six to twelve months can be expected in about 50% of cases. McCullagh and Sirridge (35) found recurrence of hyperthyroidism in 2 cases out of 6, who had been treated with methyl-thiouracil and iodine for periods of five to twelve months with complete control. Meulengracht and Kjerulf-Jensen (36) treated 190 patients with methyl-thiouracil for an average period of twelve months. An examination was subsequently made of 111 patients who had been without treatment for three months, and in 10 cases relapse had occurred. Unfavourable results have also been reported by Starr et al. (37) who treated 28 patients with propyl-thiouracil for periods up to ten months, and in nearly every case relapse occurred on discontinuing the drug. Frisk (38) in a series of 126 patients treated with methyl-thiouracil found that 14% had a remission of at least eighteen months' duration.

It is quite clear from the above figures that the tendency to relapse is considerable, but when prolonged remissions do occur several years must pass after discontinuance of treatment before the real efficacy of the thiouracil drugs can be determined. When, however, relapse does occur, the symptoms of thyrotoxicosis are usually amenable to a further course of treatment.

Radioactive Iodine

Radioactive iodine, with a mass of 131 and a half-life of eight days, is used both for the diagnosis and treatment of thyrotoxicosis. It is said to have a half-life of eight days because at the end of that period it has lost 50% of its activity. Taken by mouth, as a colourless solution in water, it is quickly absorbed from the stomach. The greater part of the absorbed radioiodine is concentrated in the thyroid. It is essential that the patient shall have taken no iodine for at least four weeks before the tests for thyrotoxicosis are made.

Diagnosis of Thyrotoxicosis. The percentage uptake of radioiodine is determined by giving by mouth a tracer dose of 30–50 microcuries of I^{131}, the percentage amount present in the thyroid being estimated by a Geiger-Müller counter at twenty-four hours. Normally the gland retains 30% to 40%, in hyperthyroidism between 40% to 90% is present in the thyroid, and in hypothyroidism the figure is between + and − 10%. There is some overlap of these values, for at times in thyrotoxicosis less than 30% is retained in the thyroid at twenty-four hours. In one of our cases of diffuse thyrotoxicosis, the B.M.R. was + 17 (Aub du Bois) and the percentage iodine uptake was 90. The diagnosis of thyrotoxicosis may also be made by the plasma clearance test. A similar tracer dose of I^{131} is given by mouth and the rate of clearance of the radioiodine from the blood is determined. Normally about 5–40 ml. of plasma are cleared of iodine per minute, in thyrotoxicosis the clearance rate is raised to about 100–1,400 ml. per minute, and in hypothyroidism the figure is low, usually less than 5 ml. per minute.

The Treatment of Thyrotoxicosis. A tracer dose of 30–50 microcuries of I^{131} is given by mouth, and the percentage uptake at twenty-four hours is determined. From this figure and the estimated weight of the thyroid the therapeutic dose is calculated. This is usually equivalent to 100–250 microcuries per gram of thyroid, the total dose being between 1–5 or 10 millicuries. The normal weight of the thyroid is about 20 grams. The beta particles of radioiodine exert their effect locally in the thyroid with a range of about 1–4 mm. The gamma rays carry a distance of about one metre and are picked up by the Geiger-Müller counter.

Special precautions must be taken when radioiodine is administered. Space does not allow detailed rules to be given here, but they are usually drawn up by the special departments concerned with the investigation and treatment of patients with radioactive substances. The patient should be in a single room. Contamination with the drug is most likely to occur through the urine, or, if the patient is sick, through the vomit. Bed clothing, night clothes, handkerchiefs, bed pans, lavatories or baths may be affected. Nurses and attendants must wear gloves, gowns and masks when attending to the patient, dealing with bed pans, or cleaning the room. Crockery must be kept separate. The urine is not thrown away until the radioactivity is considerably diminished.

Various reports on the results of treatment of patients suffering from thyrotoxicosis have been published by Hertz and Roberts (39) in 1946, by Prinzmetal et al. (40) in 1949, and by Gordon and Albright (41) in 1950. Some authorities consider that the diffuse thyrotoxic goitre is more suitable for radioiodine treatment than is the toxic adenoma. Gordon and Albright (41) treated 83 cases of diffuse goitre and 37 of nodular goitre, and found the response in both types similar. Owing to the error in estimating the size of the thyroid it appears safer to give a small dose of 3 millicuries, and after two to three months to repeat the dose if the thyrotoxicosis is not arrested. Gordon and Albright (41) found that 59 of their patients responded satisfactorily to a single dose of this size, 36 patients required 2 doses, 16 patients were given 3 doses, and 7 patients needed 4 doses. Only 2 patients had more than 4 doses.

Radioactive iodine is of value not only in the treatment of primary and secondary Graves' disease, but also in thyrotoxicosis associated with severe heart failure, in cases complicated by extreme emotional disturbances, and in multiple recurrences after what appeared to be adequate surgical removal. It should not be used during pregnancy after the fourth month, or when the goitre is large, hard, or nodular. Chapman and Evans (42) found that the degree of exophthalmos changes very little after radioiodine treatment, but the appearance of the eyes is improved from loss of chemosis, lid retraction and œdema.

Complications. It is too early to know whether carcinoma of the thyroid may develop after many years in the gland which has been treated with radioiodine. There appears to be no danger of causing sterility. In the early days of treatment radioiodine was limited to patients over the age of forty-five years, now it is given to patients of any age. Myxœdema may result from overdosage, but this can be controlled by the administration of thyroideum siccum. No damage to the kidneys has been noted.

Treatment of Carcinoma of the Thyroid. Radioiodine is only taken up by certain types of carcinoma of the thyroid. In all cases to be treated, as complete a surgical removal of the gland as possible should be made first, and then sufficient radioiodine given to induce a complete state of myxœdema, which is subsequently controlled by the oral administration of thyroideum siccum. Good results may be obtained in the treatment of secondary bony deposits of carcinoma of the thyroid. A preliminary thyroidectomy, or the administration of thyrotropic hormone, appears to assist the uptake of radioiodine by the secondary deposits.

Conclusions. It is not claimed that thiouracil or its derivatives remove the cause of thryotoxicosis, and there is little difference between the risks of medical and surgical treatment in Graves' disease. The operative mortality rate, in the best hands, is below 1%, and the chance of death from the thiouracil derivatives is possibly a little less. It is said that in the exophthalmic class of Graves' disease the chance of " cure " is as high as 80%, whereas with thyroidectomy the curative rate is higher, up to 85%. The likelihood of a permanent " cure " with thiouracil has been discussed above. The chief drawbacks of thyroidectomy are the possible complications of the operation, especially tetany, recurrent laryngeal nerve palsy and the subsequently development of exophthalmic ophthalmoplegia. Further, relapse may take place as long as twenty years after the operation. Thyroidectomy is especially indicated in toxic adenoma, and the high percentage of carcinomas which develop in fœtal adenomas of the thyroid is another point in favour of operation. Medical treatment with thiouracil derivatives is indicated in the elderly, and in patients unsuitable for surgery owing to cardio-vascular degeneration, or who have had a previous thyroid operation. Thiouracil derivatives are also useful as a preoperative treatment in those who have become iodine-fast owing to prolonged iodine treatment. They can be recommended in cases in which the goitre is not large, or in those who refuse surgery. An operation should be advised if, during thiouracil treatment, a large goitre persists despite the administration of thyroideum siccum. Finally, the cosmetic effect resulting from the removal of a large goitre cannot be achieved by thiouracil or its derivatives, the maintenance treatment is apt to be difficult with thiouracil, and there remains the never-ending possibility of the sudden development of agranulocytosis.

It is too early to assess the ultimate results of treatment with radioiodine but it may become the method of choice in the majority of cases. Elaborate equipment and a specially trained team of workers are required and so it is not suitable for use in the general wards of a hospital or in private practice.

REFERENCES

(1) Plummer and Boothby. *Journ. Iowa State Med. Soc.*, 1924, **14**, 66.
(2) Chesney, Clawson and Webster. *Bull. Johns Hopkins Hosp.*, 1928, **43**, 261.
(3) Marine, Baumann, Spence and Cipra. *Proc. Soc. Exp. Biol. N.Y.*, 1932, **29**, 772.
(4) MacKenzie, MacKenzie and McCollum. *Science*, 1941, **94**, 518.
(5) Kennedy and Purves. *Brit. Journ. Exp. Path.*, 1941, **22**, 251.
(6) MacKenzie and MacKenzie. *Endocrinology*, 1943, **32**, 185.
(7) Astwood. *Journ. Amer. Med. Assocn.*, 1943, **122**, 78.
(8) Williams and Bissel . *New Eng. Med. Journ.*, 1943, **229**, 97.
(9) Himsworth. *Lancet*, 1943, *ii*, 465.
(10) Stanley and Astwood. *Endocrinology*, 1949, **44**, 49.
(11) Himsworth. *Proc. Roy. Soc. Med.*, 1944, **37**, 693.
(12) Nussey. *Brit ourn.*, 1944, *ii*, 745.
(13) Reveno. *Journ. Amer. Med. Assocn.*, 1944, **126**, 153.
(14) Grainger, Gregson and Pemberton. *Brit. Med. Journ.*, 1945, *ii*, 343.
(15) King and Rossellini. *Journ. Amer. Med. Assocn.*, 1945, **129**, 267.
(16) Raab. *Journ. Amer. Med. Assocn.*, 1945, **128**, 249.
(17) Bartels. *Journ. Amer. Med. Assocn.*, 1944, **125**, 24.
(18) Eaton. *Lancet*, 1945, *i*, 171.
(19) Rose and McConnell. *Amer. Journ. Med. Sci.*, 1944, **208**, 561.
(20) McGavack, Gerl, Morton, Vogel and Schwimmer. *Journ. of Clin. Endocrinol.*, 1945, **5**, 259.
(21) Moore. *Journ. Amer. Med. Assocn.*, 1946, **130**, 315.
(22) Wosika and Braun. *Journ. Lab. Clin. Med.*, 1945, **30**, 779.
(23) Cargill and Lesses. *Journ. Amer. Med. Assocn.*, 1945, **127**, 890.
(24) Rothwendler and Vorhaus. *Journ. Amer. Med. Assocn.*, 1945, **129**, 739.
(25) Himsworth. *Brit. Med. Journ.*, 1948, *ii*, 61.
(26) Beierwaltes and Sturgis. *Practitioner*, 1949, **162**, 486.
(27) Bartels. *Amer. Journ. Med.*, 1948, **5**, 48.
(28) Juliar and Harris. *Journ. Amer. Med. Assocn.*, 1949, **139**, 646.

(29) Astwood. "*Progress in Clinical Endocrinology*", Soskin, 1950. Wm. Heinemann, London.
(30) Bartels. *Amer. Journ. Med.*, 1948, 5, 48.
(31) Danowski, Man, Elkington, Peters and Winkler. *Amer. Journ. Med. Sci.*, 1948, **215**, 123.
(32) Poate. *Med. Journ. of Australia*, 1948, **2**, 677.
(33) Verel. *Brit. Med. Journ.*, 1949, *i*, 892.
(34) Ravdin, Rose and Maxwell. *Journ. Amer. Med. Assocn.*, 1949, **140**, 141.
(35) McCullagh and Sirridge. *Journ. Clin. Endocrinol.*, 1949, **8**, 1051.
(36) Meulengracht and Kjerulf-Jensen. *Journ. Clin. Endocrinol.*, 1949, **8**, 1060.
(37) Starr, Petit, Meister and Stirrett. *Journ. Clin. Endocrinol.*, 1949 **9**, 330.
(38) Frisk. *Acta med. Scand.*, 1947, **129**, 164.
(39) Hertz and Roberts. *Journ. Amer. Med. Assocn.*, 1946, **131**, 81.
(40) Prinzmetal, Agress, Bergman and Simkin. *Journ. Amer. Med. Assocn.*, 1949, **140**, 1082.
(41) Gordon and Albright. *Journ. Amer. Med. Assocn.*, 1950, **143**, 1129.
(42) Chapman and Evans. *Med. Clinics North Amer.*, 1949, **33**, 1211.

CHAPTER XI

THE NERVOUS SYSTEM

Electro-encephalography

It has been known for over sixty years that electrical currents are produced in the brains of animals both at rest and during stimulation. In 1891 Gotch and Horsley (1) recorded such currents produced in the exposed brains of animals, using a string galvanometer or a capillary electrometer. Berger (2) in 1929 first showed that changes in electrical potential arising in the cerebral cortex could be demonstrated in man with electrodes applied to the scalp. He used originally a Siemen's galvanometer and the deflections were very small. There was at first some doubt as to whether the electrical changes did actually arise in the brain, but in 1934 Adrian and Matthews (3) confirmed Berger's findings and demonstrated that the waves recorded arose in the parieto-occipital region in both sides of the brain, near Vogt's area 19; all extraneous causes of change in potential, such as muscular activity, eye movements and electrode artefacts were excluded. Electro-encephalography is comparable with electro-cardiography in technique, but the potential changes led off from the scalp are often more than a hundred times smaller than those recorded from the body surface in electro-cardiography. Thus the normal scalp potential changes are in the region of 5 to 100 microvolts, but occasionally under abnormal conditions they may rise to 1 millivolt (1 microvolt = 1 millionth of a volt). The electrical potential changes on the brain surface are ten to fifty times greater than those obtained on the scalp.

The Electro-encephalograph. There are many different types of electrode, the most usual ones being either a saline pad, which may be moved about the head at will, or a solder pledget sealed to the scalp with collodion. The second is commonly used for prolonged investigation. The different techniques used have been fully described by Gibbs, Davis and Lennox (4), Kornmüller (5), Walter (6), Balado, Romero and Noiseux (7) and others.

The hair should be cut short or pushed aside under the electrodes. It should be moistened if it is very dry, and the portion of

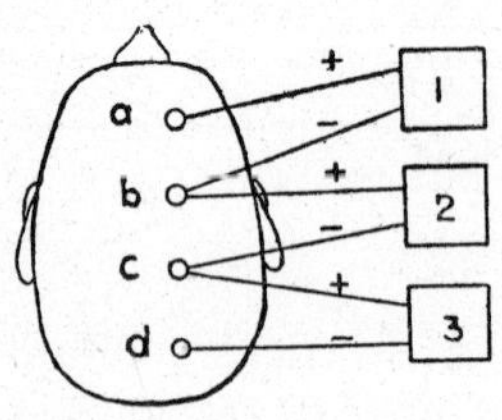

FIG. 49. Paired electrodes (after Williams and Gibbs (8)).

scalp under the electrodes should be cleaned with alcohol. Either paired electrodes or " a single scalp electrode system " may be employed. In the paired electrode system four electrodes (a, b, c and d) are placed on the scalp connected with three amplifiers (1, 2 and 3), as shown in the diagram (see Fig. 49). The amplifiers are thermionic valves, whereby an amplification of more than a millionfold can be obtained. The potentials thus amplified are led to three recording oscillographs.

Recording can also be carried out on paper by an ink-writing oscillograph or photographically by means of cathode ray tubes. As the frequencies encountered are relatively slow the ink-writing oscillograph, in virtue of its simplicity and economy of time and money, is superseding the more unstable cathode ray tube.

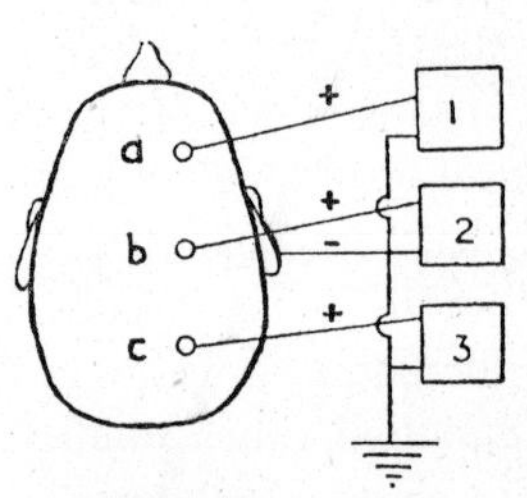

FIG. 50. Single electrode (after Williams and Gibbs (8)).

Single scalp electrodes are employed with an " indifferent " electrode placed on the ear, and earthed. The arrangement of a three single electrode system is shown in the diagram (see Fig. 50); a, b and c are electrodes placed on the scalp and 1, 2 and 3 are amplifiers.

The single scalp electrode records the potential change occurring at a single point in the brain and gives a truer reproduction of a pure wave than do the paired electrodes. It therefore records accurately the abnormal wave forms which are encountered in grand mal, petit mal and psychomotor epilepsy. The paired electrodes are used to localise foci of activity, for with paired electrodes changes in potential common to both electrodes are eliminated, and although a true picture of the electrical events occurring in the cortex is not given, the local discharges are rendered more prominent. As Williams and Gibbs (8) point out, if the potential gradient is visualised as a hill, the single scalp electrode records the height of the hill above ground level, represented by the " indifferent " electrode, whereas the paired electrodes measure the difference between the two points on the hill under examination without indicating the actual height of either point above the ground level. Thus with the single scalp electrode system, when the " hill top " or greatest change in potential is placed under one electrode, whichever way the electrode is moved, the potential will fall off as shown by the recorded

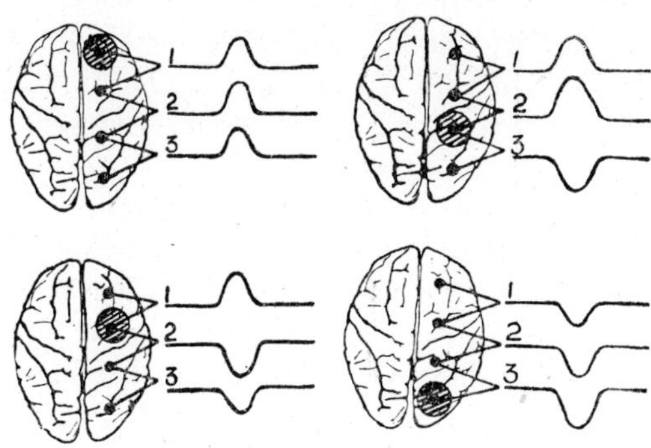

FIG. 51. Localisation of focus of activity by paired electrodes (after Williams and Gibbs (8)).

deflections. With paired electrodes, if the " hill top " is at the end of the row of electrodes the potential will fall in the same direction in each pair and will cause a deflection of each of the recorders in the same direction, the maximum deflection occurring from the electrode situated over the focus of activity. If, however, the " hill top " occurs at one of the middle electrodes the fall will be away from that electrode in both directions, and so will pass through the circuit on each side in opposite directions, making an upward signal or deflection in one, and a downward in the other; the waves are then said to be " out of phase," indicating that the focus of activity is situated under, or adjacent to, the middle electrode common to the two pairs.

The application of this method for the localisation of the focus of activity, by means of paired electrodes, is shown in the diagram (see Fig. 51).

The Alpha Waves or Berger Rhythm. Berger, placing one electrode on the frontal and the other on the occipital region.

demonstrated the occurrence of waves arising from the brain in health. They have an amplitude of 10 to 100 microvolts and a frequency of about 10 Herz (10 cycles per second). In childhood the frequency is about 6 per second and after the age of fifty the frequency diminishes. They are present when the eyes are shut and usually disappear when the eyes are open. In a few people they are not present. They are nearly sinusoidal and come and go at regular intervals (see Fig. 52A). When the eyes are shut mental concentration or a sudden noise will cause the wave to diminish in amplitude. Rarely, with sufficient mental relaxation, the waves persist even with the eyes open. The alpha waves are replaced by other wave forms during sleep. They are present in blind people, but noises or tactile stimuli may cause their disappearance. The persistence of the waves therefore appears to depend upon that part of the cerebral cortex which is concerned with the integration of the visual stimuli. They are thought to be produced by groups of neurones acting in unison, their synchronisation being due to a local pace-maker, whose activity is modified when the neurones are brought into action. Thus they are evident when cortical activity is suppressed, and abolished during functional activity. Lemere (9) has used this method to distinguish between blindness and hysterical blindness or malingering. In true blindness the alpha waves persist when the eyes are opened and the person attempts to look at an object; in feigned or hysterical blindness the alpha waves cease on opening the eyes and looking at an object. This suggests that in hysteria neither the sensory nor motor pathways, nor the cortical centres are affected.

The Beta Rhythm. Berger also described beta waves occurring in health. They are smaller than the alpha waves and have a frequency of 18 to 25 per second. They are believed to arise in the pre-frontal region of the cerebral cortex. Similar waves can be produced by contraction of the frontal and temporal muscles, and they are more prominent in records from individuals with wrinkled foreheads and raised eyebrows. Little is known about these minute waves, and their significance is not yet understood.

Changes in the Electro-encephalogram in Health

Sleep. Loomis, Harvey and Hobart (10) have shown that the alpha waves persist during the preliminary drowsy stage while the subject is still conscious. With the onset of sleep the alpha waves cease and intermittent groups of waves appear, known as " spindles," with a frequency of 14 or 15 per second. Later, in addition to the " spindles," larger and more prolonged waves, known as delta waves are seen. A dream may be accompanied by the appearance of alpha waves.

Hypnosis. The alpha rhythm is sometimes slowed during hypnosis, but the electro-encephalogram does not resemble that of natural sleep.

Cerebral narcotics cause the appearance of slower and larger waves, and basal narcotics result in quicker and larger waves.

The Electro-encephalogram in Disease

Studies have been chiefly directed to changes seen in the electro-encephalogram in increased intracranial pressure, in cerebral tumours, and in the epilepsies.

Increased Intracranial Pressure. This may be due to obstruction of the ventricular system, to cerebral tumours, concussion or meningitis. Berger (11) in 1931 showed that slow delta waves can be detected all over the skull. The waves may have an amplitude up to 100 microvolts and a frequency of 3 per second. Williams (12) has shown that the abnormal waves are not directly related to the raised intracranial pressure, but are caused by changes in the water content of the cerebral hemispheres, which is probably limited to the white matter. If the increased pressure is due to a cerebral tumour, reduction of the pressure by intravenous injection of hypertonic sodium chloride solution may enable the site of the tumour to be located, as the slow waves are now confined to the site of the tumour, as shown by Walter (6).

Cerebral Tumours. In 1933 Berger (13) demonstrated similar slow waves arising over the affected part of the brain in two cases of cerebral tumour. The waves appeared when one of the electrodes was placed over the tumour and they were not present when the tumour was midway between the electrodes. In 1935 Kornmüller (5) and Foerster and Altenburger (14) demonstrated that the potentials arise in the surrounding cerebral tissue and not in the tumour itself. Walter (15) has evolved a method for locating certain tumours by means of the electro-encephalogram.

Walter's method of localising a cerebral tumour with paired

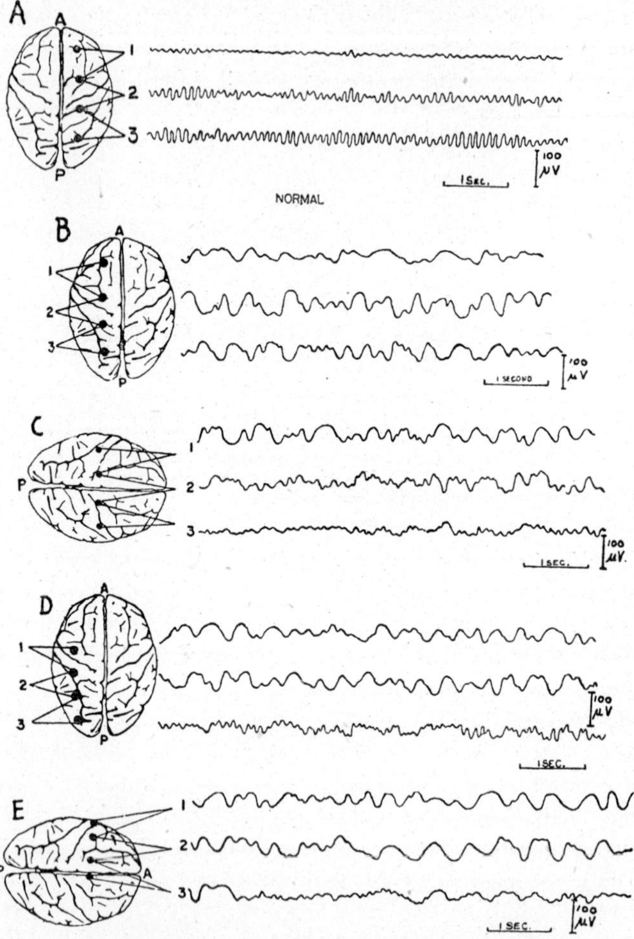

FIG. 52. Method of localisation of a cerebral tumour with paired electrodes (after Williams and Gibbs (8)).

electrodes is illustrated in the diagrams (see Fig. 52) reproduced from an article by Williams and Gibbs (8). There are five stages in the investigation : A. Right half of brain normal. B. Abnormal focus in left parietal region. C. Abnormal focus confirmed in left side of brain. D. Abnormal focus localised antero-posteriorly. E. Abnormal focus localised transversely.

Williams and Gibbs (8) investigated 50 cases, in 35 of which the lesion was demonstrated by operation or by autopsy, and in 15 the diagnosis was established by other means. A single focus was found in 36 cases and all were correctly located. In 7 cases two foci were found, in 4 of which the pathological cortical areas were confirmed. In 7 cases generalised abnormal waves were found. In 41 cases of suspected intracranial lesions the electro-encephalogram was normal, and further clinical investigations revealed no abnormality.

In general it may be stated that any tumour causing progressive destruction of cortical tissue will cause abnormally large slow waves of electrical potential to arise in the damaged cortex. Similarly, any other lesion, such as an abscess or a demyelinating disease resulting in cerebral dysfunction, will be associated with identical wave forms. It follows that discrete and non-progressive cortical lesions or deep tumours not affecting the cerebral hemispheres or the cortex itself, or cerebellar tumours are unlikely to be unmasked by indirect electro-encephalography. Walter and Dovey (16) have described a method, using a needle electrode, by which the electrical activity of the subcortical structures can be determined. This can be used to supplement conventional methods of identifying and locating subcortical tumours at operation.

Epilepsy. In 1937 Golla, Graham and Walter (17) showed that there are changes in the electro-encephalogram in 50% of patients under the age of forty suffering from convulsive epilepsy, even though no fit is seen at the time of examination. The majority of such abnormal electro-encephalograms occurred in patients suffering from grand mal. An abnormal electro-encephalogram is rarely seen in a patient who first has epileptic fits after the age of forty. The abnormality between fits consists in the occurrence of intermittent irregular slow waves. Walter states that in grand mal the focus of discharge is usually found in the region of the superior frontal gyrus on one or both sides. Krynauw (18) says that foci of discharge are also quite commonly post-central or even occipital in grand mal, and other workers have been unable to find a predilection for any particular cortical area. In petit mal the abnormal waves are widespread but the focus is usually post-central. " Seizure " waves occur during a fit, the focal discharges becoming greater and the area of discharge spreading.

The waves are then slower, but larger and more irregular. Transitory bursts of " seizure " waves are often seen in the absence of a fit and Lennox (19) has called them " subclinical seizures." An increase in the number of these outbursts often precedes a grand mal fit by days and can be used in predicting the onset of a convulsion. Gibbs, Gibbs and Lennox (20) describe the " seizure " waves in grand mal as sharp spikes occurring at twenty-five to thirty per second, in petit mal there are quick sharp spikes alternating with slow round waves, and in psycho-motor attacks (psychic variants) square flat waves occur at about three to four per second. As epilepsy is associated with the development of abnormal rhythms in the cerebral cortex they have called it a paroxysmal cerebral dysrhythmia. According to Gibbs (21) about 10% of normal people show a cerebral dysrhythmia indistinguishable from that occurring between the seizures in epilepsy, and it is possible that such individuals are suffering from asymptomatic epilepsy. Further about 5% of the near relatives of epileptics show an abnormal electro-encephalogram. Despite this, corroborative evidence of petit mal provided by an electro-encephalogram was successfully used by the defence in a murder case in England in 1942, when prolonged clinical observation of the accused in prison showed no evidence in epilepsy.

Symptomatic Epilepsy. There is no difference between the record of a fit resulting from trauma, tumour or any other lesion and that seen in idiopathic epilepsy. The fit may not necessarily be associated with any focal electrical abnormality.

Hysterical Fits. No abnormality is seen in the electro-encephalogram during the fits, and, except that unstable people are more liable to show abnormalities in the electro-encephalogram than are stable subjects, the resting record is usually perfectly normal.

Golla, McKissock and Walter (22) have shown that surgical removal of the portion of the cerebral cortex in which the delta waves originate may abolish the fits for a few months, but they ultimately recur. The actual origin of the fit therefore appears to be due to generalised cerebral changes.

Anti-convulsant drugs, such as bromides and Luminal, which are used for the treatment of epilepsy, reduce the number of abnormal electrical outbursts, or " subclinical fits," especially in grand mal epilepsy.

The types of waves met with in epilepsy are illustrated in the accompanying diagram (see Fig. 53).

Head Injuries. Williams (23) has investigated with the electro-encephalograph 74 patients suffering from acute head injuries due to war wounds. The tests were made within twenty days of the injury. He found that widespread abnormally slow waves, suppression of normal frequencies, and outbursts of high-voltage

NORMAL

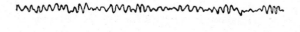

CRANO MAL PETIT MAL PSYCHOMOTOR

FIG. 53. Types of waves in epilepsy (Lennox (18)).

sine waves with a frequency of 2 or 3 per second, indistinguishable from sub-clinical epileptic attacks, occurred in the acute stage. Further, the degree of abnormality corresponded with the clinical state of the patient, and progressive changes indicated improvement or deterioration. The epileptic type of waves bore no prognostic significance as regards the occurrence of post-traumatic epilepsy. Williams (23) also investigated the electro-encephalograms in chronic post-traumatic states following head injuries. The electro-encephalogram was abnormal in 50% of cases and there was a definite relation between the electro-encephalogram, the severity of the injury, the persistence of symptoms and the presence of dural penetration.

Psychopathic Disorders. Attacks of uncontrollable anger or negativism, and behaviour disorders in children may be accompanied by cerebral dysrhythmia and an abnormal electro-encephalogram. The electro-encephalogram will also indicate whether the cerebral cortex is affected in cases of Sydenham's chorea.

Conclusions. Electro-encephalography, which started life as suspect, is now accepted as a genuine method of studying electrical changes in the cerebral cortex. It has already become a useful adjunct to other clinical methods in investigating the site of cerebral tumours and abscesses, and it has special value in giving objective proof of the presence of epilepsy and the exact type of fit in subjects whose history is inconclusive. It is of value in demonstrating impairment of function of the central nervous system in cases of head injuries. It is also helpful in the diagnosis of narcolepsy, subdural hæmatoma, cerebral trauma, meningitis, encephalitis, Schilder's disease and disorders of behaviour. Severe degrees of dementia may occur with a normal electro-encephalogram. For a more detailed discussion of electro-encephalography the reader is referred to the book edited by Hill and Parr (24).

Thymectomy in Myasthenia Gravis

In 1901 Weigert (25) recorded a case of myasthenia gravis with hyperplasia of the thymus. Since then numerous observations have been made and it appears that the thymus is always persistent, hypertrophied, or the seat of a benign tumour in myasthenia gravis. Norris (26) suggests that in myasthenia gravis the thymus shows specific histological changes, consisting of hyperplasia of the epithelial cells of the medulla. In the hyperplastic areas the normal structure of the gland may be preserved, or an undifferentiated syncytial mass of epithelium is found obliterating the round cells and Hassall's corpuscles, its structure closely resembling that of the fœtal thymus. The causal connection, which is now well established, between changes in the thymus and myasthenia gravis is unknown, but it has been suggested that a substance is formed in the thymus which inhibits the cholinergic transmission from nerve to muscle. Sauerbruch (27) in 1912 introduced the operation of thymectomy for myasthenia gravis, the patient was also suffering from hyperthyroidism. Blalock et al. (28) in 1941 reported on thymectomy in 6 cases of myasthenia gravis. One patient died, 3 were symptom-free three months after operation, one was improved but still required prostigmin, and one was unchanged two months later. Viets (29) reports on 36 patients suffering from myasthenia gravis treated by thymectomy at Massachusetts from 1941 to 1949. Seven of these patients had thymomas, and 29 showed various degrees of involution and the formation of germinal centres in the thymic tissue. Good to excellent results were obtained in about 50% of the cases. Neostigmine may be given with advantage intravenously during the operation, 0·5 mg. of neostigmine methylsulphate intravenously being approximately equivalent to 15 mg. of neostigmine bromide by mouth.

Keynes (30) has done much to lower the operative mortality of thymectomy, which should now be below 5%. He obtained the best results in cases with a short history. Of 120 patients who did not have thymic tumours 79 have shown a complete or almost complete remission of symptoms. Keynes is opposed to a transpleural operation, as even temporary collapse of the lung is harmful to the myasthenic patient. He also emphasises the danger of giving an enema to a patient after thymectomy; almost invariably the patient will collapse with syncope, and such an experiment should never again be made. Fatalities after operation are nearly always due to pulmonary complications. A myasthenic crisis may cause excessive bronchial secretion, with pulmonary consolidation, and death. Viets, however, has not seen such a myasthenic crisis, and considers that when patients drown in their own secretion it is due to excessive or ill-considered use of neostigmine. Primary operation in the case of thymomas was found to be very unsuccessful. The operation here is more difficult; and although the immediate result may be good, a serious and irrevocable relapse is very liable to occur. Such cases are best treated primarily by deep X-rays. Later it may be possible to remove the thymus with the tumour.

Conclusion. It is probable that thymectomy is indicated in rather less than 50% of all cases of myasthenia gravis. It is contra-indicated in cases well controlled by neostigmine or by tetra-ethylpyrophosphate. With neostigmine remissions may be observed equal in length to those following thymectomy. Further, tolerance to neostigmine is unlikely to occur.

REFERENCES

(1) Gotch and Horsley. *Philos. Trans.*, 1891, **182**, 267.
(2) Berger. *Arch. Psychiat. Nervenkr.*, 1929, 87, 527.
(3) Adrian and Matthews. *Brain*, 1934, **57**, 355, and *Journ. of Physiol.*, 1934, **81**, 440.
(4) Gibbs, Davis and Lennox. *Arch. Neurol. and Psych.*, 1935, **34**, 1133.
(5) Kornmüller. *Biol. Rev. Camb. Philos. Soc.*, 1935, **10**, 383.
(6) Walter. *Proc. Roy. Soc. Med.*, 1937, **30**, 579, and *Journ. Neurol. and Psych.*, 1938, N.S.I., 359.
(7) Balado, Romero and Noiseux. "*El Electro-encephalograma humano*", 1939, Buenos Aires.
(8) Williams and Gibbs. *Arch. Neurol. and Psych.*, 1939, **41**, 519.
(9) Lemere. *Journ. Amer. Med. Assocn.*, 1942, **118**, 884.

(10) Loomis, Harvey and Hobart. *Science*, 1937, **86**, 448.
(11) Berger. *Arch. f. Psych.*, 1931, **94**, 16.
(12) Williams. *Brain*, 1939, **62**, 321.
(13) Berger. *Arch. of Psych.*, 1933, **100**, 301.
(14) Foerster and Altenburger. *Deutsch. Ztschr. f. Nervenh.*, 1935, **135**, 277.
(15) Walter. *Lancet*, 1936, *ii*, 305.
(16) Walter and Dovey. *Lancet*, 1946, *i*, 5.
(17) Golla, Graham and Walter. *Journ. Ment. Sci.*, 1937, **83**, 137.
(18) Krynauw. *Brit. Med. Journ.*, 1939, *ii*, 160.
(19) Lennox. *Journ. Amer. Med. Assocn.*, 1939, **114**, 1347.
(20) Gibbs, Gibbs and Lennox. *Brain*, 1937, **60**, 377.
(21) Gibbs, *Journ. Amer. Med. Assocn.*, 1942, **118**, 216.
(22) Golla, McKissock and Walter. *See* Walter (6).
(23) Williams. *Journ. Neurol. Psychiat.*, 1941, **4**, 107 ; *ibid.*, 1941, **4**, 131.
(24) Hill and Parr. *Electroencephalography*, 1950. Macdonald & Co. Ltd., London.
(25) Weigert. *Neurol. Centralbl.*, 1901, **20**, 597.
(26) Norris. *Amer. Journ. Cancer*, 1936, **27**, 421.
(27) Sauerbruch quoted by Schumacher and Roth. *Mitt. a.d. Grenzgeb. d. Med. u. Chir.*, 1912, **25**, 746.
(28) Blalock, Harvey, Ford and Lillienthal. *Journ. Amer. Med. Assocn.*, 1941, **117**, 1529.
(29) Viets. *Brit. Med. Journ.*, 1950, *i*, 139.
(30) Keynes. *Brit. Med. Journ.*, 1949, *ii*, 611.

CHAPTER XII

THE HÆMOPOIETIC SYSTEM

Types of Anæmia and their Treatment

As our knowledge of the causation of the various anæmias increases ætiological classifications become more satisfactory. The following classification is based on that of Davidson (1).

1. *Nutritional Deficiency Anæmias.* These may be due to: (*a*) Lack of the anti-anæmic or hæmopoietic principle. This is a primary defect (the diet being adequate) in pernicious anæmia, and a secondary defect (*i.e.* resulting from a recognisable cause) in the anæmias of sprue and of dysentery, in tropical megalocytic anæmia, in the "pernicious anæmia of pregnancy", in Diphyllobothrium latum infestation, in carcinoma of the stomach and after gastrectomy. In the latter group there is also often an error in iron assimilation. There may be a deficiency of storage of the hæmopoietic factor in advanced cirrhosis of the liver. (*b*) Lack of the hæmopoietic factors, such as iron, copper, thyroxine, vitamin C and a proper salt balance in the food. This deficiency may be primary, as in simple achlorhydric anæmia and the Plummer-Vinson syndrome in which the food intake is often satisfactory but the absence of hydrochloric acid results in impaired absorption of iron, or secondary to a recognisable food or endocrine defect, as in the simple nutritional anæmia of infants, chlorosis, chronic gastritis and enteritis, cœliac disease, starvation, prolonged milk feeding as in the treatment of peptic ulcers, and in myxœdema.

2. *Post-hæmorrhagic Anæmias.* These occur after acute or chronic hæmorrhage.

3. *Hæmolytic Anæmias.* (*a*) Acute hæmolysis may result from blackwater fever, malaria, paroxysmal hæmogolobinuria, septicæmia, or toxins such as snake venoms. It also occurs in Lederer's anæmia. (*b*) A persistent hæmolysis, as in congenital or acquired acholuric jaundice, sickle-cell anæmia, Cooley's anæmia, Von Jaksch's anæmia and lead poisoning.

4. *Anæmias due to Inhibition of the Bone Marrow Function.* These may be primary, as in aplastic anæmia, or secondary, as in aplastic anæmia due to agents such as X-rays, radium, benzol,

lead or mercury. A leuco-erythroblastic anæmia results from involvement of the bone marrow in carcinomatosis, myelomatosis, Hodgkins' disease and osteosclerosis. By some writers Groups 1 and 4 in the above classification are called the dyshæmopoietic anæmias.

An alternative classification is based on the size of the red cells and their hæmoglobin content. This is of great clinical value, as it emphasises the fact that in general the macrocytic anæmias respond to liver and the hypochromic anæmias to iron therapy. Iron is, however, required in addition to liver for macrocytic anæmias if the saturation index is low. The following classification follows that of Wintrobe (2) :—

1. *Macrocytic Anæmias.* In this group the average size of the red cell is increased. The mean corpuscular volume is greater than 94 cμ. The group includes pernicious anæmia, achrestic anæmia, the anæmia associated with liver disorders and with myxœdema, the anæmia of sprue, the " pernicious anæmia of pregnancy ", the anæmia of chylous diarrhœa and of Diphyllobothrium latum infestation.

2. *Normocytic Anæmias.* Here the average size of the red cell is normal. The mean corpuscular volume is between 78 and 94 cμ. The cells may be normochromic or hypochromic. The anæmias included are aplastic anæmia, the anæmia following an acute hæmorrhage and that due to malaria.

3. *Simple Microcytic Anæmias.* There is a slight decrease in the size of the red cells. The mean corpuscular volume is less than 78 cμ. The cells are normochromic. Such anæmias may occur in chronic infections and in carcinoma.

4. *Microcytic Hypochromic Anæmias.* The red cells are smaller than normal and their hæmoglobin content is considerably reduced. The mean corpuscular concentration is less than 32%. Examples of anæmias of this class are simple achlorhydric anæmia, the anæmia of the Plummer-Vinson syndrome, the anæmia resulting from chronic hæmorrhage or from ankylostomiasis, the simple nutritional anæmia of infants and chlorosis.

The Macrocytic Anæmias

Pernicious Anæmia. The use of liver in the treatment of pernicious anæmia constitutes a therapeutic advance of similar importance to the discovery of insulin for the treatment of diabetes

There is little doubt that the origin of the idea can be found in the researches of Whipple (3) and his collaborators. These workers produced a severe secondary anæmia in dogs by bleeding, and proceeded to study the effects of various food substances on blood regeneration. They found that if liver were added in large quantities to the diet, there was a remarkable increase in the blood count which appeared to be entirely due to the liver. Shortly after the publication of these results, Minot and Murphy (4) described the application of the same principles to the treatment of pernicious anæmia. In 1926 they reported the effect of a diet rich in liver in 45 cases of pernicious anæmia. These results were very striking indeed, since they showed that one month's treatment increased the blood count by about 2,000,000 red cells. A series of publications followed, with the result that the regimen was fully upheld, and now experience has proved that the blood picture can be restored almost to normal in practically all patients.

Castle and his colleagues of Boston (5, 6) by means of a large number of experiments on the action of healthy gastric juice on beef muscle, have been able to show that the juice of the healthy stomach contains some unknown ingredient (intrinsic factor) which, through its action on an extrinsic factor contained in muscle protein, results in the formation of the anti-anæmic or hæmopoietic substance. This is able to produce a remission in pernicious anæmia equal in degree to that produced by liver extract. The identity of the intrinsic factor has not been established, but it is believed that it is quite unrelated to HCl or pepsin, and the work of Taylor et al. (7) suggests that it is probably a ferment. Formijne (8) concludes that no reaction can occur *in vitro* between the intrinsic and extrinsic factors, and he suggests that the reaction occurs in the intestinal wall. It is thermolabile and capable of acting in a "neutral" medium. These researches established the ætiological importance of the stomach and its secretion in the development of pernicious anæmia. The anti-anæmic substance, thus formed, is absorbed from the intestine and stored in the liver and to a lesser degree in the kidneys and spleen. In pernicious anæmia the intrinsic factor is absent from the gastric juice and achylia gastrica is usually present. Cohn et al. (9) have shown that the active principle is neither protein, lipoid nor carbohydrate, but is either a nitrogenous base or a polypeptide.

The Source of the Intrinsic Factor. Meulengracht (10) using the pig's stomach, found that preparations from the pyloric gland region were highly active as regards the presence of the anti-anæmic factor, whereas those from the fundus gland region were inactive. It therefore appeared probable that the " intrinsic factor" is connected with, or produced by the pyloric glands. Anti-anæmic activity was also demonstrated in preparations from the duodenum, and it was considered that this was due to Brunner's glands, which are histologically identical with the pyloric glands. The two sets of glands are called the pyloric gland organ. The cells in the fundus of the stomach which produce hydrochloric acid and pepsin would not appear from these findings to be concerned with the production of the intrinsic factor. It has been known for many years that there is atrophy of the gastric mucous membrane in pernicious anæmia, and it therefore appeared probable that the atrophy would affect the cells which produce the intrinsic factor. Almost simultaneously investigations on this point were carried out by Meulengracht (11) and by Magnus and Ungley (12). Meulengracht examined histologically the stomach and duodenum in 8 cases of pernicious anæmia, and to his surprise found that although changes were present in the fundus portion, with atrophy of glands and disappearance of the parietal and chief cells in all the cases, the glands in the pyloric region seemed relatively well preserved and no histological changes could be demonstrated in Brunner's glands. Magnus and Ungley examined the stomach from 7 cases of pernicious anæmia. In all a characteristic non-inflammatory atrophic lesion was found, localised to the region of the body mucosa, which did not affect the pyloro-duodenal region. The work of Fox and Castle (13) appears to explain this anomaly. Extracts were made from the human stomach shortly after death, and it was shown that those areas containing the fundus type of cell yielded a substance highly active in hæmopoietic properties, whereas the pyloric gland organ extracts were inactive. Man's stomach differs therefore in this respect from that of the pig. If this is so, the findings of Schenken et al. (14) are contradictory. They prepared liver extracts in cases of carcinoma of the stomach in man, and determined their anti-anæmic properties. When the carcinoma involved all the stomach except the pyloric portion, the liver extract was potent. When the pyloric portion was affected, the liver extract did not contain the anti-anæmic principle. Goldhammer (15) has shown that the volume of gastric juice is reduced in pernicious anæmia, from a normal of 150 ml. per hour to 20 ml. per hour in pernicious anæmia. The anti-anæmic activity per unit volume, however, was the same in pernicious anæmia as in health. This observation supports the view that the change in pernicious anæmia is a quantitative rather than a qualitative one.

Very little can be stated with regard to the mode of action of liver extract. The changes produced in the blood as the result of successful treatment include the restoration of a normal red cell count, return of the colour index to normal, and an increase in the number of white cells with disappearance of the relative lymphocytosis. Special attention is directed to the reticulocytes present in the blood. These are immature red cells, normally present in the blood to the extent of 0·1 to 1% of the red cells. They cannot be seen in dried stained films, but are demonstrated by "vital" staining in wet films. A blood film is made on a slide, which has previously been coated with a thin dried film of a dye, such as cresyl-blue. A cover slip is then placed on the blood film, which is examined wet (Davidson et al. (16)). The reticulocytes contain a network, granules or dots, stained blue. They probably correspond with the red cells showing polychromasia in the ordinary dry films. In untreated pernicious anæmia the reticulocytes are usually somewhat increased in number, as 2% or more of the red cells. In cases of pernicious anæmia treated with liver, in which a good response can be expected, the reticulocytes rise rapidly to 15 or 30% in a week, and then fall suddenly (reticulocyte crisis) to reach normal in about three weeks. The increase in the red cell count begins usually about the time of the reticulocyte crisis, and persists for several weeks after. The excess of bilirubin in the serum disappears early, at the time of the rise in the reticulocyte count, as shown by Dyke and Greener (17). An increase in the eosinophils after the administration of raw liver has been noted by Whitby (18) and other workers; this usually reaches a maximum, which may be as high as 26%, between the eighth and twelfth weeks of treatment. Achlorhydria persists after liver treatment.

Stomach Preparations. Following the initial papers of Castle, Sturgis and Isaacs (19) published their observations on the anti-anæmic principle contained in dried whole hog's stomach. The indications for its use are the same as those for liver and liver extract. Accounts have been published in which stomach extract has produced a remission where liver has failed. Thus Renshaw (20) describes a patient refractory to liver and liver extract, but responding readily to stomach extract. No definite explanation has been offered for their action, but the most ingenious is that of Castle, who suggests that the autolysis which occurs after death results in the interaction of the healthy gastric juice with the muscle protein of the gastric muscularis, and that by this means the necessary factor is formed. Wilkinson (21) showed that the mucous membrane and the muscle layer of the hog's stomach yield a light powder when desiccated at 40° C. *in vacuo*. Preparations from both sources are effective in the treatment of pernicious anæmia, and weight for weight are equal to, or better than, a liver diet. He also showed that normal human gastric juice, when given during meals to a patient suffering from pernicious anæmia, causes improvement. Later, Wilkinson and Klein (22) demonstrated that an active gastric extract can also be obtained by expression of the stomach juice, using a pressure of $2\frac{1}{2}$ to 3 tons per square inch and subsequently treating the juice with alcohol. This active principle they termed hæmopoietin. They regard this as the same as, or closely allied to, Castle's intrinsic factor. Wilkinson and Klein (23) further showed that when hæmopoietin is allowed to act on beef outside the body a relatively heat-resistant substance is obtained which resembles the liver active principle. Wilkinson (24) considered hæmopoietin to be an enzyme-like substance which is very easily destroyed by heat and which requires a substrate for its action. This hæmopoietin is only found in the stomach of carnivoræ.

Yeast Preparations. The beneficial effect of marmite in the treatment of certain megalocytic anæmias requires consideration and the facts observed may be briefly stated. Marmite is a yeast extract, rich in the vitamin B complex, containing the antineuritic vitamin B_1, and nicotinic acid. Wills (25), in India, found that marmite was as active as liver in causing regeneration of cells in the "pernicious anæmia of pregnancy" and in tropical macrocytic anæmia. Wills and Evans (26) have subsequently shown that tropical macrocytic anæmia does not respond to the highly purified liver extracts which cure pernicious anæmia. It does respond, however, to crude liver extract and to autolysed yeast extracts.

The active factor is not vitamin B_1, B_4, riboflavin or nicotinic acid, but it may be the extrinsic factor. It is now generally agreed, as Davidson (27) stated, that marmite alone will not cure pernicious anæmia during the acute stage. He states that many cases in the relapse stage fail to respond to vitamin B, and that marmite cannot replace liver or hog's stomach extract. Marmite is efficacious in the treatment of tropical macrocytic anæmia, the anæmia of sprue and of cœliac disease. In these diseases, however, there is no achlorhydria and the stomach produces the " intrinsic factor ", which acts on the " extrinsic factor " to form the anti-anæmic substance. In those cases of pernicious anæmia in which a response to marmite is obtained there is possibly a small amount of the " intrinsic factor " present in the gastric juice. In subacute combined degeneration of the cord associated with pernicious anæmia, marmite is not of value. Berk et al. (28) suggest that the extrinsic factor of Castle, present in food, may be closely related to vitamin B_{12}, and that the intrinsic factor in the gastric juice is necessary for the optimum utilisation of vitamin B_{12} or of chemically related substances present in various foods. Further, Bethell et al. (29) have shown that in cases of untreated pernicious anæmia, vitamin B_{12} is found in the fæces in amounts greater than are required to treat such patients by injection of the vitamin. This supports the view that pernicious anæmia results from deficient absorption of B_{12}.

Treatment of Pernicious Anæmia

In a very severe case a preliminary transfusion of 500 ml. of compatible blood given slowly is of great value, if due care is taken in matching blood.

Parenteral Administration of Liver. In addition, an intravenous injection of a liver extract, such as Neo-Hepatex or Hepastab Forte, 5 ml., should be administered slowly, or 6 to 8 ml. of Neo-Hepatex or Hepastab given intramuscularly the first day, and 2 to 4 ml. on the following days, until a reticulocyte response is obtained. For subsequent treatment a preparation such as Neo-Hepatex or Hepastab is injected intramuscularly. The maintenance dose is 2 to 4 ml. weekly until the blood is normal and there are no symptoms. Later, 2 to 4 ml. are required every two, three or even six weeks.

In America liver extracts are standardised in units, the unit being "the amount of material which when given daily to patients suffering from pernicious anæmia has produced satisfactory hæmopoietic response". In a severe case 15 units of liver extract should be given in a single or in divided doses within the first six hours. Five to 10 units should then be injected daily for a week, and subsequently 10 to 15 units weekly until the blood count is normal. A maintenance dose of 10 to 15 units every one to four weeks is required.

In 1935 Dakin and West (30) obtained the anti-anæmic principle of liver in a still more concentrated state. It is known as Anahæmin and is put up in ampoules containing 100 mg. in 1 ml. The initial dose for a severe case of pernicious anæmia is 0·5 ml., repeated daily for a week, or a single intramuscular injection of 4 ml. may be given. Subsequently a maintenance dose of 2 ml. is injected every two to four weeks. Examen or Hepastab Forte may be used instead, the dose being approximately double that of Anahæmin. Proteolysed liver was prepared in 1943 by Davis et al. (31) by digesting minced liver with papain, a proteolytic enzyme which reacts at the natural *p*H of minced liver, approximately 5·6. The product is put up as a dry powder, freely soluble in cold water. It is administered dissolved in warm water flavoured with pepper and salt, the dose being 2 dr. to 1 oz. daily. It has been found of value in cases of megaloblastic anæmia refractory to the parenteral administration of liver, including idiopathic cases and those associated with pregnancy, sprue, and the puerperium.

Hypersensitivity to Liver Extracts. A primary reaction may occur after the first injection of a liver extract, especially if a crude extract is used. There may be rise of temperature, shivering, malaise, flushing, headache, giddiness, shortness of breath, and collapse. Secondary reactions may occur with later injections, and are allergic in nature. These include skin rashes, tachycardia, dyspnœa, eosinophilia, rigors and even death. At the first sign of an allergic reaction an injection of 1 ml. of adrenaline should be given, followed by an antihistamine drug such as Benadryl mg. 50 or Anthisan mg. 50. Subsequently treatment should be maintained by the use of a stomach preparation or by vitamin B_{12}.

Folic acid must not be used in the treatment of pernicious anæmia (see p. 90). The use of vitamin B_{12} in the treatment of pernicious anæmia is considered on p. 94.

Administration of Iron and Vitamin C. If the mean corpuscular hæmoglobin is below 32%, iron should be given by mouth, in the form of ferri et ammon. cit. gr. 30 t.i.d., in addition to the liver treatment. Paræsthetic symptoms may be relieved by the iron. In some cases of refractory pernicious anæmia, as described by Wilkinson (32), ascorbic acid, 100 to 150 mg. must be given by mouth in addition to the liver in order to obtain a remission of the disease.

Oral Administration of Stomach Preparations. These are made as described above by desiccation, and are not extracts. Wilkinson (33), in 1931, showed that patients suffering from pernicious anæmia rapidly improved with 250 g. of fresh uncooked mucous membrane of hog's stomach daily. Desiccated preparations of whole hog's stomach are also available, such as Pepsac or Gastrosic. Twenty-five grams are equivalent to 100 g. of fresh whole hog's stomach. The usual dose is 10 g. three times a day. The powder must be given cold, either in soda water, cold milk, oxo, bovril, port or burgundy. Wilkinson claims that this treatment is superior to liver treatment in the speed of remission, the relief of gastro-intestinal symptoms and in the rate at which normal health is regained. Thus Wilkinson (34) has found that in seven to twelve days the reticulocytes reach a peak of 30 to 70%, followed by a rapid rise of the blood count. The maintenance dose is up to 28 g. of Pepsac daily. The stomach treatment is considerably cheaper than liver treatment. In conclusion, there are three essentials in the use of stomach preparations : (1) The preparation must be active. (2) It must be free from micro-organisms. Neglect of this simple precaution has resulted in the death of the patient. (3) The preparation must be given cold.

Parenteral administration of stomach preparations is not possible.

The Treatment of Nervous Lesions. When nervous lesions, such as subacute combined degeneration of the cord, are present, the dose of liver extract should be 2 or 3 times that given for uncomplicated cases. F. C. Wilkinson (personal communication) says that highly refined liver extracts, such as Anahæmin, may be used provided the batches have been tested and shown to be potent. The use of vitamin B_{12} in these cases is described on p. 94. Wilkinson (34) states that patients who have been bedridden owing to postero-lateral sclerosis of the spinal cord have so improved with stomach preparations that they have been able to return to work.

The Prognosis in Pernicious Anæmia. The immediate prognosis in pernicious anæmia has been revolutionised by the introduction of liver therapy. Previous to 1926 the mortality rate was nearly 100%, and death occurred in periods up to two and a half years after the diagnosis was made. Now it is very rare for a patient to die during the acute stage if adequate treatment is given. In every case the correct maintenance dose of liver or stomach preparation must be determined and controlled by regular blood examinations. The position is comparable with the administration of insulin and its control by blood sugar readings. Witts (35) has emphasised the importance of adequate after-treatment in cases of pernicious anæmia, as every patient is under the threat of subacute combined degeneration of the cord. The maintenance dose, either of a liver or stomach preparation, must be sufficient to keep the hæmoglobin over 90% and the red cells over 4,000,000 per c.mm. The blood should be examined every month. The advantage of giving intramuscular injections of liver extract every two to four weeks is that the patient is compelled to remain under medical supervision. Hill (36) has drawn attention to the fact that the death rate from pernicious anæmia fell substantially in 1928 following the introduction of liver treatment into England in 1927. Since 1931 there has, however, been a rise again in the death rate. This may be due to inadequate after-treatment, to the disease becoming refractory to treatment after a time, or to patients dying from other diseases than pernicious anæmia, especially intercurrent infections, *i.e.* to faulty certification. Wilkinson (37) writes, "In January, 1948, I have still alive 1,179 patients on stomach or liver therapy, including 1 patient of 100 years of age, 7 over 90, 99 over 80 and 396 over 70. . . . In general health they compare more than favourably with contemporary non-anæmic people."

Achrestic Anæmia (χρῆσθαι = to utilise). In 1935 Wilkinson and Israëls (38) described a type of severe macrocytic anæmia which in some respects resembles pernicious anæmia, but is resistant to liver therapy. They considered that it is due "to inability to utilise, or possibly mobilise from the storage depots (such as liver, kidney, brain), the anti-anæmic principle responsible for the correct maturation of megaloblasts; although such may be present in the body in adequate quantities ". Clinically it differs from pernicious anæmia in that the age of onset is between early adult life and old age, the sexes are equally affected, the gastric acidity is normal or almost normal, there is no disturbance of the gastro-intestinal tract or central nervous system, and no pyrexia or evidence of hæmolysis. The liver and spleen are not usually enlarged. Examination of the liver in one case showed that the anti-anæmic principle was present in sufficient amount to produce a reticulocyte crisis in a patient suffering from true pernicious anæmia. It was found in about 1% of cases thought to be suffering from pernicious anæmia. Achrestic anæmia has not met with universal acceptance ; thus some workers such as Vaughan (39) suggested that it is a megalocytic anæmia associated with liver disease, and others such as Castle and Minot (39), Zanaty (41) and Davidson and Fullerton (42) have pointed out difficulties in differentiating it from aplastic anæmia. Mahler and Greenberg (43) have reported a case of hyperchromic macrocytic anæmia refractory to liver extract, in which they say the weight of evidence strongly favours achrestic anæmia as described by Israëls and Wilkinson. Israëls and Wilkinson (44) after a further study of six new cases have strengthened their views as to the existence and nature of achrestic anæmia. They say that the only changes in the liver are fatty ones associated with a severe anæmia, and study of the bone marrow differentiates it from aplastic anæmia (see p. 328). One case of achrestic anæmia with achlorhydria was found in 1,100 cases thought to be suffering from pernicious anæmia. Bomfort and Rhoads (45) are inclined to believe that achrestic anæmia is not a specific syndrome.

Treatment. Life may be prolonged by repeated blood transfusions and by intensive anti-anæmic treatment. Liver extract, 2 ml., should be given intramuscularly t.i.d. for ten to fourteen days. Subsequently 4 to 6 ml. should be injected weekly. In addition a stomach preparation such as Pepsac, 1 oz., should be given daily by mouth. Despite treatment the disease appears to be inevitably fatal.

Macrocytic Anæmia associated with Hepatic Disorders. Wintrobe and Shumacker (46) found eleven instances of macrocytic hyperchromic anæmia among 43 cases of hepatic disorders, which included such conditions as cirrhosis, passive congestion, carcinoma and acute yellow atrophy. Free hydrochloric acid was present in the gastric juice of 6 out of 10 cases examined. The anæmia was not severe and remissions are likely to occur apart from treatment. The authors suggest that the anæmia is possibly due to impairment of storage of the hæmopoietic principle in the liver, or to a combination of partial gastric disturbance and incomplete liver damage. Rosenberg (47) investigated 48 cases of cirrhosis of the liver, mostly of an advanced type. In 43 cases there was macrocytosis, but in only 8 was the red cell count below 2·5 millions.

Macrocytic Anæmias in Myxœdema. These are of three types, simple macrocytic normochromic, Addisonian macrocytic normochromic, and macrocytic or normocytic hypochromic anæmia. In other cases of myxœdema a hypochromic or normochromic anæmia is found. Anæmia of some type is present in about 50% of all cases of myxœdema. The simple macrocytic hyperchromic anæmia can be cured by the administration of thyroid alone, as was shown by Bomford (48). The anæmia is never severe, but it may take several months to affect a cure. The Addisonian type of anæmia required thyroid and liver extract, and the hypochromic anæmia is curable with thyroid and iron.

Tropical Macrocytic Anæmia. The Anæmia of Sprue. The Anæmia of Cœliac Disease. These anæmias are probably nutritional in origin, the gastric secretion being normal. Response to treatment therefore will occur either with liver extract or with marmite. Thus Vaughan and Hunter (49) have recorded good results with marmite in the megalocytic anæmia occurring in cœliac disease.

The Nutritional Megalocytic Anæmia of Pellagra. This has been studied by Moore and his co-workers (50). The diets of their 25 patients had been very deficient in animal protein and the vitamin B complex. Free HCl was present in the gastric juice in the majority of cases, and from their experiments Moore concluded that the anæmia was not due to a deficiency of the intrinsic factor, but to a prolonged lack of Castle's extrinsic factor in the diet, associated in many cases with poor absorption from the intestines. Macrocytic anæmia due to food deficiency can therefore occur without avitaminosis.

The "Pernicious Anæmia of Pregnancy". Several types may occur in association with pregnancy and the puerperium. Thus pregnancy may complicate true Addisonian pernicious anæmia.

Osler (51) in 1919 described a "severe anæmia of pregnancy", and this is of a pernicious type. It is more common in India than in temperate zones, and usually shows itself between the sixth and eighth months of pregnancy. As described by Whitby (52) it may be plastic or hypoplastic in type. In the former case there is megalocytosis, with a high colour index and signs of blood regeneration, but in the hypoplastic or aplastic variety there is no sign of regeneration of erythrocytes, the colour index is high, and there is megalocytosis or normocytosis. A chlorotic type of anæmia, due to deficient iron supply, may also complicate pregnancy. Here the colour index is low and there is no megalocytosis. The "pernicious anæmia of pregnancy" differs from Addisonian pernicious anæmia in several respects. Thus achlorhydria is usually absent and there is a tendency to spontaneous recovery after the pregnancy is terminated. Clinically the patient has usually been in good health and there is no evidence of infection. The patient becomes deadly pale, with severe dyspnœa and often œdema or pyrexia. Hæmorrhage may occur from the nose, gastro-intestinal tract or vagina. The condition may be mistaken for an internal hæmorrhage. Davidson et al. (53) have investigated 16 cases of severe megalocytic anæmia occurring during pregnancy or the puerperium. The colour index may be below unity. Some of these were refractory to treatment by liver extract, iron and yeast, and in such cases life has to be maintained by blood transfusions until the hæmatinic treatment takes effect.

Treatment. In very severe cases blood transfusion of 500 ml. should be given at short intervals, followed by the daily administration of liver, by mouth or injection, or of stomach extract by mouth, 1 oz. daily. This treatment should be continued until the pregnancy is terminated and the anæmia is cured.

The Normocytic Anæmias

Aplastic Anæmia. In this disease there is a progressive failure of function of bone marrow. The anæmia is progressive without remissions. The colour index is usually between 0·9 and 1. There are no reticulocytes. The total white cell count is low, about 1,000, and the polymorphonuclear cells are much reduced. There is no achlorydria.

Treatment. Liver is not effective. Blood transfusions are the most hopeful line of treatment and the use of concentrated red cell suspensions, the preparation of which is described by MacQuaide and Mollison (54), and Williams and Davie (55), avoids an undue increase of the blood volume.

The Microcytic Hypochromic Anæmias

Simple Achlorhydric Anæmia (Idiopathic microcytic anæmia. Essential hypochromic anæmia). This condition was described by Faber (56) in 1914 and attention has been especially directed to it in England by Witts (57), Hartfall and Witts (58) and Davies (59), and in America by Damashek (60). It affects particularly women between the ages of thirty-five and fifty, the chief symptoms being those of flatulent dyspepsia and dyspnœa. The tongue may be smooth and red and the nails brittle or concave (koilonychia). The dietary has usually been lacking in meat and green vegetables for some time and, owing to the achlorhydria, iron absorption is deficient. The average amount of iron in a normal diet is 10 to 20 mg., of which 7 to 9 mg. are available. There is a daily loss of 5 to 20 mg. in the fæces, and 0·5 to 1 mg. in the urine.

The blood. The red cells may number 4 millions per c.mm. with a hæmoglobin percentage of only 40. Frequently there is microcytosis. There is no increase of bilirubin in the blood.

The stomach. The gastric juice contains mucus in excess and an absence of free hydrochloric acid in 70 to 80% of cases. The stomach empties rapidly or in normal time. Injection of histamine provokes some secretion of hydrochloric acid in from 15 to 25% of cases showing achlorhydria. Further, the gastric juice is not deficient in the " intrinsic factor " of Castle, for on incubation of the juice with beef protein the anti-anæmic principle is developed which is curative of pernicious anæmia. Hartfall and Witts (58) found the " intrinsic factor " below normal in some cases of simple achlorhydric anæmia, but it has not been conclusively shown to be completely absent in any case. This probably explains why the patient does not develop pernicious anæmia, although Damashek (60) suggests that the gastric juice is deficient in the power to digest organic iron.

Treatment. Iron should be given in large doses such as Ferri et ammon. cit. gr. 30, aq. chlorof. ad fl. oz. 1. Fl. oz. 1 t.d.s. In about six or eight weeks the hæmoglobin figure is usually normal.

In some cases a mixture containing Acid. hydrochlor. dil. m. 60, tnc. aurantii m. 10, aquam ad m. 120, in a glass of water t.d.s. with meals, relieves the digestive symptoms. The ferri et ammon. cit. may produce diarrhœa, in which case Blaud's pill should be substituted in doses of gr. 15 t.d.s., or Tab. Fersolate, one, t.d.s.

The Nutritional Anæmia of Infants. Mackay and Goodfellow (61) have studied this subject in the hospital type of infant in London. They estimate that 51% of artificially-fed babies and 45% of breast-fed babies are anæmic (taking as the standard of anæmia a Hb. figure 10% below normal). They consider this is due to a deficiency of iron and mineral substance in the food.

Treatment. This should be started before the age of two months, as a prophylactic measure. A mixture containing Ferri et ammon. cit. gr. 1½, aq. chlorof. ad m. 60 can be used. At first a few drops are given t.d.s. and the dose can be increased to m. 60 or 90 or more t.d.s. as required. As an alternative measure a medicated dried milk can be used, containing ferri et ammon. cit. in such proportion that between 4 and 9 grains are given daily. It was found that in the infants treated with iron the morbidity rate was halved as compared with a control series not so treated, and the weight showed a definite increase in the treated cases.

The Intravenous Administration of Iron

It was formerly thought that iron, given by mouth, is absorbed from the stomach and duodenum and excreted into the colon. It is now believed that no iron is excreted into the intestine and that the excess of iron in the fæces, which is noticed when iron is taken by mouth, is iron which has not been absorbed. Ferrous salts are more readily absorbed than are ferric ones, and iron is probably absorbed in the ferrous state. The iron is thought to combine with an acceptor substance, a protein called apoferritin, in the mucosal cells of the stomach and duodenum. This results in the formation of ferritin. The iron is released from ferritin to the blood when the plasma content falls below a certain level. The iron combines in the plasma with β_1 globulin. It has been shown that before the administration of iron there is very little ferritin or apoferritin in the mucosal cells. The absorption of iron causes the formation of apoferritin, and when ferritin yields its iron to the plasma the apoferritin disappears. It is possible that in the iron refractory types of anæmia there is a disturbance of the apoferritin-ferratin mechanism. In any case the utilisation of iron when administered by mouth is only about 14%.

Some patients suffering from iron-deficiency anæmia do not respond to the oral administration of iron even though they tolerate it, others are unable to take iron by mouth owing to gastro-intestinal disturbances. To meet the requirements of these two classes of patients, various experiments and investigations have been made to produce a preparation which can be safely administered intravenously in doses sufficiently large to cause hæmoglobin regeneration. The B.P. injectio ferri contains ferric chloride. The maximum dose for intramuscular injection is 30 minims, and this is equivalent to gr. 1/10 of iron, or gr. ½ of iron and ammonium citrate. Such a small dose is insufficient to relieve iron-deficiency anæmia.

Various ionised iron compounds, such as ferric ammonium citrate, have been used for parenteral administration, but when given intramuscularly they are painful, and when injected intravenously they are poisonous in amounts larger than 10 to 20 mg. of elemental iron.

Cappell (62), in 1930, investigating the distribution of iron in the tissues and its subsequent fate, showed that a 10% solution of saccharated oxide of iron, in amounts up to 0·3 ml. per 20 g. body weight, was well tolerated by mice on intravenous injection. There was no fear of producing hæmochromatosis, as the iron was not deposited in the pancreas. A considerable interval elapsed before these findings were applied clinically.

Goetsch and his colleagues (63) in 1946 injected colloidal ferric hydroxide or colloidal ferric oxide intravenously into 8 patients suffering from hypochromic microcytic anæmia. A single massive injection varying from 0·608 g. to 1·32 g. was used. The reticulocyte response was higher than would be expected in oral therapy, and there was good hæmoglobin regeneration. Severe toxic reactions, however, occurred in all but 2 cases, which contra-indicated the use of this measure as a therapeutic procedure. The toxic reactions are largely due to precipitation of iron in the blood, leading to pulmonary, and in some cases, to systemic emboli. There may also be gastro-intestinal disturbances, and depression of the nervous system resulting in coma and death. Nissim (64), a year later, tried the intravenous injection of colloidal ferric hydroxide and saccharated oxide of iron. The latter was a B.P.C. preparation containing about 3% of metallic iron in a sucrose solution. The saccharated oxide was found to be far less toxic than the ferric hydroxide, it is, however, a variable compound, and liable to precipitate on autoclaving. Slack and Wilkinson (65), in 1949, published the results of their experiments with various iron preparations. The most satisfactory was an iron sucrose solution obtained from anhydrous ferric chloride, sucrose, anhydrous sodium carbonate and sodium hydroxide. The final solution after filtration and autoclaving was clear, and dark brown, with a pH of about 10·5. It contained 2% elemental iron, and was given intravenously in repeated doses to over 120 people. It was found that the total dose of elemental iron required in iron deficiency anæmia is 24·5 mg. for each 1% deficit of hæmoglobin, as determined on the Haldane scale, plus 50% to restore the iron reserve in the tissues to normal. Alternatively 100 mg. of elemental iron should increase the hæmoglobin by 0·55 g. per 100 ml. The plan of dosage adopted was 25 mg. on the first day, 50 mg. on the second day, 100 mg. on the third day, and 200 mg. on the fourth and subsequent days. It is not wise to give a larger single dose than 200 mg. of this preparation. The solution used contained 2% elemental iron, with 200 mg. in 10 ml. A No. 2 stainless steel Record needle was used. The rate of injection should be 2 ml. a minute, and the same vein should not be used on consecutive days. To avoid local thrombophlebitis no pressure should be made over the vein when the needle is withdrawn, and movements of the arm should be made to encourage the rapid removal of the iron from the site of injection. Ferrivenin is another form of iron sucrose preparation used by these workers. Most of the 60 cases of iron-deficiency anæmia were treated as out-patients, and only one developed a mild reaction at the 200 mg. dose. Ten of these patients had proved refractory to full doses of iron given by mouth. It was noted that reticulocyte peak may reach 10% to 18% in seven to ten days from the beginning of the treatment. In almost all of the cases there was a rapid symptomatic and hæmatological response to treatment, and, unless chronic infection was present, nearly 100% of the injected iron appeared to be utilised. Thus a woman suffering from rheumatoid arthritis with a calculated iron deficiency of 1550 mg. required a total of 2550 mg. in three separate courses before there was a satisfactory response.

Govan and Scott (66) injected Ferrivenin in 25 cases of the anæmia of pregnancy, and found that about 40 mg. of elemental iron were required to raise the hæmoglobin by 1%. The larger amount of iron required may be due to the fœtus using some of the iron. The response to treatment was rapid, but in one case there was a severe reaction with faintness, giddiness, a sensation of bursting in the head, vomiting, slow pulse and extra systoles. The attack passed off in a few minutes, but no further injections of iron were given in this case. It is possible that the reaction was due to the fact that there had been an interval of 12 days between the previous injection and the one which proved toxic. The rapid response enables the treatment to be given during the last few weeks of pregnancy for it is at this time that the anæmia becomes severe. The necessity for a blood transfusion is thus avoided. Nissim and Robson (67), also in 1949, published their work on the methods of preparation and standardisation of saccharated iron oxide, using mice as test animals. They claimed that their preparation of iron-sucrose was less toxic than Ferrivenin, and that a dose of 300 mg. was not followed by reactions. A preparation of this nature is available under the name of Iviron, 100 mg. of iron being contained in 5 ml. Impurities in the sugar used in preparation may cause a severe anginal-like pain in the chest, arms and back. Sinclair and Duthie (68) used Ferrivenin in a series of cases of hypochromic anæmia associated with rheumatoid arthritis. A test dose of 50 mg. was injected, followed by 4 daily doses of 200 mg. Poor responses were obtained in those cases in which the sedimentation rate of the red cells was high. Ramsey (69), using Ferrivenin, tried to see if it were possible to give the amount of iron required, 300 to 800 mg., in a single intravenous injection. This somewhat bold experiment was quickly followed by a severe toxic reaction in the 11 cases so treated. The toxic reaction could be avoided by giving an initial dose of 100 mg., which is slowly increased to 200 or 300 mg.

The dose we are accustomed to employ is 50 mg. on the first day, 100 mg. on the second and third days, and 200 mg. on the subsequent days, until the calculated required dose is given. Owing to the dark colour of the iron solution it is not possible to see whether the needle is in the lumen of the vein by withdrawing a little blood into the syringe. The difficulty can be overcome by using a short glass connection, known as a "sightfeed", with a metal adaptor at each end, between the syringe and needle. A little blood withdrawn from the vein can be clearly seen in the glass connection. The blood serves as a buffer for the iron solution. The injection must be made slowly, about 2 ml. a minute, as rapid injection appears to cause venospasm. If the needle becomes displaced from the lumen of the vein during the injection the skin around is quickly stained a slate-grey colour. The injection must then be stopped immediately. The iron solution must never be mixed with saline, as an unstable preparation may be produced. If it is wished to administer the iron slowly by drip transfusion, as in a case of a child in which it has been necessary to cut down on the vein, the calculated amount of the iron solution is added to 900 ml. of 5% dextrose solution and run in at the rate of 30 to 45 drops a minute. In this way 35 or 40 ml. of iron solution (700–800 mg. iron) may be run in during the course of eight or nine hours.

Agranulocytic Angina and Malignant Neutropenia

The term "agranulocytic angina" was applied by Schultz (70) in 1922 to describe the illness of patients exhibiting severe progressive oral sepsis with marked prostration and neutropenia. Schilling (71) in 1929 suggested the alternative name of malignant neutropenia. Two varieties of acute cases are now described—primary agranulocytic angina and secondary malignant neutropenia. In the former, occasionally without any known cause, the patient is taken ill with fever, severe prostration and ulcerative lesions in the mouth or other mucous membranes, such as the vagina. There is a total reduction of the white cells, often to below 1,000 per c.mm. and a very low polymorphonuclear count. Many of these cases are now thought to be due to amidopyrine or to an amidopyrine and barbiturate compound, to which the patient has become susceptible by a preliminary sensitising dose.

Plum (72), in Copenhagen, recorded seven cases of agranulocytosis due to amidopyrine, and since 1933 many cases of agranulocytosis have been recorded developing after the therapeutic administration of amidopyrine preparations, such as Pyramidon, Gardan and Amidophen, or to barbiturates containing amidopyrine, such as Allonal, Cibalgin, Compral, Somnosal, Veramon and Veropyron. Agranulocytosis has also followed the administration of dinitrophenol, dinitrocresol, benzol, arsenic preparations, Sedormid, bismuth and gold salts. A fatal case following the administration of prontosil flavum has been recorded in Holland by Borst (73), and in America death has followed the use of sulfanilamide as recorded by Schwartz and his co-workers (74), and by Berg and his co-workers (75). It has also resulted from the use of other sulphonamide drugs, especially if improperly given in small doses for prolonged periods, or in amounts totalling more than 25 to 30 g., and from the use of thiouracil. Both types of disease, if untreated, in the majority of cases pursue a rapidly fatal course. The blood changes in malignant neutropenia resemble those of agranulocytic angina, but they are secondary to some infection such as pneumonia, sinusitis, osteomyelitis, staphylococcal septicæmia or liver abscess. Further, chronic cases of neutropenia have been described by Doan (76), in which the white cells from time to time fall below 4,000 per c.mm., owing to a reduction of the granulocytes, with accompanying symptoms of ill-health and a liability to septic infections. Barsby and Close (77) describe a case of a recurrent agranulocytosis in which the symptoms recurred for three to seven days after the menstrual periods for four years, and during the last seven months of the patient's life, were accompanied by a neutrophil agranulocytosis.

Treatment. In 1924, Jackson (78) demonstrated the existence in normal human blood of pentose nucleotides. Jackson and his co-workers (79) in 1931 and 1932 reported the effect of treatment of cases of agranulocytic angina and malignant neutropenia with a preparation called "nucleotide K.96". This is now available as "pentnucleotide" and is put up in ampoules of 10 ml. containing 0·7 g.

In very acute cases 0·7 g. of pentnucleotide in 100 ml. of saline is injected slowly intravenously every morning for four days, and 0·7 g. of pentnucleotide in 10 ml. of distilled water is injected in the evening intramuscularly. The intramuscular injections are continued subsequently twice daily until the white cell count has definitely risen, and then an injection is given once a day until the white count has been essentially normal for three consecutive days. If there is myocardial degeneration the intravenous injection should not be given, owing to risk of hear failure from the reaction of dyspnœa and palpitations which is often provoked. In the average case only the daily intramuscular injections are given. The patient may appear worse during the first days of the treatment, but the improvement is usually definitely noted by the fourth or fifth day and the blood count returns to normal by the eighth or tenth day. In addition to the injections a careful search should be made for ulceration of the mucous membranes, or local abscesses elsewhere, and these should be appropriately treated. Blood transfusions are of doubtful value, but if the patient is intolerant of pentnucleotide, as shown by symptoms of cardiac distress after a trial dose, a small transfusion (500 ml.) should be given. The use of penicillin in the treatment of agranulocytosis is described in Chapter II.

Results. Jackson and his co-workers (80) have reported sixty-nine cases treated by pentnucleotide by themselves and other physicians, with a recovery rate of 74%. In cases treated previously by various other methods a cure was only effected in 25% of cases. Cases successfully treated in England by pentnucleotide have been recorded by Bulmer (81), Marriott (82), Wilkinson and Israëls (83), and by Smith (84), and we have also treated a severe case of malignant neutropenia with good results. Fairley and Scott (85) report a fatal case of agranulocytic angina, in which there was a complete absence of response to nucleotide K.96 injections. It must, however, be remembered that the American observers report a recovery rate of only 74%. Israëls and Wilkinson (86) say that pentnucleotide has little effect in chronic neutropenia. For the latter Gupta and Witts (87) recommend the intramuscular injection of liver. It should be noted that pentnucleotide is useless in the treatment of aplastic anæmia, of leukæmia or of sepsis without neutropenia and leucopenia. We have also successfully treated with penicillin a case of agranulocytosis due to thiouracil.

Sternal Puncture

Ghedini (88) of Genoa, in 1908, introduced the method of human bone marrow biopsy by puncturing the shaft of the tibia and withdrawing a small amount of marrow for microscopical examination. Seyfarth (89), in 1923, recommended that the sternum should be trephined rather than the tibia, and Arinkin (90), in 1927, advised that a thick needle should be used for sternal puncture. Peabody (91), in 1927, investigated bone marrow, obtained by trephine from the tibia, in cases of pernicious anæmia. Salah (92), in 1937, described the needle which now forms the model of that used for sternal puncture. He used "a lumbar puncture needle (made of hard steel) with its stillet (*sic*) cut to 3 cms. length, its point sharpened but made broad so that it will not break. A movable shield is made to fit round the needle with a screw to fix it at the required distance."

The figures for the normal range of marrow cells have been worked out by Nordenson (93), Young and Osgood (94), Vogel, Erf and Rosenthal (95) and by Hynes (96). In some cases, especially in aplastic anæmia and myelosclerosis, it is necessary to know the histological structure of bone marrow, which can be done by removing a disc of bone with a 1 cm. trephine.

Method. A Salah or Klima pattern needle is sterilised in hot oil. The patient is given an injection of morphine, gr. $\frac{1}{4}$, or aspirin, gr. 10 and nepenthe, m. 15, by mouth, half an hour before the operation. The skin over the manubrium sterni is sterilised with alcohol or iodine. The skin, subcutaneous tissues and periosteum are infiltrated with about 1 ml. of 2% procaine hydrochloride solution, in the mid-line at the level of the third costal cartilage, using a fine intradermic needle with a short bevel. The patient lies on his back with a pillow between the shoulders. The Salah needle is then passed through the skin down to the sternum. The adjustable stop is fixed 5 mm. above the skin, and the needle is forced through the outer table of the bone by means of gentle taps with a small hammer. When it is felt to enter the medullary cavity the stylet is withdrawn and a dry 1 ml. syringe is attached. Marrow juice is

TABLE 1

Cells.	Neutrophil per cent.	Eosinophil per cent.	Basophil per cent.
Segmented polymorphs	9 –30	0–3	0–0 5
Non-segmented polymorphs	20 –40	0–2	0–1
Metamyelocytes	2 5–12	0–2 5	—
Myelocytes	2 – 8	0–1	—
Premyelocytes	0 5– 5		
Myeloblasts	0 – 2·5		
Lymphocytes	5 –20	Total cell count 25,000	
Plasma cells	0 – 1	to 100,000 per c.mm.	
Monocytes	0 – 5		
Normoblasts	7 –19	Myeloid-erythroblastic	
Erythroblasts	2 – 7	ratio	
Megaloblasts	0 – 4	2 : 1 to 8 : 1.	

then sucked into the syringe. This produces a sensation of discomfort or even of actual pain. Hynes (96) recommends that 0·25 ml. of marrow fluid be withdrawn and placed in a tube containing Wintrobe's dry oxalate mixture. The tube is prepared by placing in it 0·1 ml. of a solution of 0·2% potassium oxalate and 0·3% ammonium oxalate and drying it in the incubator. Smears are then prepared, stained by Leishman's method, and a differential count is made of 400 or 500 cells.

Dangers. Death from perforation of the right ventricle during sternal puncture has been recorded by Scherer and Howe (97) and by Bardhan (98). In Scherer and Howe's case the needle penetrated the sternum to a depth of ¾ in., and in Bardhan's 2 cases the screw-guard was fixed at a level of 8 mm. and 11 mm. Hæmophilia is usually regarded as a contra-indication, although successful cases have been recorded by Limarzi et al. (99).

Normal Marrow Findings

The normal ranges in the bone marrow differential count, as described by Hynes (96), are shown in Table I. The cells in the lymphocyte series include the lymphoblast, when it is possible to distinguish it from the myeloblast, and a variety of intermediate forms. The first six types of cell in the table are myeloid in nature and the last three are erythroblastic.

Abnormal Marrow Findings

Leukæmia. Sternal puncture is of great value in the diagnosis of aleukæmic (leucopenic) leukæmia. The marrow changes here are similar to those found in leukæmia with leucocytosis.

The Acute Leukæmias. The marrow is very cellular, 70 to 99% of the marrow cells being primitive white cells either of the myeloid or lymphatic series. The proportion of primitive red cells is low, but the erythroblasts almost equal in number the normoblasts. There is no premature hæmoglobinisation of the erythroblasts such as occurs in the bone marrow in pernicious anæmia. This maturation defect is probably associated with the macrocytic anæmia which is so often present in leukæmia.

Chronic Lymphatic Leukæmia. Here 40 to 90% of the marrow cells are lymphocytes, which may be normal small lymphocytes or show abnormalities in the size and structure of the nucleus. The myeloid cells and the erythroblasts show a maturation defect.

Chronic Myeloid Leukæmia. The marrow in early cases shows an increase in myeloblasts, premyelocytes and myelocytes. Lymphocytes and monocytes are few or absent. There is a maturation defect in the nucleated red cells. In the final stages of the disease the marrow resembles that found in acute myeloid leukæmia.

Pernicious Anæmia. In untreated cases 25 to 45% of the marrow cells are megaloblasts and erythroblasts, and premature hæmoglobinisation is present. The polymorphs are greatly decreased, but the number of earlier myeloid cells is not affected.

Aplastic Anæmia. The bone marrow should be studied by histological section and not by needle puncture. The marrow is usually hypoplastic, showing a lack of mature cells, particularly of the myeloid type, and an increase of primitive cells resembling small lymphocytes. In other cases the marrow is hyperplastic with many primitive cells. Israëls and Wilkinson (100) state that megaloblasts are not found.

Achrestic Anæmia. Israëls and Wilkinson (100) found megaloblastic hyperplasia resembling that of pernicious anæmia. Hynes (96) examined the marrow in one case and recorded an increase in the early hæmoglobinised erythroblasts and also in the normoblasts. The megaloblasts were normal. Mahler and Greenberg (101) found increased megaloblastic activity with diminished numbers of normoblasts.

Other Macrocytic Anæmias. In sprue and in carcinoma of the stomach marrow changes are found similar to those in pernicious anæmia.

Secondary Anæmias. Young and Osgood (94) demonstrated an erythroblastic reaction in the bone marrow in the anæmia which accompanies hæmorrhage, toxæmias and infections.

Polycythæmia. In some cases there is an increase in the erythroblasts and myeloid cells in the marrow. In others the only change found is an increase in the segmented polymorphs.

Acholuric Jaundice. In chronic cases the marrow is usually normal; in the acute phases, however, there is an increase of the normoblasts, erythroblasts and megaloblasts.

Agranulocytosis. In some cases there appears to be a

maturation defect, the bone marrow having its normal number of cells, but all the myeloid cells being myeloblasts. In others there is an aplasia of the marrow, lymphocytes and plasma cells being the only white cells present.

Gaucher's Disease. The typical Gaucher's cells are present in the marrow.

Kala-azar. The Leishman-Donovan bodies are seen in the monocytes in the marrow.

Malaria. Parasites are more numerous than in the blood, being seen in the red cells and leucocytes in the marrow.

Myelomatosis. An excess of plasma cells may be present in the marrow.

Carcinomatosis. In secondary carcinoma of bone, carcinoma cells, in groups or isolated, are found in some instances in the marrow.

The appearances of the bone marrow in the abnormal conditions described above are largely based on the article of Hynes (96).

Conclusions. Sternal puncture is chiefly of value in the diagnosis of leukæmia with leucopenia, enabling a confident opinion to be expressed which cannot be done by blood examinations alone. It is also of value in the diagnosis of obscure cases of anæmia and certain other diseases, as described above.

Bone Marrow Transfusion

In some cases it is extremely difficult, if not impossible, to introduce fluids into the body by the direct intravenous route. This is likely to be so in adults if the veins are collapsed owing to shock, or if they are compressed by œdema of the subcutaneous tissues. Similar difficulties are met with in young children profoundly dehydrated as the result of gastro-enteritis, and in infants whose veins are either too small to receive the cannula or too tender to retain it even if successfully introduced.

That fluid may pass from the bone marrow cavity through the emissary veins into the general circulation was demonstrated by Tocantins and O'Neill (102) in America in 1936. Experimenting on the transplantation of marrow from animal to animal, they observed that if two needles were inserted into the marrow cavity of the rabbit's femur, one at either end of the bone, and 5 ml. of saline injected through the proximal needle, only about 2 ml. of fluid would come up through the needle at the distal end. Further investigations proved that the fluid passed direct from the bone marrow into the general circulation. Tocantins and O'Neill were not slow in applying their experimental results to clinical medicine, and, using the bone marrow of the sternum, the lower end of the femur and the upper end of the tibia, successfully infused citrated blood, citrated plasma, 5% dextrose solution and physiological saline into the general circulation both of adults and of children. These workers considered that the method was likely to prove of value in patients suffering from extensive burns, mutilating wounds, generalised œdema, circulatory collapse or where the veins are poorly developed or have been rendered useless by repeated punctures or by injections of hypertonic saline. A case of diabetic coma was successfully treated by infusion of insulin and dextrose solution into the bone marrow, attempts at intravenous injection having failed, as the patient was pulseless and the veins were collapsed.

Hamilton Bailey (103) in 1944 reported on his experiences of the method in England and concluded that not only is the medullary cavity of the sternum as good a receptor as a vein for all kinds of infusions and for Pentothal, to induce anæsthesia, but it is particularly valuable for the resuscitation of the very shocked and the very young. Again in 1946 (104) he recorded how a patient was rapidly revived after a severe surgical operation by the injection of over a pint of saline into the sternal marrow cavity, the infusion being completed within three minutes using a sternal puncture trocar and cannula and Record syringes.

Sternal Transfusion. Strict aseptic precautions must be taken to prevent the likelihood of osteomyelitis developing as a complication. In the method described by Hamilton Bailey (103) the patient lies flat and 2 ml. of 1% procaine hydrochloride solution are infiltrated into the skin, subcutaneous tissues and periosteum in the midline just above the manubrio-gladiolar junction, the site of the injection then being massaged with a sterile swab so that the bony landmark can be clearly felt. The special trocar and cannula for sternal puncture is now pushed with a boring movement through the outer plate of the bone just above the manubrio-gladiolar junction, and directly the outer plate is felt to be penetrated the direction of the instrument is changed, the point being directed upwards towards the patient's head and the wings now prevent the point from piercing the inner plate of the bone. The trocar is withdrawn, and a Record syringe, half-filled with 3·8% sodium citrate solution, is attached to the cannula, a little citrate solution injected into the marrow cavity, and, on slowly withdrawing the piston, the syringe is seen to fill with the red bone marrow. Some more citrate is now injected, the syringe disconnected, and the cannula joined to the transfusion apparatus, the tubing of which must be free from air bubbles. The wings of the cannula, and the tubing are held in position by strapping attached to the chest wall, and the transfusion allowed to proceed. The container holding the fluid should be between 4 and 6 feet above the level of the sternum; if the pressure is too high pain will ensue. The flow of blood can be aided by oxygen pressure or by the use of a blood-saline mixture.

Tibial Transfusion. This is the method of choice for infants and young children. The leg must be maintained in a semi-externally rotated position by means of a splint, the other leg being loosely tied to the side of the cot to prevent dislocation of the cannula by kicking. Gunz and Dean (105) found that the legs were most satisfactorily controlled by firmly bandaging the soles of the feet to a padded splint, the feet being about 9 inches apart and the ends of the splint tied to the sides of the cot. Gimson (106) has devised four needles and stylets of different length and size for tibial transfusion in infants and young children (see Fig. 54). The flange is fixed and each needle has its own stylet. The needles measure below the flange, $\frac{1}{4}$ inch, $\frac{3}{8}$ inch,

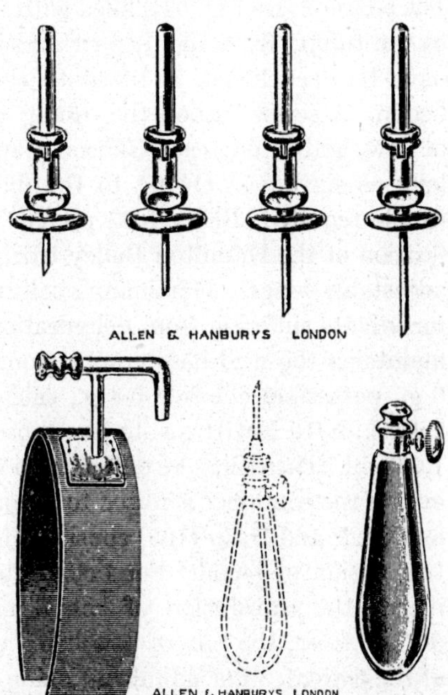

FIG. 54. Needles, etc., for bone marrow transfusion.

$\frac{1}{2}$ inch and $\frac{5}{8}$ inch. The two shorter needles are size 18 S.W.G., the two longer ones 16 S.W.G. The $\frac{1}{4}$ inch needle is for premature infants and the newborn, the $\frac{1}{2}$ inch and $\frac{5}{8}$ inch needles for children of about 5 years, but the size of the child and the amount of subcutaneous fat must be taken into consideration in selecting the needle. The handle (see Fig. 54) is screwed on to the stylet, and the needle and stylet inserted, after preliminary cleaning of the skin and anæsthetisation with procaine, into the subcutaneous surface of the tibia, and at right-angles to the subcutaneous bony plate. The site selected is inferior and medial to the anterior tibial tuberosity, below the epiphyseal line and above the nutrient artery. The flange rests on the skin, the point of the needle being in the marrow cavity. The stylet is withdrawn and a small amount of marrow wells up or is sucked up into a syringe partly filled with saline attached to the needle. A little saline is injected into the marrow cavity to make sure that the needle is in position. The adaptor (see Fig. 54), filled with transfusion fluid and connected to the tubing from the dripper and bottle from which air bubbles have been excluded, is fitted to the needle and the transfusion begun. A screw clip on the tubing can be used to adjust the rate of flow, and in one case Gimson maintained the transfusion for as long as six days. Owing to the difficulty in judging the size of needle required, Behr (107) prefers for tibial transfusion a modification of the Hamilton Bailey trocar and cannula, furnished with adjustable wings. Hartmann's solution is valuable as a transfusion for infants suffering from dehydration due to gastro-enteritis, as it maintains the acid-base equilibrium. It contains sodium chloride 6 g., potassium chloride 0·4 g., calcium chloride 0·2 g., lactic acid 2·4 ml., N/10 NaOH q.s. to neutralise the lactic acid, and water to 1,000 ml. There may be difficulty in transfusing blood, if undiluted, even if the container is raised to as much as 7 feet above the needle, and Gunz and Dean (105) considered the method unsuitable for the transfusion of blood. For dehydrated infants Behr (107) recommends the transfusion of half strength Hartmann's solution in 5% dextrose, the rate of flow being varied according to the weight of the patient. For infants weighing less than 5 lbs. the flow should be 4 drops a minute, if under $7\frac{1}{2}$ lbs. 6 drops a minute, under 10 lbs. 8 drops a minute, and under 15 lbs. 12 drops a minute. The drops apply to a drip-bulb delivering 1 ml. in 16 drops.

Massey (108) has reviewed the literature of bone marrow infusions, and concludes that the intra-tibial method is very satisfactory for the administration of parental fluids in infants when difficulty is found with the intravenous method.

HEPARIN

McLean (109), in 1916, extracted from dog liver a substance which retards the coagulation of blood *in vitro*. Further investigations were carried out by Howell and Holt (110) in 1918 and the anti-coagulant substance was called heparin. In 1923 Howell and Holt (111) described an improved method for its preparation and defined the unit of heparin as being that weight of substance which would prevent 1 ml. of cat blood from clotting for twenty-four hours when kept in the cold. McHenry and Glaister, at Best's suggestion, subsequently prepared small quantities of heparin from beef liver, and Charles and Scott (112), in 1933, evolved a process by which it could be prepared in much larger quantities from liver. They also obtained a blood anti-coagulant, presumably heparin, from skeletal muscle and lung. In 1936 the same workers (113) prepared a crystalline barium salt of heparin having a high potency of about 500 units per mg. They gave the empirical formula of heparin as $C_{25}H_{65}O_{50}N_2S_5$. By treating the crystalline barium salt with excess of ammonium carbonate solution at 65°C. the barium was removed, the heparin was then precipitated by acetic acid, centrifuged down, washed with ether and dried. For use a solution is prepared to which tricresol is added, and it is sterilised by passing through a Berkefeld filter. Jorpes and Bergstrom (114) classified heparin as a mucoitin polysulphuric acid, closely related to chondroitin-sulphuric acid. Best (115) has suggested as a standard that the unit is the activity contained in 0·01 mg. (10γ) of the barium-free material, *i.e.*, 100 units in 1 mg. There is evidence to suggest that heparin is either formed in, or stored in the mast cells, as had been shown by Jorpes, Holmgren and Wilander (116).

Mode of Action. It is believed by Howell that heparin is normally present in the blood. Howell and Holt (110) showed that heparin has no effect in preventing coagulation when added to mixtures of thrombin and fibrinogen, and differs in this respect from hirudin. They suggested that it delays coagulation by inhibiting the activation of prothrombin to thrombin. Mellanby

(117) considered that heparin acts as an antithrombase and says it is improbable that heparin is responsible for the normal fluidity of blood. He suggests that heparin is concerned with the prevention of localised thrombosis in the immediate neighbourhood of disintegrating tissue. Best (118), in 1939, upheld the view that heparin apparently combines with the antithrombin of the serum albumin fraction and thus acts as an anti-coagulant by increasing the affinity of this substance for thrombin.

Clinical Applications. Heparin has been used in surgery, in medicine and in blood examinations. Heparin is available in sterile solution in rubber-capped vials of 3 ml. ($\frac{1}{2}$% = 5 mg. per ml.); of 5 ml. (1% = 10 mg. per ml.), and of 5 ml. (5% = 50 mg. per ml.). This preparation contains 500 units per mg. Heparinised tubes (10 ml.), each containing 1 mg., are available for collection of blood samples. In man 1 mg. of heparin per kg. body weight, when given intravenously, prolongs the coagulation time to approximately forty minutes. For clinical use the average dose for an adult is 75 to 150 mg., given intravenously in the form of a 5% solution. This dose is repeated every third or fourth hour, four or five times a day, and the effect should be checked by determination of the coagulation rate, which should be kept at about fifteen to twenty minutes by the Lee and White method (normal four to seven minutes).

Surgical. Murray et al. (119), after showing that heparin will prevent thrombosis resulting from mechanical and chemical injury to blood vessels in dogs, first administered heparin to a patient in a surgical ward of the Toronto General Hospital in 1935. The solution was injected into the brachial artery under local anæsthesia, and samples of blood from the veins of the injected arm showed a rise in clotting time from the normal of six minutes to that of eighteen minutes. Subsequently heparin was administered post-operatively as a prophylactic measure against thrombosis. The injections were commenced two to three hours after the operation and were continued for twenty-four to 120 hours. An effort was was made to keep the clotting time at fifteen to twenty minutes. The operations included appendicectomy, herniotomy, resection of colon, etc. Heparin has also been used in arteriotomies for embolism. Crafoord (120) advises that in these cases it may be necessary to start heparinisation during the operation. When heparin has thus been given, or when hæmorrhage unexpectedly sets in during the course of heparin treatment, the original coagulation time of the blood may be restored by the injection of protamine. Chargaff and Olson (121) described this neutralising effect on heparin, and Jorpes et al. (122) state that 60 mg. of protamine (Clupein) instantaneously neutralise the effect of 100 mg. of heparin. They say, however, that the protamine injection should only be used as a last resort, and a blood tranfusion will usually effect the necessary hæmostasis. Richmond (123) records a case which shows that the intravenous injection of heparin to prevent post-operative thrombosis is not devoid of danger. An intravenous injection of 20 mg. of heparin in normal saline was given to a girl aged eleven years after removal of a twisted ovarian dermoid. Massive hæmaturia occurred sixteen hours later, the blood coagulation time being seventeen minutes. The patient was very collapsed, but recovered with bladder irrigations and a blood transfusion.

Medical. Ploman (124) used heparin in the treatment of acute thrombosis of the central vein of the retina. Intravenous injections of a 5% heparin solution were given with a fine needle. Four injections were made daily, the first three of 50 mg. and the last of 100 mg. Marked improvement or full restoration of vision was obtained. Magnusson (125) recorded a case of thrombosis of the posterior inferior cerebellar artery in a woman aged forty-eight. Intravenous injections of a 5% solution were used; 150 mg. in the morning and afternoon of the first day, and the same amount three times a day for five days. He states that the case was a severe one and that improvement was more rapid than would be expected normally. Kelson and White (126) have reported some favourable results in the treatment of subacute bacterial endocarditis by the combined use of heparin and sulphapyridine. Their method is as follows: The contents of a 10 ml. vial of heparin (10,000 units) are added to 500 ml. of normal saline and the solution is given by continuous intravenous drip for fourteen days. The rate of flow, usually 15 to 25 drops per minute, is regulated to maintain as well as possible the venous clotting time at approximately one hour. Sulphapyridine, g. 4–6 daily, is given by mouth for a week before, during and a week after the heparin treatment. Blood transfusions are given if there is an anæmia of 3·5 million red cells or lower. All patients are saturated with ascorbic acid, 200 mg. being given by mouth four times a day for three days and subsequently 100 mg. a day.

We have used this method in 2 cases of subacute bacterial (streptococcus viridans) endocarditis without benefit, the patients dying a few weeks later. If the sulphapyridine, which is given before the heparin, fails to sterilise the blood, there appears to be an increased risk of the occurrence of vascular accidents, such as cerebral hæmorrhage. McLean, Meyer and Griffith (127), reviewing 67 cases treated by this method, report very unfavourably on it.

Heparin has also been used in the treatment of thrombophlebitis, including the migratory type, in pulmonary embolism and in coronary thrombosis. Murray (128) states that in phlebitis the effect of heparin is most noticeable when given early in the disease. In the migratory type, although the heparin will probably relieve the symptoms of thrombosis, it will not affect the cause of the disease. In an average case of thrombophlebitis, heparin is given for ten days. After the first three to four days the patient is encouraged to move actively in bed, and he should get up by the tenth to twelfth day. Murray (128) records that 22 cases of massive pulmonary embolism have been treated with heparin with pleasing results; no patient died from the embolism, and dyspnœa and distress were rapidly relieved. Some cases of coronary thrombosis have been treated, but experimental results indicate that heparin may prevent the occurrence of mural thrombosis with subsequent risk of peripheral embolus formation. Stansfield (129) treated successfully a case of puerperal cerebral thrombophlebitis with heparin, using an intravenous drip of 5% dextrose saline, containing 200 mg. heparin in each pint. The coagulation time was prolonged to forty minutes by this treatment. Other cases of recovery have, however, been recorded without the use of heparin. Massive hæmaturia has resulted from the treatment of a case of cavernous sinus thrombosis with sulphathiazole and heparin, as described by Ershler and Blaisdell (130). The evidence given in the article indicates that the bleeding was due to the heparin and not to the sulphathiazole.

Blood Transfusions. Hedenius (131), in 1937, reported on the use of heparin in blood transfusion. A 5% solution is used, 1 mg. per kg. body weight being injected intravenously into the donor. The blood coagulation time is prolonged rapidly at first and returns to normal in one and a half hours. Ten minutes after the injection blood is removed from the donor with any standard equipment, and the whole blood in its natural state injected into the recipient. If syringes are used the plunger should be moistened with a drop of sterile paraffin to prevent cell destruction and kinase production. The coagulation rate of the recipient is not affected. The technique employed in citrate transfusions may also be used, heparin being added to the drawn blood instead of citrate, using 20 mg. heparin (0·4 ml. of a 5% solution diluted with 10 ml. sterile saline) for 500 ml. of blood. These methods have also been reported on favourably by Sappington (132) in America.

Blood Examinations. Heparinised blood may be used for biochemical and cytological examinations, but is not suitable for performing the Wassermann reaction. The blood is placed in a 10 ml. tube containing 1 mg. of heparin, which is distributed as a smear on the inside of the tube. A leucocyte count should be carried out within two hours of collecting the blood.

Conclusions. It is evident that the administration of heparin is not devoid of danger from cerebral or renal hæmorrhage, and its use seems only to be justified in cases in which the treatment is very carefully controlled.

Plasma Transfusion

Clinically many occasions arise where plasma is preferable to whole blood for transfusion. They occur where there is marked fluid loss but no loss of red cells, as in post-operative shock and in shock following burns and wounds. It may also be used to restore blood volume after a hæmorrhage, should no blood be available. In burn shock with marked hæmoconcentration, the hæmatocrit reading is a useful guide in treatment. Infusion of plasma until the plasma–cell ratio is normal and constant greatly reduced the mortality.

Whilst plasma has the advantage of being easily and quickly administered to any patient without matching, and requires no special storage, the risk of transmitting the virus which produces serum hepatitis, with the possible complication of liver necrosis and cirrhosis, must be borne in mind. (See Chapter VI.) At first large pool plasma batches (*i.e.* at least 300 donors) were used, with varying reports for the incidence of serum hepatitis. In the series of Brightman and Korns (133) it was 4·5% and Havens (134) reported it as high as 16%. It is now recommended that only small pool batches (*i.e.* not more than 10 donors) should be used, when the incidence falls to a rate comparable with that of whole blood transfusion. In the series of Lehane and others (135) the incidence from small pools was 1·3% and from whole blood 0·8%.

The early claims that irradiation with ultra-violet light would destroy the virus have been disproved by the reports of Rosenthal, Bassen and Michael (136), James, Korns and Wright (137) and others.

In 1943 Grönwall and Ingelman (138) in Sweden began work on a plasma substitute named Dextran which is now available. It is a non-antigenic polysaccharide built entirely of glucose molecules; a 6% solution having a viscosity similar to that of plasma. It is metabolised within five days of administration and carries no risk of transmitting serum hepatitis.

Dextran produces very heavy rouleaux formation. Therefore blood samples required for grouping and matching should be taken before the administration of Dextran.

The Rhesus Blood Group System

In 1940 Landsteiner and Wiener (139) showed that the antibody produced by the immunisation of rabbits with the blood of the Macacus rhesus monkey agglutinated the red cells of 85% of the white population of New York. Those persons whose cells are agglutinated are termed Rh positive and the remainder Rh negative. Wiener and Peters (140) described antibodies which reacted in the same way as the anti-Rh rabbit sera in 3 patients who developed transfusion reactions from the administration of homologous ABO blood. In 1941, Levine, Katzin, Burnham and Vogel (141) demonstrated that erythroblastosis fœtalis is due to rhesus incompatibility between mother and child.

Further antibodies agglutinating 80%, 70% and 30% of test cells were discovered and in 1943 Fisher (142) suggested that the rhesus system consisted of 3 pairs of allelomorphic genes which he called C and c, D and d, E and e. Allelomorphic genes are alternative genes, capable of occupying the same locus on a chromosome. These 3 allelomorphic pairs give rise to eight phenotypes.

Fisher's notation	*Convenient "shorthand" notation*
CDe	R_1
cDE	R_2
cDe	R_0
Cde	R′
cdE	R″
CDE	R_z
CdE	R_y
cde	r

Further alleles, some very rare, have since been described, increasing the number of Rh phenotypes. Three alleles of C and c are C^w, reported by Callender and Race (143), and C^u and c^v by Race, Sanger and Lawler (144). Stratton (145) described D^u, an allele of D and d. Recently two alleles of E and e were reported, E^u by Armytage, Ceppellini, Ikin and Mourant (146) and e^x by Gilbey (147).

However, from the clinician's point of view, the important factor in most cases is whether or not the patient is D positive or D negative.

Production of Rhesus Antibodies. These antibodies are immune and rarely, if ever, occur naturally. They occur either from stimulation due to multiple pregnancies or from repeated blood transfusions. During pregnancy some of the fœtal red cells escape into the mother's circulation via the placenta, and should they carry an Rh antigen derived from the father but not possessed by the mother, they may act as a foreign substance, sensitise the mother and cause the production of antibodies in her serum. Generally the first pregnancy sensitises the mother and antibodies appear in future pregnancies. These antibodies return to the fœtus via the placenta, destroy fœtal red cells and produce erythroblastosis fœtalis. Similarly, transfusion of blood of heterologous Rh group, may sensitise the patient, with the production of antibodies at subsequent transfusions. As small a volume as 1 or 2 ml. of blood may be sufficient to sensitise, even if given in early childhood.

Obviously blood of a different Rh type to that of the patient is frequently transfused, and many mothers carry a fœtus of another Rh type to that of themselves, and yet antibody production is much less frequent than might be expected. The explanation is that the genes have varying antigenic potency; *i.e.*, varying ability to produce an antibody if introduced into the circulation. D is by far the most powerful antigen, followed by C, and the great majority of Rh antibodies are anti-D or anti-C + D. E and c are weaker antigens and antibodies to either are not often encountered, while e and d are very weak antigens and only two examples of anti-d have been reported. Thus erythroblastosis mainly affects infants of Rh negative mothers and seldom those of Rh positive mothers. For the same reason it is important that Rh negative persons, particularly young girls and women in the childbearing period, should be transfused with Rh negative blood only.

People vary in their ability to produce antibodies and this may explain why only 1 in 10 or 15 of Rh negative women married to Rh positive men have infants affected by erythroblastosis fœtalis. In Great Britain approximately 1 in every 200 infants at birth have their red cells sensitised by maternal antibodies; not all are clinically affected, a positive direct Coombs' test on the infant's red cells at birth sometimes being the only evidence of sensitisation *in vivo*.

In assessing the prognosis for future pregnancies in a family where a child has suffered from erythroblastosis, it is an advantage to know the Rh genotype of the husband. Taking as a common

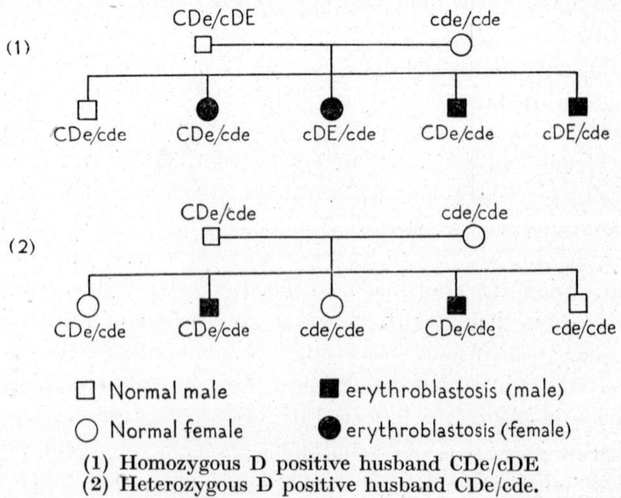

(1) Homozygous D positive husband CDe/cDE
(2) Heterozygous D positive husband CDe/cde.

example an Rh negative mother who has produced anti-D, should the husband be homozygous D positive all future children will almost certainly be affected, but if the husband is heterozygous D positive only half the children may be affected.

How is it possible for a child to suffer from erythroblastosis when both parents have been reported as Rh positive? In routine work, because the full genotyping sera are very rare and as D is the most powerful antigen, blood is examined for the presence or absence of the D antigen only, with anti-D serum. Therefore a mother (R_1R_1) (CDe/CDe) and father (R_2r) (cDE/cde) would both be reported Rh positive, but the mother might develop anti-E or anti-c as she lacks both these antigens, while the fœtus will carry either or both of them.

Anthropological Value of Blood Group Systems. The blood group frequencies vary in races throughout the world and are valuable in anthropological studies. As people migrate and intermarry with local populations, frequency differences tend to merge, but small racially " pure " communities may still be found. The Hungarian gipsies are known to have come from India many generations ago and a study of their ABO groups helps to confirm this. Their frequency for A and B is very close to that of the Indian Hindus but quite different from that of the ordinary Hungarian population.

Group B increases in frequency towards the East. In Great Britain it has a frequency of 8%, in Eastern Europe, Poles 20%, Russians 23%, and in the Peking Chinese it is 35%.

Even in Britain the frequencies show significant variations. Travelling from Southern England to Northern England the value for O steadily increases and that for A decreases. The Icelandic people have an ABO frequency similar to that found in Northern Scotland, suggesting a common ancestry. Changes occur also in the Rhesus distribution. The Basques have the highest Rh negative frequency known, while the North American Indians and Chinese are almost entirely Rh positive. The latter are said to develop erythroblastosis fœtalis only very rarely.

ABO Grouping. To each of 2 tubes, one containing a volume of anti-A serum and the other a volume of anti-B serum, add a volume of a 2% saline suspension of the washed unknown cells. Similarly add a volume of the unknown serum to each of two tubes, one containing a volume of known A cells and the other a volume of known B cells. Tap the tubes to mix the contents and leave at room temperature (about 20°C.) for one to two hours. The tests may then be read macroscopically, and if apparently negative, microscopically by transferring the contents on to a glass slide. Known A, B and O cells must be added to tubes containing anti-A and anti-B to act as controls for the tests.

Determination of Rh groups. A volume of the unknown cell suspension is added to two tubes each containing a volume of different anti-D sera, as some D positive red cells will not react with all anti-D sera. The tubes are incubated at 37°C. for two hours and then the cells are gently transferred on to a glass slide and read microscopically. Rh agglutinates are fragile and rough-handling will break them up and cause errors. Both D positive and D negative red cells must be used as controls. This method gives the most accurate results but two rapid methods are described. That of Chown (148) requires the mixing of a high-titre anti-D serum with the unknown cells in their own serum in a capillary tube and incubating at 37°C. for fifteen to twenty minutes. In the method of Diamond and Abelson (149) a drop of high-titre anti-D serum is mixed with test cells in their own serum on a slide which is warmed and rocked on a special box for three minutes. Not all anti-D sera are suitable for these two rapid methods.

Rhesus Antibodies. These antibodies are immune (*i.e.*, result from iso-immunisation) and in common with other immune blood-group antibodies react most strongly at 37°C. Two forms exist—complete and incomplete.

Complete antibodies are saline agglutinating antibodies; *i.e.*, a serum containing a complete antibody will agglutinate red cells carrying the appropriate antigen when they are suspended in saline. Incomplete antibodies are also termed blocking antibodies or albumin agglutinating antibodies. An incomplete antibody will not agglutinate appropriate red cells suspended in saline, but will so affect them that they can no longer be agglutinated by a saline agglutinating antibody, *i.e.*, the cells are " blocked ". However, incomplete antibodies will agglutinate appropriate red cells if they are suspended in 20% bovine albumin.

Coombs' Test. *Direct.* This test depends on the presence of an antibody on the red cell receptors and the fact that such cells will agglutinate in the presence of Coombs' reagent, and is valuable in testing newborn children suspected of suffering from erthroblastosis fœtalis and in cases of acquired hæmolytic anæmia. Coombs' reagent (rabbit anti-human globulin serum) can be prepared by immunising a rabbit with serum from a group O person, or with purified globulins.

To perform the test, the red cells are washed 3 times in saline to remove any trace of plasma proteins and then mixed on a slide with the Coombs' reagent. Should any antibody (globulin) be attached to the cell envelope agglutination will occur.

Indirect. The indirect test will detect incomplete antibody in a patient's serum. The unknown serum is incubated with cells of known group at 37°C. for one hour or more. The cells are then washed three times and mixed with Coombs' reagent as in the direct test. Both in the direct and indirect test red cells of known type must be tested concurrently to act as controls.

Detection of Antibody. Samples of blood from persons requiring transfusion and who have had previous transfusions or borne children, and from pregnant women who have an obstetric history suggestive of hæmolytic disease should be examined for the presence of immune antibodies. Their serum should be incubated at 37°C. with cells of known Rh type suspended in saline and albumin, and an indirect Coombs' test performed. By noting the reactions with cells of known genotype the particular type of antibody may be identified. The identification of the rarer antibodies can generally be done only in special laboratories.

Matching Blood for Transfusion. Donor's cells mixed on a slide with the patient's serum is not a satisfactory test of compatibility for transfusion purposes. This method will not detect immune antibodies in most cases, as they normally react at 37°C. and are often incomplete (albumin agglutinating).

The patient's serum should be incubated at 37°C. for one hour in tubes with the donor's cells suspended both in saline and albumin. This method will detect any incompatibility and it is most important that such a method be used in all cases of transfusion.

Only in cases of the direst emergency, where any delay in transfusing may endanger the life of the patient, is it permissible to use blood without matching, and in these cases blood known to be group O Rh negative should be used, unless the patient has been previously grouped.

Blood Transfusion Hazards. (1) *Pyrogens.* Pyrogens may cause mild pyrexia, rigors and backache. These reactions can be reduced to a minimum by the use of pyrogen-free water for solutions and by scrupulous aseptic technique in use and cleaning of materials.

(2) *Overloading the Circulation.* Great care is essential in the transfusion of patients with cardiovascular disease and/or chronic anæmia. A rising pulse rate and falling blood pressure, together with a persistent rise in venous pressure may herald the onset of pulmonary œdema or congestive cardiac failure. Generally this type of patient should be slowly transfused with small volumes of packed red cells.

(3) *Incompatible Transfusions.* These may be due to the following :—

(*a*) Presence of cold agglutinins.
(*b*) Mistaking rouleaux formation for agglutination.
(*c*) Failure to cross-group with patient's serum.
(*d*) Errors in grouping technique or interpretation.
(*e*) Clerical errors in laboratory or ward.
(*f*) Failure to carry out a satisfactory matching test.

The first three pitfalls will be avoided if the cells to be tested are washed in saline and the grouping done as described above.

If the matching of the donor's cells and recipient's serum is carried out at 37°C. with saline and albumin as suspending fluids, and, when necessary, with the use of the indirect Coombs' test, then incompatible transfusions rarely occur.

Homologous blood should always be used. Very rarely a person of group O may have an extremely high anti-A titre and, if this blood should be transfused to a person of group A, a reaction may well occur. The indiscriminate use of group O blood throws an unnecessarily heavy strain on group O blood donors.

(4) *Transmittible Disease.* The virus causing serum hepatitis is the greatest danger and Lehane and others (135) reported 0·8% as the incidence following whole blood transfusion. It is possible also to transmit both syphilis and malaria by blood transfusion. Donors who have had any of these diseases should be

rejected. A bottle of blood opened and not used within twelve hours should be discarded as bacteria may have been introduced.

Paternity Testing. In English law it is only possible to use blood grouping tests to exclude paternity, and Race and Sanger (150) have shown that about 60% of men wrongfully accused of paternity could be exonerated provided the tests could be carried out against all the blood group systems for which anti-sera are available.

Secretion. The A, B, H and, rarely, O antigens are secreted in various body fluids, particularly saliva, of some persons, and this ability to secrete is inherited as a Medelian dominant character. Grubb and Morgan (151) showed that about 77% of the London population are secretors. Grubb (152) observed a close relationship between secretion and the Lewis blood groups. Briefly, Lewis positive persons are non-secretors of A, B, or H substances and the majority of Lewis negative persons are secretors of A, B and H.

MNS Blood Group System. In 1927 Landsteiner and Levine (153, 154) described the M and N antigens which give rise to three genotypes, MM, MN, and NN. An antibody, now called anti-S, was discovered in 1947 by Walsh and Montgomery (155). S is closely associated with M and N and increases the genotypes to 6, MMS, MsMs, MNS, MsNs, NNS and NsNs. (s denotes cells which do not react with anti-S.)

Anti-M and anti-N occur both as natural and immune antibodies while anti-S sera are usually immune. They rarely are the cause of hæmolytic reactions. Anti-s has so far not been demonstrated.

Blood group system	First reported	Frequency in Britain	Nature of antibody	Cause of haemolytic reactions
P . .	Landsteiner and Levine 1927 (154)	P 74% +ve	usually natural	very rarely
Kell .	Coombs, Mourant and Race 1946 (156)	K 10% +ve	immune	occasionally
Lewis .	Mourant 1946 (157)	Le[a] 22% +ve	usually natural	very rarely
Lutheran	Callender and Race 1946 (158)	Lu[a] 7·5% +ve	immune	very rarely
Duffy .	Cutbush, Mollison and Parkin 1950 (159)	Fy[a] 65% +ve	immune	very rarely

Further Blood Group Systems. Five other blood group systems are very briefly described in the table on the previous page. All are weak antigens and so rarely stimulate antibody production. Any antibody which they may stimulate can be detected by the use of saline and albumin as suspending fluids for the red cells, except in the case of the Duffy antibodies, the majority of which can be demonstrated only by the use of the indirect Coombs' test.

Kidd System. This blood group system was described in 1951 by Allen et al. (160). It was discovered during the investigation of a maternal serum, the child of the mother having suffered from typical erythroblastosis fœtalis. 77% of Americans were shown to be Kidd positive (Jk^a+ve.).

REFERENCES

(1) Davidson. *Trans. Med. Chir. Soc. of Edin., Edin. Med. Journ.*, 1932, **39**, 105.
(2) Wintrobe. *Proc. Soc. Exp. Biol. and Med.*, 1930, **27**, 1071.
(3) Whipple and Robscheit-Robbins. *Amer. Journ. Physiol.*, 1925, **72**, 395.
(4) Minot and Murphy. *Journ. Amer. Med. Assocn.*, 1926, **87**, 470.
(5) Castle. *Amer. Journ. Med. Sci.*, 1929, **178**, 748.
(6) Castle, Townsend and Heath. *Amer. Journ. Med. Sci.*, 1930, **180**, 305.
(7) Taylor, Castle, Heinle and Adams. *Journ. Clin. Invest.*, 1938, **1**, 335.
(8) Formijne. *Arch. Int. Med.*, 1940, **66**, 1191.
(9) Cohn, McMeekin and Minot. *Journ. Biol. Chem.*, 1930, **87** (*Proc.*), xlix.
(10) Meulengracht. *Acta med. Scand.*, 1934, **82**, 352.
(11) Meulengracht. *Amer. Journ. Med. Sci.*, 1939, **197**, 201.
(12) Magnus and Ungley. *Lancet*, 1938, *i*, 420.
(13) Fox and Castle. *Amer. Journ. Med. Sci.*, 1942, **203**, 18.
(14) Schenken, Stasney and Hall. *Amer. Journ. Med. Sci.*, 1940, **200**, 11.
(15) Goldhammer. *Amer. Journ. Med. Sci.*, 1937, **193**, 23.
(16) Davidson, McCrie and Lovell Gulland. *Lancet*, 1928, *i*, 847. Davidson and McCrie *Ibid.*, 1928, *ii*, 1014.
(17) Dyke and Greener. *Lancet*, 1928, *i*, 1068.
(18) Whitby. *Lancet*, 1928, *i*, 285.
(19) Sturgis and Isaacs. *Journ. Amer. Med. Assocn.*, 1929, **93**, 747.
(20) Renshaw. *Brit. Med. Journ.*, 1930, *i*, 334.
(21) Wilkinson. *Brit. Med. Journ.*, 1930, *i*, 230.
(22) Wilkinson and Klein. *Lancet*, 1932, *i*, 719.
(23) Wilkinson and Klein. *Lancet*, 1933, *ii*, 629.
(24) Wilkinson. *Proc. Roy. Soc. Med.*, 1933, **26**, 1341.
(25) Wills. *Brit. Med. Journ.*, 1931, *i*, 1059.
(26) Wills and Evans. *Lancet*, 1938, *ii*, 416.
(27) Davidson. *Lancet*, 1931, *ii*, 1935.
(28) Berk, Castle, Welch, Heinle, Anker and Epstein. *New Engl. Journ. of Med.*, 1948, **239**, 911.
(29) Bethell, Meyers and Neligh. *Journ. Lab. Clin. Med.*, 1948, **33**, 1477.

(30) Dakin and West. *Journ. Biol. Chem.*, 1935, **109**, 489.
(31) Davis, Davidson, Riding and Shaw. *Brit. Med. Journ.*, 1943, *i*, 655.
(32) Wilkinson. *Practitioner*, 1942, **149**, 284.
(33) Wilkinson. *Brit. Med. Journ.*, 1931, *i*, 85.
(34) Wilkinson. *Clin. Journ.*, 1934, **63**, 449 ; *Liverpool Med. Chir. Journ* 1933, **41**, 163.
(35) Witts. *Brit. Med. Journ.*, 1933, *i*, 1091.
(36) Hill. *Lancet*, 1935, *i*, 43.
(37) Wilkinson. *Lancet*, 1949, *i*, 336.
(38) Wilkinson and Israëls. *Brit. Med. Journ.*, 1935, *i*, 139 and 194 ; Israëls and Wilkinson. *Quart. Journ. Med.*, 1936, **29**, 69.
(39) Vaughan. " *The Anœmias* ", 2nd Edit., 1936. Oxford University Press, London.
(40) Castle and Minot. " *The Pathological and Physiological Description of the Anœmias* ", 1936. Oxford University Press, London.
(41) Zanaty. *Lancet*, 1937, *ii*, 1365.
(42) Davidson and Fullerton. *Quart. Journ. Med.*, 1938, **31**, 43.
(43) Mahler and Greenberg. *Journ. Amer. Med. Assocn.*, 1939, **112**, 1150.
(44) Israëls and Wilkinson. *Quart. Journ. Med.*, 1940, **32**, 163.
(45) Bomford and Rhoads. *Quart. Journ. Med.*, 1941, **34**, 175.
(46) Wintrobe and Shumacker, Jr. *Bull. Johns Hopkins Hosp.*, 1933, **52**, 387.
(47) Rosenberg. *Amer. Journ. Med. Sci.*, 1936, **192**, 86.
(48) Bomford. *Quart. Journ. Med.*, 1938, **31**, 495.
(49) Vaughan and Hunter. *Lancet*, 1932, *i*, 829.
(50) Moore, Vilter, Minick and Spies. *Journ. Lab. Clin. Med.*, 1944, **29**, 1226.
(51) Osler. *Brit. Med. Journ.*, 1919, *i*, 1.
(52) Whitby. *Journ. Obstet. and Gynœc. of Brit. Empire*, 1932, **39**, 267.
(53) Davidson, Davis and Innes. *Brit. Med. Journ.*, 1942, *ii*, 31.
(54) MacQuaide and Mollison. *Brit. Med. Journ.*, 1940, *ii*, 555.
(55) Williams and Davie. *Brit. Med. Journ.*, 1941, *ii*, 641.
(56) Faber. *Berl. klin. Woch.*, 1913, **50**, 958.
(57) Witts. *Lancet*, 1932, *i*, 495.
(58) Hartfall and Witts. *Guy's Hosp. Rep.*, 1933, **83**, 3 and 24.
(59) Davies. *Quart. Journ. Med.*, 1931, **24**, 447 ; *Lancet*, 1931, *ii*, 385.
(60) Damashek. *Journ. Amer. Med. Assocn.*, 1933, **100**, 540.
(61) Mackay and Goodfellow. *Med. Res. Counc. Rep.*, 1931, No. 157.
(62) Cappell. *Journ. Path. Bact.*, 1930, **33**, 175.
(63) Goetsch, Moore and Minnich. *Blood*, 1946, **1**, 129.
(64) Nissim. *Lancet*, 1947, *ii*, 49.
(65) Slack and Wilkinson. *Lancet*, 1949, *i*, 11.
(66) Govan and Scott. *Lancet*, 1949, *i*, 14.
(67) Nissim and Robson. *Lancet*, 1949, *i*, 686.
(68) Sinclair and Duthie. *Lancet*, 1949, *ii*, 649.
(69) Ramsey. *Brit. Med. Journ.*, 1950, *i*, 1109.
(70) Schultz. *Deutsch. med. Woch.*, 1922, **48**, 1495.
(71) Schilling. " *The Blood Picture* ", 1929. C. V. Mosby, St. Louis.
(72) Plum. *Lancet*, 1935, *i*, 14.
(73) Borst. *Lancet*, 1937, *i*, 1519.
(74) Schwartz, Garvin and Koletsky. *Journ. Amer. Med. Assocn.*, 1938, **110**, 368.

(75) BERG, NEWARK and HOLTZMAN. *Journ. Amer. Med. Assocn.*, 1938, **110**, 370.
(76) DOAN. *Journ. Amer. Med. Assocn.*, 1932, **99**, 194.
(77) BARSBY and CLOSE. *Lancet*, 1942, *i*, 99.
(78) JACKSON. *Journ. Biol. Chem.*, 1924, **59**, 529.
(79) JACKSON, PARKER, RINEHART and TAYLOR. *Journ. Amer. Med. Assocn.*, 1931, **97**, 1436.
(80) JACKSON, PARKER and TAYLOR. *Amer. Journ. Med. Sci.*, 1932, **184**, 297.
(81) BULMER. *Lancet*, 1933, *i*, 1119.
(82) MARRIOTT. *Lancet*, 1934, *i*, 448.
(83) WILKINSON and ISRAËLS. *Lancet*, 1934, *ii*, 353.
(84) SMITH. *Lancet*, 1934, *ii*, 1219.
(85) FAIRLEY and SCOTT. *Lancet*, 1933, *ii*, 75.
(86) ISRAËLS and WILKINSON. *Quart. Journ. Med.*, 1937, **30**, 85.
(87) GUPTA and WITTS. *Brit. Med. Journ.*, 1937, *i*, 1197.
(88) GHEDINI. *Clin. med. Ital.*, 1908, **47**, 724.
(89) SEYFARTH. *Deutsch. med. Woch.*, 1923, **49**, 180.
(90) ARINKIN. *Vestn. Khir.*, 1927, **10**, 57.
(91) PEABODY. *Amer. Journ. Path.*, 1927, **3**, 179.
(92) SALAH. *Journ. Egypt. Med. Assocn.*, 1934, **17**, 846.
(93) NORDENSON. *Stockholm Thesis*, 1935.
(94) YOUNG and OSGOOD. *Arch. Int. Med.*, 1935, **55**, 186.
(95) VOGEL, ERF and ROSENTHAL. *Amer. Journ. Clin. Path.*, 1937, **7**, 436.
(96) HYNES. *Lancet*, 1939, *i*, 1373.
(97) SCHERER and HOWE. *Journ. Lab. Clin. Med.*, 1945, **30**, 450.
(98) BARDHAN. *Indian Med. Gaz.*, 1947, **82**, 459.
(99) LIMARZI, PONCHER and BIRCH. *Journ. Lab. Clin. Med.*, 1946, **31**, 777.
(100) ISRAËLS and WILKINSON. *Quart. Journ. Med.*, 1940, **33**, 163.
(101) MAHLER and GREENBERG. *Journ. Amer. Med. Assocn.*, 1939, **112**, 1150.
(102) TOCANTINS and O'NEILL. *Surg. Gynec. Obstet.*, 1941, **73**, 281.
(103) BAILEY. *Brit. Med. Journ.*, 1944, *i*, 181.
(104) BAILEY. *Brit. Med. Journ.*, 1946, *i*, 661.
(105) GUNZ and DEAN. *Brit. Med. Journ.*, 1945, *i*, 220.
(106) GIMSON. *Brit. Med. Journ.*, 1944, *i*, 748.
(107) BEHR. *Lancet*, 1944, *ii*, 472.
(108) MASSEY. *Brit. Med. Journ.*, 1950, *ii*, 197.
(109) MCLEAN. *Amer. Journ. Physiol.*, 1916, **41**, 250.
(110) HOWELL and HOLT. *Amer. Journ. Physiol.*, 1918, **47**, 328.
(111) HOWELL and HOLT. *Amer. Journ. Physiol.*, 1922, **63**, 434.
(112) CHARLES and SCOTT. *Journ. Biol. Chem.*, 1933, **102**, 425, 431 and 437.
(113) CHARLES and SCOTT. *Biochem. Journ.*, 1936, **30**, 1927.
(114) JORPES and BERGSTROM. *Zeits. f. physiol. Chem.*, 1936, **244**, 253.
(115) BEST. *Brit. Med. Journ.*, 1938, *ii*, 977.
MURRAY and BEST. *Journ. Amer. Med. Assocn.*, 1938, **110**, 118.
(116) JORPES, HOLMGREN and WILANDER. *Z. mikr.-anat. Forsch.*, 1937, **42**, 279. Quoted in BEST. *Proc. Mayo Clinic*, 1939, **14**, 81.
(117) MELLANBY. *Proc. Roy. Soc.*, 1934, B, **116**, 1.
(118) BEST. *Proc. Mayo Clinic*, 1939, **14**, 81.
(119) MURRAY, JAQUES, PERRETT and BEST. *Surgery*, 1937, **2**, 163.
(120) CRAFOORD. *Acta Chir. Scand.*, 1937, **79**, 407. *Ibid.*, 1939, **82**, 319.
(121) CHARGAFF and OLSON. *Journ. Biol. Chem.*, 1938, **122**, 153.
(122) JORPES, EDMAN and THANING. *Lancet*, 1939, *ii*, 975.

(123) Richmond. *Journ. Amer. Med. Assocn.*, 1942, **118**, 609.
(124) Ploman. *Acta Ophthalmol.*, 1938, **16**, 502.
(125) Magnusson. *Lancet*, 1938, *i*, 666.
(126) Kelson and White. *Journ. Amer. Med. Assocn.*, 1939, **113**, 1700.
(127) McLean, Meyer and Griffith. *Journ. Amer. Med. Assocn.*, 1941, **117**, 1870.
(128) Murray. *Brit. Journ. Surg.*, 1940, **27**, 567.
(129) Stansfield. *Brit. Med. Journ.*, 1942, *i*, 436.
(130) Ershler and Blaisdell. *Journ. Amer. Med. Assocn.*, 1941, **117**, 927.
(131) Hedenius. *Lancet*, 1937, *ii*, 1186.
(132) Sappington. *Journ. Amer. Med. Assocn.*, 1939, **113**, 22.
(133) Brightman and Korns. *Journ. Amer. Med. Assocn.*, 1947, **135**, 268.
(134) Havens. *Penn. Med. Journ.*, 1949, **52**, 1653.
(135) Lehane, Kwantes, Upward and Thomson. *Brit. Med. Journ.*, 1949, *ii*, 572.
(136) Rosenthal, Bassen and Michael. *Journ. Amer. Med. Assocn.*, 1950, **144**, 224.
(137) James, Korns and Wright. *Journ. Amer. Med. Assocn.*, 1950, **144**, 228.
(138) Grönwall and Ingelman. *Acta Phys. Scand.*, 1944, **7**, 97.
(139) Landsteiner and Wiener. *Proc. Soc. Exp. Biol. N.Y.*, 1940, **43**, 223.
(140) Wiener and Peters. *Annal. Int. Med.*, 1940, **13**, 2306.
(141) Levine, Katzin, Burnham and Vogel. *Amer. Journ. Obstet. and Gyn.*, 1941, **42**, 925.
(142) Fisher, cited by Race. *Nature*, 1944, **153**, 771.
(143) Callender and Race. *Annal. Eugen.*, 1946, **13**, 102.
(144) Race, Sanger and Lawler. *Nature*, 1948, **161**, 316.
(145) Stratton. *Nature*, 1946, **158**, 25.
(146) Armytage, Ceppellini, Ikin and Mourant. *Boll. Ist. Siero Milanese*, 1950, **29**, 123.
(147) Gilbey. *Brit. Journ. Exp. Path.*, 1950, **31**, 695.
(148) Chown. *Amer. Journ. Clin. Path.*, 1944, **14**, 114.
(149) Diamond and Abelson. *Journ. Lab. Clin. Med.*, 1945, **30**, 204.
(150) Race and Sanger. "*Blood Groups in Man*", 1950. Blackwell Scientific Publications, Oxford.
(151) Grubb and Morgan. *Brit. Journ. Exp. Path.*, 1949, **30**, 198.
(152) Grubb. *Nature*, 1949, **162**, 933.
(153) Landsteiner and Levine. *Proc. Soc. Exp. Biol. N.Y.*, 1927, **24**, 600.
(154) Landsteiner and Levine. *Proc. Soc. Exp. Biol. N.Y.*, 1927, **24**, 941.
(155) Walsh and Montgomery. *Nature*, 1947, **160**, 504.
(156) Coombs, Mourant and Race. *Lancet*, 1946, *i*, 264.
(157) Mourant. *Nature*, 1946, **158**, 237.
(158) Callender and Race. *Annal. Eugen.*, 1946, **13**, 102.
(159) Cutbush, Mollison and Parkin. *Nature*, 1950, **165**, 188.
(160) Allen, Diamond and Niedziela. *Nature*, 1951, **167**, 482.

CHAPTER XIII

BIOCHEMICAL METHODS

THE essential requirements of methods used for routine analyses are accuracy, speed and ease of operation. Generally colorimetric methods are used, as satisfying these conditions: for certain types of analysis however volumetric or gravimetric procedures, or the use of special apparatus, are recommended.

COLORIMETRY

Photoelectric colorimeters are now generally used instead of direct vision colorimeters, as they have a wider field of application and eliminate the personal error: there is very little to choose between the different commercial makes of single cell machines. It is essential however to use a double cell null-point instrument for those analyses where it is inconvenient or not possible to prepare a standard for each analysis, and where a calibration curve must be used.

THE COLLECTION AND STORAGE OF BLOOD SPECIMENS

The first prerequisite of an accurate blood analysis is a representative blood sample. The collection of blood by capillary puncture is not to be recommended, except in skilled hands, because of the difficulty of avoiding adulteration of the blood by tissue fluid. On the other hand, venepuncture affords a convenient method of withdrawing blood samples ample in volume for any series of estimations.

The technique of blood withdrawal by venepuncture is a matter of common knowledge in the medical field. Not so well known, however, are the limitations set by chemical considerations, factors which, sometimes overlooked by the uninitiated, can vitiate the most careful analysis.

A most frequent source of error lies in the choice of anticoagulant, or indeed in making a decision whether an anticoagulant should be used at all. For example, fluoride, a specific enzyme inhibitor, is useless for any estimation involving the use or assay of an enzyme (*e.g.* urease in urea estimations or for the estimation of phosphatase activity). Paradoxically, it is just this property of fluoride which makes it pre-eminently suitable for the collection of blood samples for inorganic phosphate determination, where failure to inactivate the blood phosphatase will lead to the liberation on standing of phosphate from organically bound phosphorus yielding a falsely high result. Fluoride is best known for its use to prevent glycolysis where a sugar has to be estimated.

Potassium oxalate is probably the most effective common anticoagulant; fluoride is commonly used mixed with oxalate as fluoride alone is a poor anticoagulant. For obvious reasons, both these anticoagulants, potassium oxalate or sodium fluoride, are quite unsuitable for use when sodium or potassium themselves are being estimated, and since oxalate or fluoride precipitate calcium they also invalidate this analysis.

For certain analyses, namely chloride, bicarbonate and blood gases it is essential that the specimen be collected under liquid paraffin to avoid loss of gas from the sample and consequent ionic shift.

As far as possible the tendency nowadays is to use serum for as many analyses as possible for the use of any solid anticoagulant will alter the water distribution between cells and plasma, and wherever there is any choice serum is to be used.

Haemolysed specimens should always be treated with reserve, especially when estimating the serum or plasma content of any substance known to be present in much higher concentration in the erythocytes; *e.g.* potassium or the phosphatases.

For the collection of specimens where anticoagulant is required a suitable concentration of potassium oxalate is 2 mg./ml. of final sample, and where fluoride is desired this is added as well as the oxalate to a concentration of 0·7 mg./ml. Suitable concentrated solutions of these substances may be prepared and the appropriate amount of solution placed into a bottle; the amount calculated for an average sample of 10 ml. of blood. The solution is run over the sides of the bottle which is then dried in an oven, at a temperature not exceeding 110° C., leaving the anticoagulant distributed in a finely divided easily soluble form.

Physiological Normals

(By methods described in text)

A. Blood

(Values as mg./100 ml. unless otherwise stated.)

	Whole Blood	Plasma or Serum
Alkali Reserve (as HCO_3') .	—	24–35 mEq/l
Amino-acid nitrogen . .	4–8	3–7
Bilirubin (Van den Bergh) .	—	0·1–0·8
Calcium (total) . . .	5–7	9–11
Calcium (diffusible) . .	—	4·2–5·6
β-Carotene	—	0·05–0·3
Chloride (as Cl′) . . .	76–87 mEq/l (270–310)	96–105 mEq/l (340–370)
Cholesterol (total) . .	110–230	140–280
Creatine	2–8	0·2–0·8
Creatinine	0·5–2·5	0·5–2·5
Iron	—	0·08–0·18
Liver Function tests :		
Colloidal gold . . .	—	0–1 units
Thymol turbidity . .	—	0–4 units
Oxygen : Males :		
arterial . .	15–24 ml./100 ml.	—
venous . .	11–17 ml./100 ml.	—
Females : 2 ml.% less in each case.		
Phosphatase (acid) . .	—	1–3 K–A units/100 ml.
Phosphatase (alkaline) . .	—	3–13 K–A units/100 ml.
Phosphate (inorganic) (as P) .	2·5–5·0	2–4·5
(as HPO_4'') .	(1·5–2·9)	(1·2–2·6 mEq/l)
Potassium (as K·) . .	38–64 mEq/l	4·4–5·6 mEq/l
Protein : total . . .	—	5·5–8·0 g./100 ml.
Albumin	—	3·5–6·0 g./100 ml.
Globulin	—	1·5–3·0 g./100 ml.
A/G Ratio	—	'1·5 : 1–3·5 : 1'
Fibrinogen	—	0·2–0·4 g./100 ml.
Prothrombin time . .	—	14″–16″
Concentration . . .	—	70%–140%
Sodium (as Na·) . . .	74–98 mEq/l	139–150 mEq/l
Sugar (as glucose) :		
" Total fasting " :		
venous or capillary .	60–110	60–110
after a meal :		
venous	up to 150	up to 150
capillary	up to 180	—
Urea	15–40	15–40
Uric acid	1–4	1·5–6

B. Urine

(Values as g./24 hrs. unless otherwise stated.)

Calcium	0·1–0·5
Chloride (as Cl′)	6–9
Corticoids	1–4 mg./24 hrs.
Creatine	0–0·05
Creatinine	1·0–2·0
Diastase (amylase)	2–50 units/ml.
17-Ketosteroids (total neutral)	
Males	15–25 mg./24 hrs.
Females: post menopause	4–10 mg./24 hrs.
premenopause	6–18 mg./24 hrs.
Phosphate (as P)	0·5–2·0
Potassium (as K·)	1·5–4·0
Pregnanediol:	
Males: and females (follicular phase)	0–0·5 mg./24 hrs.
Females: (luteal phase)	1–10 mg./24 hrs.
Sodium (as Na·)	2–6
Urea	10–40
Uric acid	0·1–2·0
Vitamin C	0–80 mg./24 hrs.

C. Fæces

Total fat	10–25% of dried fæces
Split fat: fatty acids	3–10% of dried fæces
soaps	3–10% of dried fæces
Unsplit (neutral fat)	3–8% of dried fæces
Trypsin	200–2000 units per g. wet fæces
Urobilinogen (= stercobilinogen)	0·05–0·3 g./24 hrs.

D. C.S.F. (Values as mg./100 ml.)

	Lumbar	Ventricular
Chloride (as NaCl)	720–760	720–760
Protein	10–40	5–15
Sugar (as glucose)	40–80	50–100

Flame Photometry

Flame photometry is an analytical technique now being applied to clinical biochemistry. The principles of flame photometry are (1) certain elements on suitable excitation emit light of characteristic wavelength, (2) the intensity of the light emitted is proportional to the concentration of the appropriate element in the material tested. By means of an appropriately designed burner atomiser system operating under controlled conditions it is possible to provide stable and reproducible means of excitation and consequently of estimation of certain metals (see Fig. 55).

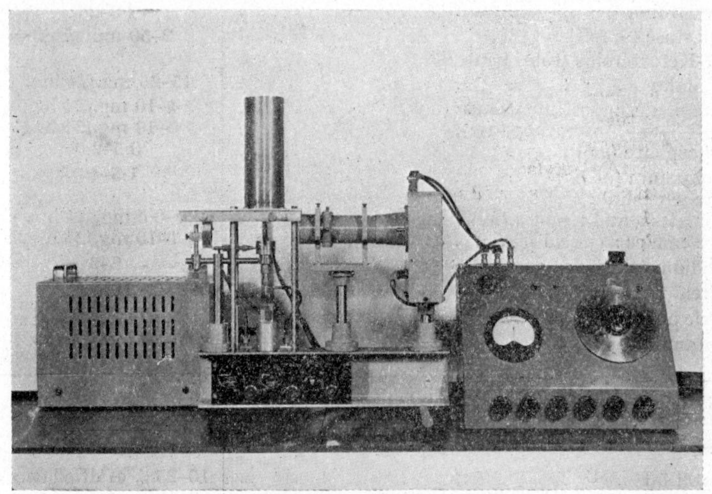

FIG. 55. The Flame Photometer

The Courtauld Institute Flame Photometer was constructed for the routine estimations of sodium and potassium in biological fluids.

The aspirator situated at the centre of the burner draws the solution from the beaker, atomises it in the stream of oxygen and passes it into the flame. The intensity of the light produced is measured by means of emission-type photo cells, appropriate filters being used to separate the sodium and potassium radiations. A bridge amplifier system modified from that described by Bills et al. (1) is employed to measure the photo cell current.

The burner atomiser system used is a modified form of that of Weichselbaum and Varney (2) with the novel feature that it may be completely dismantled for cleaning, being constructed from only two pieces of metal. Other features include the elimination of back-firing (troublesome in the original design) and injection mixing of the fuel (butane and oxygen).

In routine use the photometer illustrated gives readings consistent to $\pm 1{\cdot}5\%$. The range of concentration in the aspirated solution normally employed for sodium estimations is 0·004–0·4 mEq/l and for potassium 0·002–0·2 mEq/l. At these concentrations the calibration is for practical purposes linear. The final volume of the material used is limited by the size of the beakers convenient to handle (2 ml. fluid in a 5 ml. beaker).

The layout of the instrument is as follows. The various optical components, burner and photo cell compartments are mounted on an optical bench. The compartment on the left houses the pressure gauges and needle valves that indicate and regulate the pressure of the fuel and oxygen. The burner on the left is water cooled (as is the chimney). The optical system and filter slide are mounted on the right of the instrument and on the extreme right is the photo cell compartment carrying two photo cells, one for potassium and one for sodium. These cells are mounted side by side and are easily interchangeable. Output from the photo cells is led by screened cables to the amplifier. On the extreme left is the stabilised power supply. The photo cell current is measured by the large calibrated dial which is attached to a potentiometer. A detailed description of the working of this instrument is not given here because it is not commercially available and different makes of instruments would naturally have to be differently operated. For those laboratories not possessing a flame photometer a suitable method for the estimation of serum sodium is that of McCance and Shipp (3) and for the estimation of serum potassium that of Jacobs and Hoffman (4), which may be suitably modified for the estimation of urinary sodium and potassium.

Gasometric Analysis

Alkali Reserve Estimation (macro-method)

Method of Peters and Van Slyke (5).

Reagents. (1) *Lactic acid* 1*N*. Take one volume of lactic acid, S.G. 1020, and dilute with nine volumes of distilled water. Place into a flask and draw a stream of air through the solution for at least one hour. The incoming air should be freed from carbon dioxide by means of a soda lime tube.

(2) *Lactic acid* 0·1*N*. Dilute the above solution ten times with distilled water and again aerate.

Method. The blood is collected into a plain tube and covered with a layer of liquid paraffin. If an urgent estimation is required it is permissible to use an oxalate bottle and carry out the analysis on plasma. Upon receiving the specimen at once centrifuge, and transfer the serum to a lusteroid plastic test tube. For the analysis the sample must be equilibrated with carbon dioxide at the concentration present in alveolar air. To do this slowly blow through the serum a stream of air containing 5% carbon dioxide (this mixture can be obtained commercially in cylinders).

Whilst the blood is being gassed inspect the apparatus and test for leaks. To test for leaks run about 10–15 ml. of distilled water into the shaking chamber ; seal the top cock of the chamber with mercury, lower the mercury level in the chamber to the 50 ml. mark and shake for three minutes to remove the air from the water. Raise the water level to the 2 ml. mark and read the level of the mercury in the manometer tube. Re-lower the mercury level, again shake for one minute, raise to the 2 ml. mark and read the manometer. Repeat this process three or four times. If there are no leakages then a constant reading will be obtained: a slight difference between the first two readings is permissible.

For the analysis a drop of caprylic alcohol is placed into the cup and the reservoir placed in position 1. Open cocks C and D. Allow the mercury to rise into the cup. Close cocks D and C. Place reservoir in position 2. Open cock C. Slowly open cock D until the caprylic alcohol is in the capillary of the stopcock D. Close D, raise reservoir to position 1. Close C. Lower reservoir to position 2. Measure 1·5 ml. of 0·1N lactic acid into the cup. 1 ml. of gassed serum is drawn up into a volumetric 1 ml. pipette with the tip protected by a rubber cuff, and the pipette is inserted into the cup as shown in Fig. 56 (Method 2). When the pipette is in position open cock D and let the serum flow into the chamber by turning cock C. (Cock C is used instead of cock D as the flow of mercury is more easily controlled than the flow of serum.) The delivery is continued until the serum has entirely left the pipette and a minute bubble of air has followed the serum into the capillary at the bottom of the cup ; close cock D. The bubble should float to the top; if this does not happen then remove the bubble using a piece

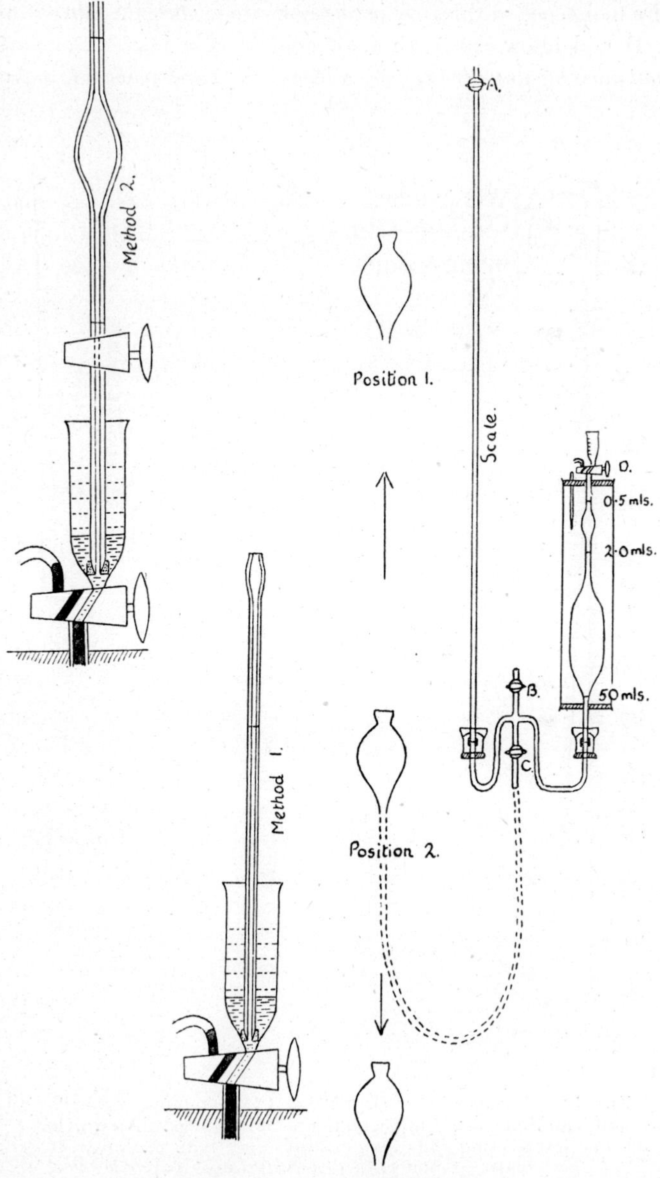

FIG. 56. The Van Slyke Apparatus

of wire moistened with caprylic alcohol. Open cock C. Slowly open cock D and allow the 1·5 ml. of acid to flow into the chamber *without allowing any air to enter.* Close cock D and place a few drops

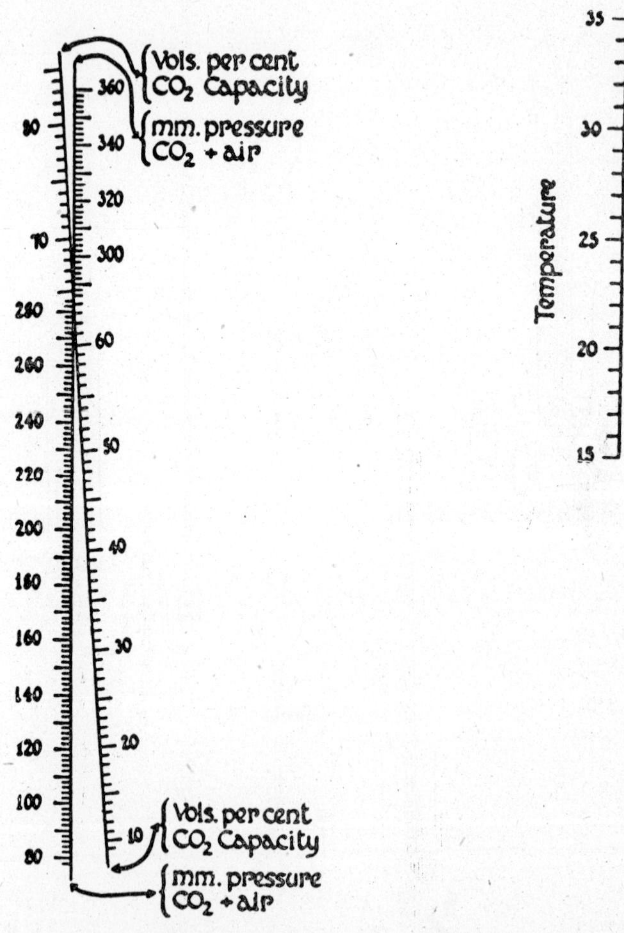

FIG. 57. *Nomogram* for calculating CO_2 combining capacity of Van Slyke and Cullen manometric readings. A straight line intersecting the 'temperature' and 'mm. pressure CO_2 + air' scales at points of observed values cuts the 'vols. per cent CO_2 capacity' scale at the point showing the CO_2 capacity of the plasma, when the plasma sample analysed is 1 ml. (5).

of mercury in the cup. Slowly open cock D and fill the capillary of the cock with mercury. Close cock D. Lower the reservoir to position 3 and close cock C when the mercury reaches the 50 ml. mark. Return the reservoir to position 2. Shake the chamber for two minutes at a speed of three movements per second. After shaking allow the fluid to drain, then slowly open cock C and by careful control allow the fluid level to rest on the 2 ml. mark. Read the gas pressure on manometer scale (= P_1). Open cock C and bring the reservoir level with the fluid in the chamber, in order to bring the gas pressure to slightly above atmospheric. Close cock C and open cock D; if the previous manipulation has been correctly performed no movement of the gas should occur. Raise the reservoir to position I. By the cautious adjustment of cock C expel the gas through cock D, and fill the cock with fluid. Place some mercury in the cup, fill the cock with mercury by lowering the reservoir, and close cock D. Lower the reservoir to position 3 and close cock C when the fluid level is exactly at the 2·0 ml. mark. Read the gas pressure on the manometer (= P_0.) Take the temperature of the water jacket. $P_1 - P_0$ = corrected pressure. Read Vols. % CO_2 on the nomogram of corrected pressure against temperature (see Fig. 57).

Alkali Reserve Estimation (micro-method)

Reagent. (1) 0·01*N Lactic acid.* Dilute 0·1N lactic acid ten times with distilled water and aerate as in the macro-method.

Method. The serum or plasma is gassed with 5% carbon dioxide in air exactly as for the macro-method. For the analysis a drop of octyl alcohol and 0·20 ml. of the saturated serum or plasma are run into the chamber of the apparatus followed by enough 0·01N lactic acid to bring the volume of the solution in the chamber down to the 2·0 ml. mark. The same analytical technique is used as in the macro-method; the reading of the pressure of the extracted gases being made at 0·5 ml. volume. The pressure observed is applied to the nomogram as in calculating the results of the macro-determination, and the final result is multiplied by 1·26 to give the correct capacity.

This correction is necessary to compensate for the different volume of reading and the re-adsorption difference.

Blood-gas Analysis by Haldane's Method

After Douglas & Priestley (6)

The general form of the apparatus is shown in Fig. 58. The gases liberated from or taken up by the blood in the small, thin walled bottle A, which is connected to the rest of the apparatus by narrow-bore rubber pressure tubing, are measured in the burette C (a 1 ml. measuring pipette, graduated to 0·01 ml. and capable of being read to 0·001 ml.). The second thin walled glass bottle B with its connecting tube, having the same volume as the analytical bottle and connecting tube serves as a thermo-barometer to allow for

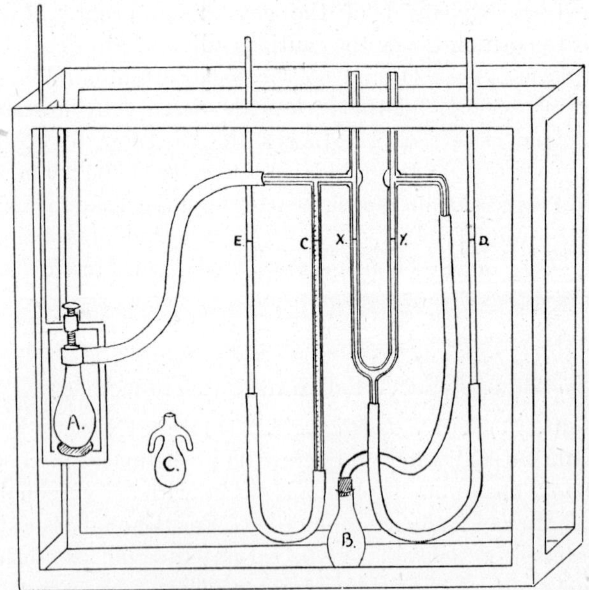

Fig 58. Haldane Apparatus

compensation of changes of temperature during the course of an experiment and should contain about 2 ml. of water to ensure that the air in it is always saturated with aqueous vapour. The two bottles A and B are connected through 3-way taps to the gauge tubes X and Y respectively, which unite with one another below, and are in communication with a levelling tube D. X, Y and D are partly filled with water containing a trace of sodium taurocholate to lower the surface tension and ensure free movement.

The burette C is connected by rubber tubing to a levelling tube E, which also contains water plus trace of sodium taurocholate. At the start of an analysis the two water menisci are brought to a levelling mark on tubes X and Y by raising or lowering the levelling tube D while the 3-way taps are open to air. The taps are now turned so that the bottles A and B communicate only with X and Y, but are shut off from the air, and the analysis is begun.

If during the course of the analysis the volume of gas in A is altered by a change of external temperature or barometric pressure a similar change will occur in the compensator bottle B and the meniscus in Y will be displaced from the mark; this change can be compensated by suitable movement of the levelling tube D, and as this levelling tube communicates with X as well as with Y, the compensation will also be applied through X to the bottle A, provided that the meniscus in X is also brought back exactly to its mark by adjustment of E. If these precautions are taken every time a reading of the burette has to be made all the readings will be strictly comparable with one another, without further corrections for changes of external temperature or pressure.

The whole apparatus (including bottles A and B) is immersed to the level of the taps in a stirred glass fronted tank of water maintained at a constant uniform temperature. To keep the water tank free of moulds the use of methyl-*p*-hydroxy-benzoate, $\frac{1}{4}$ oz. to a gallon, is advised.

Reagents. (1) *Borate solution.* Add 12·404 g. of pure dry boric acid to 100 ml. of N caustic soda and dilute to 1 litre.

(2) *Borate buffer pH* 10. Add 300 ml. of the above solution to 200 ml. 0·1N caustic soda.

(3) *Saponin ferricyanide solution.* Dissolve 0·3 g. of saponin of known high lytic power and 0·6 g. of potassium ferricyanide in 10 ml. of water.

Method

Oxygen Unsaturation

Place in bottle A 3 ml. of buffer solution and cool in the tank. 3 ml. of blood which has been collected into heparin, under paraffin, is drawn up into an Ostwald Van Slyke pipette and carefully delivered under the buffer. The amount of blood used is determined by the degree of unsaturation of the sample; for the brighter red, less unsaturated samples (*e.g.* arterial blood) 4 or 5 ml. should be used. Connect the bottle to the apparatus with the taps open to the air, immerse, adjust the menisci in tubes **X** and **Y** to the marks, the pipette reading to about 0·7 ml., and close the taps. If the apparatus is suitably designed flush it through with carbon dioxide free air, to reduce the time necessary for equilibrium by obviating absorption of carbon dioxide from the gas by the buffer. Allow to stand when no further change in the pipette reading is noted, return the menisci to their marks and read the pipette. Shake bottle A to oxygenate the blood : complete saturation has occurred when no further change is registered on the pipette or the levelling tube **X**, which usually takes about 10 minutes. Readjust the menisci **X** and **Y** and take pipette reading.

Calculation.

$$\frac{\text{ml. } O_2 \text{ absorbed}}{\text{ml. blood used}} \times 100 \text{ (correct to S.T.P.)} = \text{ml. oxygen absorbed}$$

per 100 ml. blood.

Oxygen Capacity

Oxygenate the blood sample provided by rotating it in a separating funnel. Place into bottle C 2 ml. of buffer followed by 1 ml. of blood. Into the side arm of bottle C place 0·5 ml. of saponin ferricyanide solution. Adjust the menisci as for determination of unsaturation except that the fluid level in the pipette is set at 0·3 ml. Close the taps and shake the bottle until equilibrium is reached taking care not to mix the contents of the bottle with the side arm. Adjust the menisci **X** and **Y** and note pipette reading " a ". Tilt the bottle to run the saponin-ferricyanide solution into the blood buffer mixture. Shake again to expel all the oxygen from the blood and until a steady reading is obtained on the pipette, and this usually takes about ten minutes : readjust the menisci **X** and **Y** and take the pipette reading " b ".

Calculation. $(b - a) \times 100$ (Correct to S.T.P.) = ml. O_2 capacity per 100 ml. blood.

Some Colorimetric Methods

Estimation of Amino Acids in Blood

Adapted from the methods of Kravel (7) and Wilson & Eyles (8)

Reagents. 1. 0·05*N Caustic soda.*

2. *Phenolphthalein.* A 0·25% alcoholic solution.

3. *Sodium biborate.* A 2% aqueous solution.

4. *Amino acid reagent.* A 0·5% aqueous solution of sodium-beta-naphthoquinone-4-sulphonate prepared within five minutes of using.

5. *Acetate buffer solution.* 100 ml. 50% acetic acid + 100 ml. 5% sodium acetate.

6. *Sodium thiosulphate.* A 4% aqueous solution.

7. *Stock standard.* Take 536 mg. of glycine dried to constant weight over sulphuric acid *in vacuo* and dissolve in 0·07N hydrochloric acid containing 0·2% sodium benzoate and make up to 1 litre with this solution. 1 ml. = 0·1 mg. nitrogen.

8. *Working standard.* Dilute 2 ml. of the stock standard to 50 ml. with distilled water.

9. *Dilute tungstic acid solution.* Take 4 ml. 10% sodium tungstate + 4 ml. 2/3N. sulphuric acid and dilute to 100 ml. with distilled water. (This solution must be prepared and used within three hours.)

Method. To 6 ml. dilute tungstic acid in a 15 ml. centrifuge tube add 0·2 ml. blood. Allow to stand for five minutes and centrifuge. Into a graduated tube place 5 ml. filtrate and into another tube 5 ml. water for blank. Add 1 drop phenolphthalein to each tube and neutralise to a faint pink colour with 0·05N caustic soda. To each tube add 1 ml. 2% sodium borate and 0·4 ml. of amino acid reagent, mix and place in a boiling water bath for exactly three minutes. Cool the tubes immediately in running water and add to them 1 ml. of acetate buffer and 1 ml. 4% thiosulphate. Dilute to the 10 ml. mark with distilled water and compare the colour of the " unknown " with the colour produced from the range of standards described below, setting to zero with the reagent blank, and using a blue filter maximum transmission 450 mμ. The reading of the standard taken should be that nearest the reading of the unknown. Prepare standards taking 1, 2, 3, 4 and 5 ml. of working standard, making up in each case to 5 ml. with water, and treating as the 5 ml. of filtrate above. After experience with the method it is sufficient to use only the standards prepared from 2 and 5 ml.

Calculation.

1 ml. standard	=	2·5 mg.	amino acid nitrogen/100 ml. blood.
2 ml. ,,	=	5·0 mg.	,, ,, ,, ,,
3 ml. ,,	=	7·5 mg.	,, ,, ,, ,,
4 ml. ,,	=	10.0 mg.	,, ,, ,, ,,
5 ml. ,,	=	12.5 mg.	,, ,, ,, ,,

$$\text{Blood amino acid concentration} = \frac{\text{Reading of unknown}}{\text{Reading of standard}} \times \text{concentration of standard.}$$

Estimation of Serum Iron

Modified from Høyer (9) and Dahl (10)

Reagents. 1. *Water doubly redistilled* from glass.

2. *Concentrated hydrochloric acid.*

3. *Concentrated nitric acid.* Reagents 2 and 3 are the constant boiling pure acids prepared by redistilling A.R. concentrated acids.

4. 25% *trichloroacetic acid.* This is prepared from A.R. trichloroacetic acid, further distilled using an all-glass air cooled still, and the redistilled acid dissolved in glass distilled water.

5. *Approx.* 5*N potassium thiocyanate solution,* prepared by dissolving 10 g. of A.R. thiocyanate in 20 ml. of redistilled water. This solution must be prepared on the day of the test.

6. *Stock standard iron solution* (1 ml. = 100 micrograms iron). 0·864 g. of A.R. ferric ammonium sulphate is dissolved in about 100 ml. of redistilled water. 10 ml. of pure hydrochloric acid (2) are added, and the mixture is made up to a litre. From this solution suitable dilutions can be made, and a calibration curve constructed covering the range 0–400 micrograms of iron/100 ml.

7. *Sodium acetate solution.* A 20% solution of A.R. sodium acetate in redistilled water.

All these reagents must be stored in pyrex bottles.

Precautions. The estimation is carried out on serum which has been collected with special care to avoid contamination with free iron : at least 12 ml. of blood are needed which should be taken with a dry all-glass syringe using a new stainless steel needle. The blood is allowed to clot and the serum separated ; a minimal amount of hæmolysis does not interfere with the estimation. All glassware used for the test must be specially cleaned (soaked in dichromate, and finally rinsed with doubly-distilled water) to ensure its being iron-free.

Method. Into a 15 ml. conical centrifuge tube place 5 ml. of serum and 1 ml. of 5N hydrochloric acid: stir with a clean glass rod and allow to stand for about fifteen minutes. Add 1 ml. of sodium acetate followed by 3 ml. of 25% trichloroacetic acid, shake and allow to stand for five minutes. Place in a gently boiling water-bath for about one minute to complete precipitation of the protein. Cool and centrifuge at about 3,000 r.p.m. for half an hour.

Place 6 ml. of *clear* supernatant fluid in a test-tube, followed by 0·1 ml. of concentrated nitric acid, shake and allow to stand for five minutes, then add 2 ml. of 5N potassium thiocyanate with gentle shaking.

Blank. To 5 ml. of redistilled water, in place of the serum, add 1·0 ml. of hydrochloric acid and proceed exactly as for the test.

Reading. Read blank and unknown in a null point colorimeter using a blue filter maximum transmission 500 mμ. The unknown and the blank reading are converted to serum iron concentration by means of the calibration chart. If the blank gives a reading greater than 25% of the total, then the test is unsatisfactory because the reagents contain overmuch iron.

The Estimation of Urinary Corticoids

Adapted from the method of Heard and Sobel (11) and Pincus (12).

Reagents. Dilute immediately before use the *phosphomolybdic acid* reagent (described for blood sugar estimation on page 372), with an equal volume of glacial acetic acid. The precipitate that forms readily redissolves.

Method. Adjust to approximately pH 1 with concentrated hydrochloric acid a twenty-four hour urine specimen, collected without any preservative. Stand the acidified urine at room temperature for twenty-four hours to seventy-two hours. Extract the total sample four times in a separating funnel each time with a quarter of its volume of chloroform. Combine all the chloroform extracts in a separating funnel and wash them with 3 × 100 ml. of ice-cold 0·1N caustic soda solution, followed by washing with 3 × 100 ml. of ice-cold water. Dry the washed chloroform extract by means of anhydrous sodium sulphate, evaporate the washed, dry chloroform extract to dryness in an all-glass vacuum distillation apparatus keeping the temperature below 50° C., and dissolve the gummy residue in 10 ml. of dry chloroform. Take an aliquot of this chloroform solution (containing 0·01 to 0·1 mg. of " corticoid " material) and evaporate to dryness in a test tube (0·2 ml. is usually a convenient amount). Dissolve it in 0·1 ml. of glacial acetic acid and use another 0·1 ml. of acid in another tube for the " blank ". To each add 2 ml. of phosphomolybdic acid reagent. Plug the tubes very tightly with cotton wool wrapped in filter paper to prevent ingress of water vapour and immerse the lower third of the tubes in a gently boiling water bath for sixty minutes. Cool the tubes for two minutes in running water and dilute each with a further 8 ml. of phosphomolybdic acid reagent; mix and allow to stand for two minutes for gas bubbles to rise.

The colour density is read on a null point colorimeter against the blank determination (which should be colourless to the naked eye if the reagents are pure) using red filters with maximum transmission at 650 mμ.

The colorimeter reading is converted to mg. of " corticoid " present in the tube by means of a calibration curve.

A calibration curve is prepared using as the standard material 0·01 to 0·1 mg. of deoxycorticosterone, in suitable steps. This method gives a straight line calibration curve so it is legitimate and convenient to use a factor multiplying the colorimeter reading to give mg. deoxycorticosterone equivalent to the " corticoids " present in the estimation tube.

NOTE.—This method, although giving consistent figures, is not now considered to estimate the true urinary corticoid content.

Estimation of Total Neutral 17-Ketosteroids

Adapted for rapid clinical estimations from the method of Talbot et al (13).

Reagents. 1. *Sodium hydroxide solutions:* (*a*) 1*N solution*, (*b*) 2·5*N solution.*

2. *N/2 hydrochloric acid.*

3. *Absolute ethyl alcohol.* Aldehyde content must be lower than 0·0025 %.

4. *Diethyl ether.* Peroxide free—A.R. quality.

5. *Benzene* (crystallizable).

6. 2·5*N potassium hydroxide* in absolute ethyl alcohol solution. The solution is made fresh daily by dissolving 1·4 g. A.R. potassium

hydroxide in 10 ml. of absolute alcohol using a mechanical shaker. Filter through hardened filter paper (Whatman No. 50 or 54). The solution should be crystal clear.

7. *Meta-dinitrobenzene.* This material must be very pure. The compound as supplied commercially is further purified as follows :—Dissolve 20 g. of *m*-dinitrobenzene in 750 ml. of 95% alcohol and warm to 40° C. Add 100 ml. of 2N sodium hydroxide. After five minutes cool the solution and add 2,500 ml. of water. Collect the precipitated *m*-dinitrobenzene on a Buchner funnel, wash thoroughly with water, suck dry and recrystallize twice in succession from 120 ml. and 80 ml. of absolute alcohol by dissolving in the quantity of alcohol stated and evaporating off alcohol until crystallization commences.

The purified material must be well crystallized, almost colourless needles, of melting point 90·5 to 91° C. A mixture of a 1% alcoholic solution of the compound with an equal volume of aqueous 2N caustic soda should give no colour after an hour.

Use a 2·5% solution of purified *m*-dinitrobenzene in absolute alcohol as the reagent. Store in a dark bottle at 0° C. This solution keeps for approximately one month, but each time before use the excess solid should be brought into solution by gentle warming.

Method. *Hydrolysis and extraction.* Measure the urine volume. Into a 500 ml. round-bottomed flask place an aliquot of the mixed specimen (100 ml. is suitable) add 15 ml. of concentrated hydrochloric acid and 50 ml. benzene. Boil in a 500 ml. ground glass flask for thirty minutes under a reflux condenser. Cool fairly rapidly. Transfer to a separating funnel, withdraw the benzene and re-extract the aqueous phase with two further 50 ml. amounts of benzene.

Combine the three benzene extracts and transfer to a separating funnel and wash consecutively with 2 × 25 ml. of N. sodium hydroxide followed by washing with 2 × 25 ml. of N/2 hydrochloric acid, and finally washing with 3 × 25 ml. of water. Evaporate off the benzene from the washed extract by distilling on a water bath under reduced pressure. By means of about 20 ml. of petrol ether transfer the ketosteroid extract quantitatively to a test tube, making several rinses (the petrol ether insoluble material is non-steroid pigment). Carefully evaporate to dryness in a water bath and dissolve the residue in 1 ml. of *absolute* alcohol.

Select two glass stoppered tubes of approximately 15 ml. capacity and pipette in respectively 0·2 ml. of alcoholic solution and 0·2 ml. alcohol for the " blank ". Into each tube pipette 0·2 ml. of 2·5% alcoholic *m*-dinitrobenzene solution and 0·2 ml. of 2·5N alcoholic potassium hydroxide solution. Mix and place the tubes in a water-bath at 25° C. for one hour. Add 10 ml. of absolute alcohol to each tube. Mix and read in a null point colorimeter within five minutes of dilution using yellow-green filters of maximum transmission 550 mμ. If the unknown gives an optical density reading above the range of the calibration curve repeat the colour development using a smaller quantity of alcoholic solution.

A calibration curve is prepared using as the standard material iso-dehydro-androsterone. For calibration purposes a suitable range to construct is from zero to 0·4 mg. of sterone per 0·2 ml. of alcohol.

Patterson Reaction for Iso-Dehydro-Androsterone

Method of Patterson (14)

Evaporate to dryness 0·2 ml. of the neutral alcohol extract obtained from the estimation of 17-ketosteroids. Add 1 ml. of concentrated sulphuric acid and shake until the steroid gum completely dissolves. Place into a water bath at 25° C. for twenty minutes. Cool by immersing in cold water and add 1 ml. of distilled water drop by drop with constant shaking. Heat the mixture in a boiling water bath for one minute during which time a blue colour develops if the test is positive.

Other Routine Analytical Methods

In this section are listed the methods necessary for the clinical-biochemistry laboratory which are not fully described above and which comply with the essential requirements of routine analysis (page 350). Useful modifications of the standard procedures are described under the appropriate headings.

The method generally used for the estimation of serum *calcium* is that of Clarke and Collip (15) (A). This involves the precipitation of calcium as an oxalate, which is suitably washed and titrated with potassium permanganate. It can be adapted for the estimation of urinary *calcium*, provided a double precipitation technique is used. For this purpose take 2 ml. of slightly acidified urine, add 1 ml. of 20% sodium acetate and one drop of 0·02% alcoholic methyl red. Add strong ammonia until just alkaline, then acidify with glacial acetic acid and add 1 ml. of ammonium oxalate solution. After allowing to stand, centrifuge. Discard the supernatant fluid and dissolve the precipitate in 1 ml. of normal hydrochloric acid. Titrate at 60° C. with decinormal potassium permanganate until the solution has a distinct pink colour. Add one drop of 3% hydrogen peroxide, 1 ml. of sodium acetate solution, and 1 ml. ammonium oxalate solution. Centrifuge, wash the precipitate and titrate exactly as for the serum calcium.

The *ionised calcium* (Maclean and Hastings (16)) is obtained by estimating the serum total calcium as given by the method of Clark and Collip (15) and the serum total protein by any suitable method.

Knowing both of these values the percentage of ionised calcium can be read off the nomogram shown (see Fig. 59).

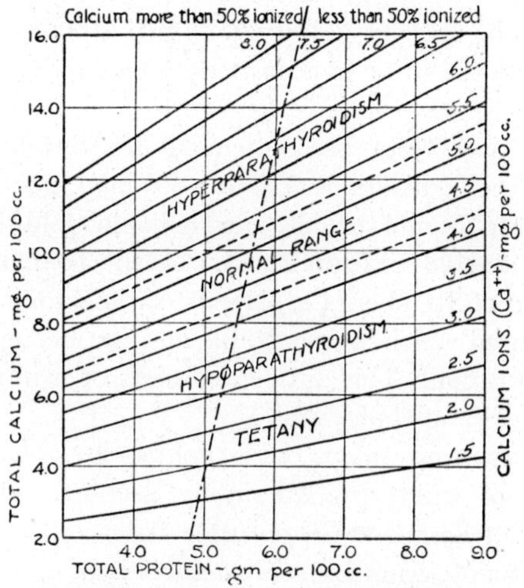

FIG. 59. Chart for calculation of Ca^{++} concentration from total protein and total calcium of serum or plasma.

Serum *carotenoids* are estimated by the method of Connor (17). For this method a working standard curve is prepared from potassium dichromate, calibrated by comparison with pure β-carotene (obtainable from the National Institute of Medical Research).

To estimate *chlorides* in urine, blood or cerebro-spinal fluid the method of Van Slyke and Hiller (18) (B) is recommended. The advantage of this method is that it can be adapted for the analysis of as little as 0·04 ml. of material.

Serum or plasma *cholesterol* is best estimated by a method, based on the original technique of Bloor (19), such as that of Schoenheimer and Sperry (20) (B). The disadvantage in the use of these methods is that they tend to give higher results than those in which the material to be extracted is first absorbed on to sodium sulphate or filter paper. The only points of technique worth noting are that water must be excluded during the development of the colour and any filter papers used must first be rendered lipoid-free by extraction with chloroform.

For the estimation of *creatine* and *creatinine* the best method is that of Peters (21). This method may also be adapted for urine estimations by suitable dilution of the urine based upon its specific gravity: dilute the urine 4 × the last two figures of the specific gravity (*e.g.* S.G. 1006, dilute twenty-four times), and the urine is then treated exactly as for the blood method.

The flocculation tests recommended for investigating liver function are the *cephalin-cholesterol*, *colloidal gold* and *thymol turbidity*. For the thymol turbidity and colloidal gold the methods of Maclagan (22 and 23) are preferred. In the cephalin-cholesterol test the method of Steinberg (24) is most satisfactory as a chemical "antigen" is used which is very stable and can be kept for months without deterioration. This antigen consists of a mixture of pure desoxycholic acid and cholesterol.

The serum *bilirubin* may be estimated by several different methods none of which are absolutely accurate: a satisfactory method is that of King and Coxon (25).

The estimation of serum *bromsulphthalein* is best achieved by the method of Rosenthal and White (26). As we find that the colour of permanent alkalised bromsulphthalein tends to fade it is advisable to prepare a calibration curve. The standard curve is constructed by taking a pooled normal sample of serum which has bromsulphthalein added to it to a concentration of 10 mg. per 100 ml. This concentration is considered as 100% and suitable dilutions are then made with more serum to obtain concentrations equivalent to 10,

20, 30, 40, 50, 60, 70, 80 and 90%, and these, after being made alkaline, read on a null-point colorimeter.

For the *galactose tolerance test,* Maclagan (27) has described a method of estimating the blood galactose, after glucose has been removed by yeast fermentation, by a modification of the Schaffer-Hartman blood sugar technique.

Para-aminosalicylic acid in serum may be estimated by the method of Tarnoky and Brews (28): the *p*-aminosalicylic acid is decarboxylated and the *m*-aminophenol estimated by a diazotisation procedure.

Numerous methods are available for the estimation of the serum phosphatases. For *acid phosphatase* a standard procedure is that of Gutman and Gutman (29) (A), and for *alkaline phosphatase* that of King et al. (30) (A) is probably the best method.

Quinaldine red is a reagent which has recently been proposed for the estimation of *inorganic phosphorus* by Soyenkoff (31). A method, using this reagent, which forms an insoluble dye phosphomolybdate complex, which remains in suspension, can be used with very small quantities of blood (or other material), to give very reliable results.

The standard method for the estimation of *plasma proteins* is by means of the Kjeldahl technique of nitrogen assay (C). This procedure has been used for many years and is probably still the most accurate. Its main disadvantage is the limitation of the number of analyses which may be performed at the same time and other procedures, such as the method of Kingsley (32) (B) based on the biuret reaction, have been proposed. The biuret methods enable more analyses to be made at the same time but these methods do not possess the same degree of accuracy as does the Kjeldahl method. The fractionation of the proteins is usually achieved by means of sodium sulphate, sodium sulphite or ammonium sulphate and most laboratories standardise on one procedure, and have their own normal values, although such salting-out methods do not necessarily agree with the pattern of the plasma proteins given by electrophoresis.

Aggeler et al. (33) and Biggs and MacFarlane (34) have proposed methods for the estimation of *prothrombin time and concentration.* The essential point of these methods is the preparation of the brain thromboplastin as a fine granulated powder. This is done by macerating fresh human brain from the post-mortem room (or rabbit brain if human is not obtainable) with acetone and repeatedly extracting with further quantities of acetone and finally drying at 37° C. The powder is stored in small quantities in an evacuated desiccator over calcium chloride in a refrigerator. It is standardised by testing against at least a dozen normal plasma speicmens, and determining the necessary quantity of brain powder and concentration of calcium ion to yield a prothrombin time, in normal plasma, between fourteen and sixteen seconds. A standard curve is compiled by pooling the normal samples which fall within this standard range and diluting the (theoretically 100% prothrombin) pooled batch with physiological saline to contain 50, 30, 20, 10 and 5% of plasma, then plotting the graph of prothrombin time against concentration. This graph must be reconstructed for each fresh batch of thromboplastin and also checked monthly against known normals.

The old and well-tried method of Folin and Wu (35) (B) is still one of the best for the routine estimation of *blood sugar*. A modification which may be made is that after the final colour has been developed with phosphotungstic acid, the mixture should be again heated in the boiling-water bath for three minutes, then cooled, diluted and read in a colorimeter. This re-heating technique renders the coloured material more stable over the period of reading. The same method may be used for the estimation of *urinary sugar* after the urine has been diluted to bring the concentration of sugar to between approximately 0·1% and 0·2%. It is also advisable to remove interfering substances from the urine before dilution: this is best done by adding to 1 ml. of the urine, 1 ml. N/10 sulphuric acid, 0·2 g. of Lloyd's alkaloidal reagent, 1 g. of permutit and 8 ml. of water in a stoppered tube, vigorously shaking for five minutes, filtering and diluting the filtrate as necessary.

The Barrett urease method (36) (A) for the estimation of *blood urea* is satisfactory, and his recommended technique of adding a few drops of 10% sodium hypochlorite solution to the Nessler's solution (Koch & McMeakin (37)), is well worth the extra time involved; the modification has the advantage that any trace of organic material present in the original solution does not interfere and cause a cloudiness of the final coloured solution. The same method may be adapted for the estimation of *urinary urea*, dilution of the urine being effected by a calculation based on the specific gravity: 1 ml. of urine is diluted to 5, 10, 25 or 50 ml., the final volume being the figure nearest the last two figures of the specific gravity, *e.g.* Urine S.G. 1021, dilute 1 ml. of urine to 25 ml.

This method of diluting urine may be used for numerous estimations such as *urinary phosphate, urea or uric acid.*

Apart from slight modifications no real advances have been made on the method of Folin (38) (B) for the estimation of *uric acid*, and for clinical use this method is still quite satisfactory. If used for urine it is first necessary to employ the silver precipitation technique (38) (B) where the urine is buffered, silver nitrate added and the precipitate redissolved in the urea cyanide reagent.

The components of cerebro-spinal fluid which are estimated as a routine are chloride, sugar and protein. The chloride may be assayed by the same method as already outlined for serum chloride, namely that of Van Slyke and Hiller (18) (B) although some laboratories prefer to titrate the chloride direct with silver nitrate using dichlorofluorescein as the indicator (Rose (39)). Sugar is estimated exactly as for blood sugar whilst the protein level is obtained by the method of King and Haslewood (40), a method also of use for *urinary protein* estimation. The standards necessary for these protein methods may be purchased commercially.

For the routine estimation of *fæcal fats* the method of Cammidge (41) still gives satisfaction although a more accurate estimation may be obtained by one of the methods where a prolonged Soxhlet extraction is employed (Harrison (C)).

Estimations of *fæcal trypsin* are based on the digestion of different substrates by means of the enzyme in alkaline solution. Anderson and Early's method (42) relies upon the liquefaction of a standard amount of gelatin by varying the amount of fæces mixed with sodium bicarbonate solution. The result is expressed in units representing the reciprocal of the limiting dilution necessary to digest a given amount of gelatin, *e.g.* limiting dilution 1 g. of fæces/100 g. of sodium bicarbonate solution—result 100 units/g. wet fæces. It should be noted that this analysis may only be carried out on fresh fæces, as trypsin rapidly decomposes. The method may also be used for the assay of *trypsin in duodenal juice.*

The estimation of *fæcal urobilinogen* is now coming into more general use and a suitable method for its estimation is that of Maclagan (43). In this method an artificial standard is used consisting of a alkaline solution of phenolphthalein and this is compared with an extract of fæces which has been treated with alkaline ferrous sulphate to reduce any urobilin present to urobilinogen, before reacting it with Erhlich's aldehyde reagent.

For the routine clinical estimation of *urinary ascorbic acid* the use of 2 : 6 : dichloroindophenol is still the simplest technique. Harris and Ray (44) have produced a method based on this reaction, but if a more accurate estimation is required or if it is desired to estimate the ascorbic acid in blood use should be made of one of the methods where the ascorbic acid is reacted with 2 : 4 : dinitrophenolhydrazine (Roe and Kuether (45)).

When estimating *urinary diastase* by the method of Wohlgemuth (46) it is essential that the urine should first be suitably buffered at pH 6·1 with phosphate buffer (B, page 812).

The estimation of *urinary galactose* may only be required for the galactose tolerance test. The method for blood galactose is satisfactory after suitable dilution.

After the intravenous injection of sodium benzoate where it is desired to estimate the excretion of *hippuric acid* the method of Quick et al. (47) is eminently suitable. The most difficult point in this technique is to obtain the crystals of hippuric acid from the concentrated acidified urine. Friction is the best method to initiate their formation from the urine after it has once been cooled although, in cases of extreme difficulty, it is permissible to seed with a very small crystal of pure hippuric acid.

Urinary pregnanediol is best estimated by slight modification of the method of Somerville and Marrian (48), where the urine is hydrolysed by boiling with hydrochloric acid and extracting with toluene as one operation. The toluene is washed with caustic soda to remove impurities, evaporated under dryness and the pregnanediol precipitated from an alcoholic solution of the gum under carefully controlled conditions with caustic soda. The precipitated material is then reacted with concentrated sulphuric acid to give the yellow colour by which it is estimated, in comparison with a previously constructed calibration curve prepared from pure pregnane 3 α 20 α diol.

REFERENCES

(1) Bills, McDonald, Niederman and Schwartz. *Anal. Chem.*, 1949, **21,** 1076.
(2) Weichselbaum and Varney. *Proc. Soc. Exp. Biol. and Med.*, 1949, **71,** 570.
(3) McCance and Shipp. *Biochem. Journ.*, 1931, **25,** 449 and 1845.
(4) Jacobs and Hoffman. *Journ. Biol. Chem.*, 1931, **93,** 685.
(5) Peters and Van Slyke. *Quantitative Clinical Chemistry* (Methods), 1932, **2,** 296. Baillière, Tindall & Cox, London.
(6) Douglas and Priestley. *Human Physiology,* 3rd Edit. 1948, 150. Clarendon Press, Oxford.
(7) Kravel. *Journ. Lab. Clin. Med.*, 1944, **29,** 222.
(8) Wilson and Eyles. *Amer. Journ. Dis. Child.*, 1946, No. 3, 72.
(9) Høyer. *Nord. Med.*, 1943, **18,** 801.
(10) Dahl. *Brit. Med. Journ.*, 1948, *i*, 731.
(11) Heard and Sobel. *Journ. Biol. Chem.*, 1946, **165,** 687.
(12) Romanoff, Player and Pincus. *Endocrinol.*, 1949, **45,** 10.
(13) Talbot, Wolfe, MacLachlan and Berman. *Journ. Biol. Chem.*, 1941, **139,** 521.
(14) Patterson. *Lancet*, 1947, *ii*, 580.
(15) Clark and Collip. *Journ. Biol. Chem.*, 1925, **63,** 461.
(16) McLean and Hastings. *Amer. Journ. Med. Sci.*, 1935, **189,** 601.
(17) Connor. *Journ. Biol. Chem.*, 1928, **77,** 619.
(18) Van Slyke and Hiller. *Journ. Biol. Chem.*, 1947, **167,** 107.
(19) Bloor. *Journ. Biol. Chem.*, 1916, **24,** 227.
(20) Schoenheimer and Sperry. *Journ. Biol. Chem.*, 1934, **106,** 745.
(21) Peters. *Journ. Biol. Chem.*, 1942, **146,** 179.
(22) Maclagan. *Brit. Journ. Exp. Path.*, 1944, **25,** 234.
(23) Maclagan. *Brit. Journ. Exp. Path.*, 1946, **27,** 370.
(24) Steinberg. *Journ. Lab. Clin. Med.*, 1949, **34,** 1049.
(25) King and Coxon. *Journ. Clin. Path.*, 1950, **3,** 248.
(26) Rosenthal and White. *Journ. Amer. Med. Assocn.*, 1925, **84,** 1112
(27) Maclagan. *Quart. Journ. Med.*, 1940, **9,** 151.
(28) Tarnoky and Brews. *Biochem. Journ.*, 1949, **45,** 508.
(29) Gutman and Gutman. *Journ. Biol. Chem.*, 1940, **136,** 201.
(30) King, Haslewood, Delory and Beall. *Lancet*, 1942, *i*, 207.
(31) Soyenkoff. *Journ. Biol. Chem.*, 1947, **168,** 447.
(32) Kingsley. *Journ. Biol. Chem.*, 1940, **133,** 731.
(33) Aggeler, Howard, Lucia, Clark and Astaff. *Blood*, 1946, **1,** 220.
(34) Biggs and MacFarlane. *Journ. Clin. Path.*, 1949, **2,** 33.
(35) Folin and Wu. *Journ. Biol. Chem.*, 1929, **82,** 83.
(36) Barrett. *Lancet*, 1936, *i*, 84.
(37) Koch and McMeakin. *Journ. Amer. Chem. Soc.*, 1924, **46,** 2066.
(38) Folin. *Journ. Biol. Chem.*, 1933, **101,** 111.
(39) Rose. *Biochem. Journ.*, 1936, **30,** 1140.
40) King and Haslewood. *Lancet*, 1936, *ii*, 1153.
41) Cammidge. *The Fæces of Children and Adults.* 1914, 516, John Wright & Son Ltd., Bristol.
(42) Anderson and Early. *Amer. Journ. Dis. Child.*, 1942, **63,** 891.
(43) Maclagan. *Brit. Journ. Exp. Path.*, 1946, **27,** 90.

(44) Harris and Ray. *Lancet*, 1935, *i*, 71.
(45) Roe and Kuether. *Journ. Biol. Chem.*, 1943, **147**, 399.
(46) Wohlgemuth. *Biochem. Zeit.*, 1908, **9**, 1.
(47) Quick, Ottenstein and Weltchek. *Proc. Soc. Exp. Biol. and Med.*, 1938, **38**, 77.
(48) Sommerville and Marrian. *Lancet*, 1948, *ii*, 89.
(A) Beaumont and Dodds. *Recent Advances in Medicine*, 12th Edit., 1947. J. &. A. Churchill Ltd., London.
(B) Hawk, Oser and Summerson. *Practical Physiological Chemistry*, 12th Edit. 1947, J. & A. Churchill Ltd., London.
(C) Harrison. *Chemical Methods in Clinical Medicine*, 3rd Edit. 1947. J. & A. Churchill Ltd., London.

INDEX

Richmond Hill Printing Works Ltd., Bournemouth.